Word-Finding Intervention Program

SECOND EDITION

Diane J. German

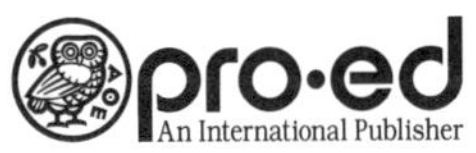

8700 Shoal Creek Boulevard
Austin, Texas 78754-6897
800/897-3202 Fax 800/397-7633
www.proedinc.com

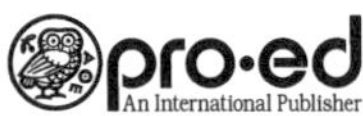

Published by PRO-ED, Inc.
8700 Shoal Creek Boulevard
Austin, Texas 78754-6897
800/897-3202 Fax 800/397-7633
www.proedinc.com

Editor: Lynda Miller, PhD

Designer: Cinqué Hicks

ISBN 1-4164-0124-5

Printed in the United States of America

1 2 3 4 5 6 7 8 9 10 09 08 07 06 05

The WFIP–2 is dedicated to my husband, Arthur E. German. I thank him for his unwavering support of my work in word finding. Together we make this contribution to individuals with word-finding difficulties in hopes that it will assist them in improving their communication skills.

CONTENTS

SECTION 3 Goals, Objectives, and Lesson Plans • 55

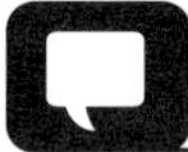

FIGURES

PREFACE

When the *Word Finding Intervention Program* (WFIP) was published in 1993, it was a welcome addition to the intervention of child word finding. It offered clinicians and special education teachers a three-pronged approach to treating children with word-finding difficulties that was applicable in both academic and work contexts. Over the last 12 years, the WFIP has been well-received in the field and has been used in numerous schools, centers, and hospitals by speech–language pathologists, special education personnel, and reading teachers.

Like the WFIP, the *Word-Finding Intervention Program–Second Edition* (WFIP–2) provides professionals (i.e., specialists and teachers) with specific intervention steps to take after assessment of a learner's word-finding skills. Retrieval strategies are matched to learners' word-finding error patterns, and learners are presented with activities that encourage generalization of these strategies at school, home, work, or play. The lesson plans also guide the learners in the use of methods to modify word-finding demands present in the classroom. The word-finding self-advocacy program component guides learners in the use of methods to self-monitor their word-finding abilities across communication contexts. Important changes and additions were incorporated in the WFIP–2. These changes were motivated by the author's own observations and feedback from the users of this program. Like the WFIP, the WFIP–2 provides the user with a three-pronged approach to word-finding intervention: retrieval strategy instruction, self-advocacy instruction, and word-finding accommodations. In addition, the second edition is improved in its organization, user-friendly presentation, retrieval strategy selection, word-finding accommodations, lesson plans, specialist's forms, and integration of technology recommendations throughout. Specific improvements are as follows:

- New research-supported mnemonic retrieval strategies
- New assessment discussion of the differential diagnosis of word-finding error types
- New organization according to error patterns typically observed in individuals with word-finding difficulties
- Link to assessment, with retrieval strategies matched to the learner's word-finding error patterns
- Retrieval strategies applied to social studies, math, and science vocabulary as well as baseball, football, golf, tennis, soccer, hockey, and swimming vocabulary
- Benchmarks and long-term objectives for retrieval strategy instruction, self-advocacy instruction, and word-finding accommodations

- Technology recommendations for both retrieval strategy instruction and word-finding accommodations
- User-friendly lesson plans for retrieval strategy instruction, self-advocacy instruction, and word-finding accommodations
- User-friendly student study forms for retrieval strategy practice
- New Word-Finding Self-Assessment Survey
- New Classroom Observation Form to identify needed word-finding accommodations
- New Recommended Word-Finding Accommodations Form to individualize word-finding accommodations
- Differentiated instruction and assessment for oral classroom participation, vocabulary instruction, classroom work, homework, examinations, reading, and written language
- Technology recommendations for retrieval strategy instruction, oral presentations, and written language

ACKNOWLEDGMENTS

As author of the *Word-Finding Intervention Program–Second Edition* (WFIP–2), I feel extremely fortunate in having had the support and feedback from many fine professionals. In particular, I want to thank Diane Edger, PhD, CCC-SLP, and Lynda Miller, PhD, CCC-SLP, for their helpful and thoughtful reviews of the WFIP–2; Cinqué Hicks for his distinctive cover and page design; Dolly Jackson and Becky Shore for their copyediting support; Jan Schwanke, MA, CCC-SLP, and the children at Oak Grove School in Oak Grove, Illinois; and Elaine Boeman, MA, CCC-SLP, and the children at Cherokee School in Lake Forest, Illinois, for their assistance in conducting our intervention studies. I would also like to thank Cara Benes, MA, CCC-SLP, and Beth Cohen, MA, CCC-SLP, for their assistance in creating the completed Syllable-Dividing and Same-Sounds Syllable Cue Study Forms; Sandy Hilmert for her clerical assistance; and the many National-Louis University students who offered valuable suggestions during the development of the WFIP–2. Finally, I would like to express my appreciation to Shirley and Pat Ryan for their support of my work on behalf of children challenged with word finding.

SECTION 1

Introduction to Word Finding, Word-Finding Difficulties, and Word-Finding Intervention

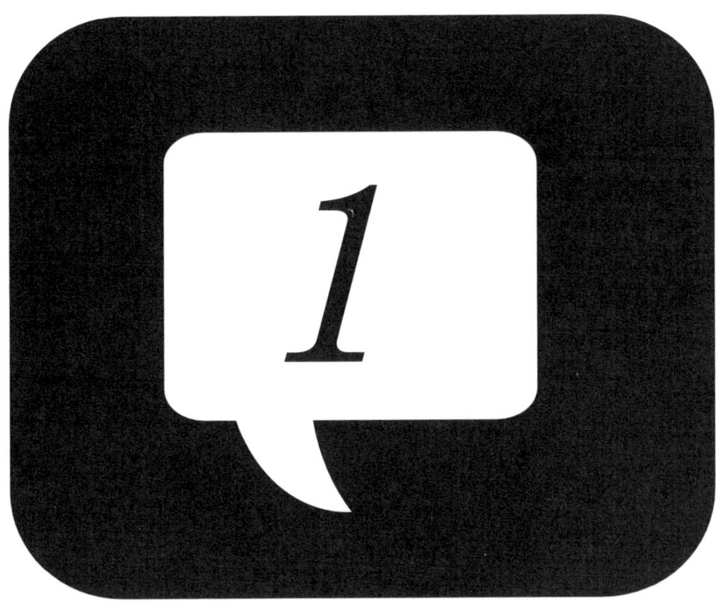

Introduction

Word finding refers to the ability to retrieve a desired word in single-word or discourse contexts. Difficulties in word finding can result in significant expressive language problems that can profoundly affect one's life. In young people, word-finding difficulties can impede learning and interfere with interpersonal communication. If left untreated, word-finding problems continue into adulthood and impede fluent expression in personal, social, and professional situations.

Learners with word-finding difficulties need a specific dual-focused approach to vocabulary instruction if they are to become automatic in their word usage. To become fluent in the usage of names and words studied in classes or associated with their personal, academic, or social activities, learners need both (a) vocabulary instruction focused on establishing and storing meanings of target words and (b) instruction in retrieval strategies.

The *Word-Finding Intervention Program–Second Edition* (WFIP–2) is designed to aid practitioners in planning for individuals challenged with word finding in schools and clinics. It provides the specific mnemonic strategies they need embedded in their vocabulary instruction to enhance word learning. These word-finding strategies are focused on supporting retrieval of words in both single-word naming and discourse contexts.

The WFIP–2 is based on a threefold model for word-finding intervention drawn from the literature in the fields of speech and language, learning disabilities, and cognitive science. The model includes the following:

1. Retrieval strategy instruction
2. Word-finding self-advocacy instruction
3. Word-finding accommodations

The primary goal of the WFIP–2 is to help learners improve their word-finding skills when communicating at home, at school, at work, and in social interactions. Because the WFIP–2 has a "life-based" focus, objectives, materials, and contexts are relevant and applicable to the daily life of the learner. Applications to everyday situations are embedded in the WFIP–2 lesson plans.

WFIP–2 PROGRAM AREAS FOR SERVICE DELIVERY

Programming in word finding must be comprehensive with respect to its focus and its application. The WFIP–2 directs the practitioner to focus in three program areas for service delivery:

- retrieval strategy instruction,
- word-finding self-advocacy instruction, and
- word-finding accommodations.

Effectiveness of word-finding intervention is dependent on teaching and learning retrieval strategies, coupled with an understanding and self-application of these strategies by the learner (word-finding self-advocacy) and facilitated by modifications of both school and home communication environments (word-finding accommodations). The primary goal of each of the three areas of programming is to facilitate word re-

trieval in school and at home. Each area focuses on different aspects of the intervention process and all three areas should be implemented for a comprehensive word-finding intervention program. The three components of the WFIP–2 intervention model are described in the following sections and shown in Figure 1.1.

RETRIEVAL STRATEGY INSTRUCTION

The purpose of retrieval strategy instruction programming is to provide learners with strategies that will improve their retrieval of words they comprehend. These strategies may be used in isolation or in combination. Six types of retrieval strategies are presented in the WFIP–2:

- Mnemonic cueing strategies (German, 1993, 2001, 2002; Higbee, 1993; Mastropieri, Sweda, & Scruggs, 2000; McNamara & Wong, 2003; Nelson, 1998)
- Alternate-word strategies (Harrell, Parenté, Bellingrath, & Lisicia, 1992)
- Segmenting strategies (Catts, 1999; German, 2002; VanKleeck, 1990; VanKleeck, Gillam, & McFadden, 1998)
- Pausing strategy (Harrell et al., 1992)
- Self-monitoring and self-correction (Hanson, 1996; Levelt, Roelofs, & Meyer, 1999; Paul, 2001)
- Rehearsal (Conca, 1989; German, 2002; Wiig, 1984)
- Attribute-cueing strategies (McNamara & Wong, 2003; Rubin, Bernstein, & Katz, 1989; Wiig & Semel, 1984; Wing, 1990)

WORD-FINDING SELF-ADVOCACY INSTRUCTION

The purpose of word-finding self-advocacy instruction is to empower learners to advocate for themselves. Using the WFIP–2, they learn to apply retrieval strategies to aid their word finding and to request classroom accommodations that will improve their learning in school. Specific goals that underlie this portion of the WFIP–2 include the following:

1. To help learners self-monitor (Hallahan & Kauffman, 2000; Hanson, 1996) and self-correct their word-finding errors
2. To teach learners to self-assess their word-finding skills across various domains
3. To help learners self-apply their retreival strategies and request corresponding accommodations to facilitate their communication

- Word-Finding Intervention Program–Second Edition
  - Retrieval Strategy Instruction
    - Mnemonic Cueing Strategies
    - Alternate-Word Strategies
    - Segmenting Strategies
    - Pausing Strategy
    - Self-Monitoring and Self-Correcting
    - Rehearsal
    - Attribute-Cueing Strategies
  - Word-Finding Self-Advocacy Instruction
    - Cognitive Modification
      - Self-Monitoring and Self-Correction
    - Word-Finding Self-Assessment
      - Speaking Settings
      - Language Circumstances
      - Retrieval Contexts
      - Language Contexts
      - Subject of Words
      - Lexical Factors
    - Self-Application
      - Retrieval Strategies
      - Requests for Accomodations
  - Word-Finding Accomodations
    - Modification of Language Environment
      - School
      - Home
      - Recreation
      - Social Experiences
    - Use of Support Materials
      - Technology Applications
      - Resource Notebooks
      - Cue Cards

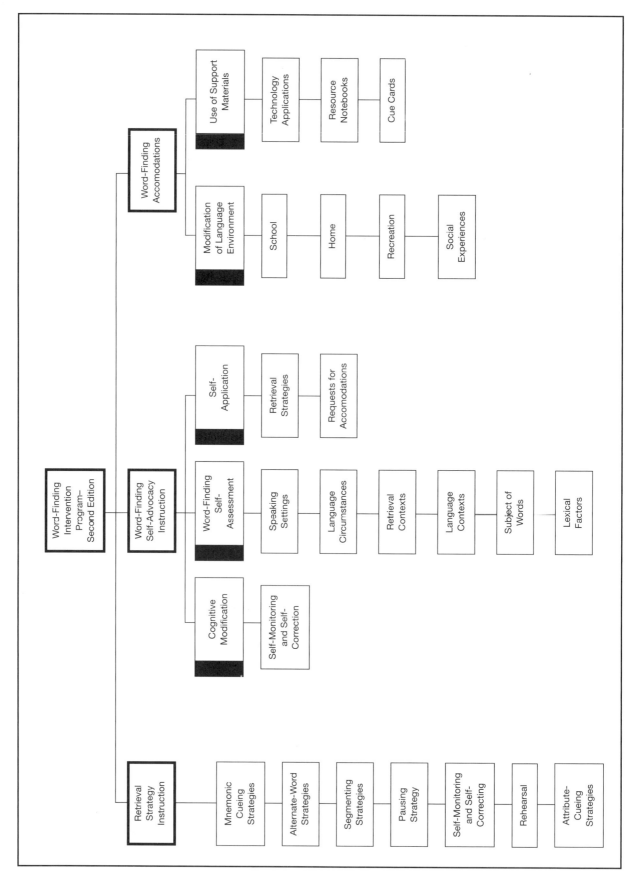

Figure 1.1. The three components of the WFIP–2 intervention model.

WORD-FINDING ACCOMMODATIONS

The purpose of word-finding accommodations is twofold:

1. To present methods for modifying the school, home, and work language environments to facilitate the learning of students with word-finding difficulties
2. To provide support materials to aid learners with word-finding difficulties when they are participating in classroom discussions, taking exams, or completing homework assignments

The emphasis in word-finding accommodations is on reducing the retrieval load inherent in classroom oral discourse, classroom activities, homework, and exams in academic areas such as reading, written language, math, science, and language arts. Word-finding accommodations in the WFIP–2 involve specialist–teacher dialogue, classroom observations, identification of appropriate modifications for oral work (e.g., multiple choice, cueing, extending time), and teacher–learner collaboration. Recommended support materials include technology applications, resource notebooks to be used during evaluations and when doing homework, and cue cards to aid retrieval of procedural information in math and science (see Figure 1.1).

FEATURES OF THE WFIP–2

The scope and structure of the WFIP–2 offer several important features to aid the user (see Figure 1.2).

SCOPE AND STRUCTURE OF THE WFIP–2

- Theoretically and evidence based intervention for word-finding difficulties
- Strategic instruction to teach word retrieval strategies
- Procedures for teaching word-finding self-advocacy
- Procedures for implementing word-finding accommodations for selected content areas
- Technology recommended for learners with word-finding difficulties
- Vocabulary lists and sentences related to curriculum, recreation, and everyday life activities
- Curriculum-based instructional activities
- Curriculum-based generalization activities
- IEP goals and benchmarks for students with word-finding difficulties

Figure 1.2. WFIP–2 scope and structure.

RESOURCE TOOL

The WFIP–2 can serve as a collection of procedures for improving word-finding skills, and the practitioner can build upon these procedures to develop a customized library of successful methods. Specifically, the WFIP–2 manual provides retrieval strategies that can be used with individuals within a wide age range and that can be applied to different types of vocabulary. Thus, as an individual's needs change and different types of vocabulary emerge as important to the learner, the practitioner can continue to apply the WFIP–2 methods. For example, if the vocabulary provided in the WFIP–2 is not of interest to the learner or if he or she has gained word-finding facility with the vocabulary lists presented, other lists can be developed and used with the WFIP–2 retrieval strategies. Blank master worksheet forms are provided for this purpose in the appendixes of this manual. Therefore, as a resource tool, the WFIP–2 can facilitate improvement of an individual's word-finding skills with any vocabulary selected.

FLEXIBILITY

Although the WFIP–2 provides the user with lesson plans for retrieval strategies, word-finding self-advocacy instruction, and word-finding accommodations, the practitioner is not expected to use all the lesson plans provided. Rather, specialists are encouraged to design a program specific to the needs of their learners, selecting only those retrieval strategies that are appropriate for the learners' word-finding error pattern (i.e., strategic retrieval strategy instruction). The WFIP–2 lessons also may be implemented at home, school, or work and may be adapted for a variety of instructional formats, including one-to-one, small group, and classroom situations.

WIDE AGE RANGE

The WFIP–2 retrieval strategies are designed for use with children, adolescents, and adults who exhibit characteristics of word-finding difficulties. Thus, the intervention principles, retrieval strategies, and lesson plans may be applied to a wide age group. Even though the WFIP–2 provides the user with vocabulary lists (see Appendix A), the WFIP–2 can be used with other vocabulary lists, making it appropriate for clients of any age.

LINK TO ASSESSMENT

The WFIP–2 is organized according to diagnostic error patterns typically observed in individuals with word-finding difficulties. WFIP–2 retrieval strategies are not to be applied randomly but are to be matched to the learner's word-finding error pattern. The practitioner begins with findings from an individual's differential diagnosis. For example, lesson plans are recommended for those students who are slow, inaccurate responders and who manifest word-finding blocks yet respond to phonemic cueing (Error Pattern 2; commonly called "tip of the tongue" errors). Other lessons are for slow, inaccurate responders who produce phonologic errors and do not respond to the phonemic cue (Error Pattern 3; commonly referred to as "twist of the tongue" errors).

LESSON PLANS

The WFIP–2 includes comprehensive lesson plans for each of the three program components:

- Retrieval strategies
- Word-finding self-advocacy
- Word-finding accommodations

OVERVIEW OF THE WFIP–2

This WFIP–2 manual is the major source describing the underlying principles, instructional components, and specific procedures for implementing the WFIP–2. The manual consists of 10 chapters and three appendixes.

- Chapter 1 provides the user with descriptions of the WFIP–2 features, model, and applications.
- Chapter 2 describes the processes of interpreting assessment results, developing intervention goals, and planning intervention with the WFIP–2.
- Chapter 3 presents practical guidelines for implementing the three components of the WFIP–2 in individual and group settings, as well as in the classroom. Suggestions for using the WFIP–2 specialist and learner study forms (see appendixes) are also presented in this chapter.

- Chapter 4 presents the retrieval strategy instruction component of the WFIP–2, including a presentation of instructional principles and retrieval strategies for improving word-finding skills.
- Chapter 5 presents specific goals and benchmarks for retrieval strategy instruction, self-advocacy instruction, and word-finding accommodations. It also introduces the format of the lesson plans for each component.
- Chapters 6, 7, and 8 contain specific lesson plans for teaching retrieval strategies that address Error Patterns 1, 2, and 3, respectively.
- Chapter 9 presents the word-finding self-advocacy instruction component of the WFIP–2. This chapter describes principles and gives specific lesson plans for implementing this part of the program.
- Chapter 10 presents the word-finding accommodations component of the WFIP–2. This chapter includes principles and lesson plans for identifying and implementing the accommodations needed in school and home environments.

The WFIP–2 appendixes include the forms used to implement the program. These forms may be reproduced for use with learners.

- Appendix A contains the forms used to teach the word-finding retrieval strategies:
  - Retrieval Strategy Lesson Plan
  - Vocabulary and Retrieval Strategy Practice Form
  - Syllable-Dividing and Same-Sounds Syllable Cue Study Form
  - Completed Syllable-Dividing and Same-Sounds Syllable Cue Study Forms
  - Model Sentences for Selected WFIP–2 Vocabulary
  - Dual-Focus Vocabulary Instruction Form

- Appendix B contains the Word-Finding Self-Assessment Survey, which is used in teaching the WFIP–2 word-finding self-advocacy part of the program.

- Appendix C contains the forms used in teaching the word-finding accommodations component of the WFIP–2:
  - Classroom Observation Form
  - Recommended Word-Finding Accommodations Form

APPLICATIONS ACROSS SERVICE DELIVERY MODELS

The WFIP–2 was designed to provide professionals (i.e., specialists and teachers) with specific intervention steps to take after assessment of a learner's word-finding skills. Whereas testing sheds light on the nature and severity of an individual's word-finding challenge, the WFIP–2 provides the specialist or teacher with the next step: a carefully designed set of methods and lesson plans designed to improve a learner's word-finding skills. The WFIP–2 uses a flexible service delivery model that encourages WFIP–2 implementation in several settings.

- **Speech and language settings.** The program provides a comprehensive selection of lesson plans ideal for use in one-to-one and small-group settings.
- **Classroom settings.** The WFIP–2 uses vocabulary from the classroom as the curriculum for the retrieval strategies lessons. As a student is learning the retrieval strategies in the WFIP–2, he or she is taught to apply these strategies when having word-finding difficulties during academic activities in the classroom. The WFIP–2 also provides generalization activities focused on applying retrieval strategies in the classroom. The student's academic activities serve as the context for teaching and reinforcing the retrieval strategies introduced in the WFIP–2. The word-finding self-advocacy component teaches the student to self-monitor his or her word-finding skills in the classroom, and the WFIP–2 word-finding accommodations component provides the specialist, learner, and classroom teacher with methods to reduce retrieval demands in the learner's language environment.
- **School, home, work, or recreation settings.** The WFIP–2 provides the learner with activities that encourage generalization of strategies at school, home, work, or play. The lesson plans also guide the learner in the use of methods to modify word-finding demands present in these speaking situations. Further, word-finding self-advocacy instruction guides learners in the use of methods to self-monitor their word-finding abilities across these four communication contexts.

Linking Assessment to Intervention

Planning an individualized word-finding intervention program requires linking the information obtained in word-finding assessment and observation with the goals and benchmarks, or objectives, established for word-finding intervention. This chapter describes what constitutes a word-finding error, provides an outline of important information to gather during the observation and assessment process, and discusses how to establish relevant goals and objectives for word-finding intervention based on assessment results.

What Is a Word-Finding Error?

German (2000a) defined word-finding errors as those failures (or significant delays) that learners make when they attempt to say a word, the meaning of which they comprehend and which they may have spoken previously. Although the learner possesses both the semantic and syntactic features (known as the *lemma*) and the phonological features (the *form*) of the target word and demonstrates an ability to construct and execute the motor plan for the word, the learner is unable to retrieve the word for spontaneous usage (Dapretto & Bjork, 2000).

Theoretically, word finding involves four stages of lexical access (see German, 2000a, for a more complete discussion of lexical access in children).

The Four Stages of Word Retrieval

Stage 1. The stimulus (e.g., a picture or question) elicits the conceptual structure or underlying concepts associated with a target word (Bierwisch & Schreuder, 1991).
Stage 2. The conceptual structure accesses the target word's semantic and syntactic features (referred to as the lemma) from among neighboring entries (Garrett, 1991; Levelt, Roelofs, & Meyer, 1999).
Stage 3. The lemma accesses the entry's corresponding phonological features (i.e., its syllabic frame and sound units) to create a complete phonological schema (Levelt, 1991; Levelt et al., 1999).
Stage 4. A motor plan is created and forwarded to lower level articulation processes to produce the word.

The most important part of understanding the nature of learners' word-finding difficulties is that the semantic and phonological aspects of words are believed to be accessed from two different lexical components (Stages 2 and 3 in the preceding list; Garrett, 1991; Gordon, 1997; Levelt, 1989, 1991; Levelt et al., 1999). This assumption suggests two potential underlying causes for a failure in lexical access: Either (a) the semantic aspects of a target word are inaccessible to a learner, making the phonological features unavailable also, or (b) the semantic features are accessible while subsequent retrieval of the word's phonological features are blocked.

Other researchers have reported that children's retrieval errors may be related to disruptions at lexical Stages 2 and 3. For example, McGregor and Appel (2002) and Lahey and Edwards (1999) described semantic and phonological naming errors suggestive of two distinct stores in the mental lexicon (Stages 2 and 3), and Elbers (1985) reported evidence of a 2-year-old child demonstrating "tip of the tongue" errors (a disruption at the juncture between Stages 2 and 3) during discourse.

FROM ASSESSMENT TO INTERVENTION

Implementing a program in word finding follows a process from screening to assessment to intervention.

SCREENING FOR WORD-FINDING DIFFICULTIES IN THE CLASSROOM

The first step in gathering information about learners with word-finding difficulties is screening through focused observation and referral. Using focused observation, specialists can collaborate with classroom teachers, family members, and other school personnel (e.g., special education teacher, psychologist) to identify those learners who may need further assessment in the area of word finding. German & German (1992) developed a screening checklist for this purpose: the *Word-Finding Referral Checklist.* A sample completed checklist is shown in Figure 2.1.

Use of this screening checklist provides a list of specific language behaviors that are characteristic of learners who have word-finding difficulties. Distributing the checklist to designated observers is recommended. When working with students, specialists may distribute the checklist to teachers and other professionals at the beginning of, at the end of, or during the school year.

Observers are asked to pay particular attention to the oral language of their students with respect to the word-finding behaviors listed on the checklist. Learners who display many of the word-finding behaviors on the checklist are referred to specialists for deep assessment in the area of word finding.[1]

DEEP ASSESSMENT IN WORD FINDING: IDENTIFYING WORD-FINDING ERROR PATTERNS

The screening process is designed to help identify learners who need diagnostic assessment in the area of word finding. The actual in-depth diagnostic assessment provides the specific information needed to develop an individualized word-finding intervention program. Diagnostic assessment of word-finding skills should yield information about the

---

[1] See German's (2001) book, *It's on the Tip of My Tongue: Word-Finding Strategies to Remember Names and Words You Often Forget,* for a similar checklist for adults. Adults who are judged to manifest a high number of word-finding behaviors on the checklist are administered an in-depth word-finding assessment by the speech–language specialist.

WORD-FINDING REFERRAL CHECKLIST

Name of Child/Adult Art Age 10 (yrs) 2 (mos)

School/Home Address Lincoln Elementary

Observer Shirley Date 9/25

Relationship to Child/Adult Classroom teacher

Does the child usually	YES	NO
1. Know the word he/she wants to say, but cannot think of it?	☑	☐
2. Have good understanding of spoken language used in class or at home?	☑	☐
3. Have difficulty remembering names of people, places or objects that he/she knows?	☑	☐
4. Substitute		
a. a real word or nonsense word that sounds like the word he/she can't remember (such as, says "custard" for mustard; "geophy" for geography)	☑	☐
b. the function of the word he/she can't remember (such as, "cutting" for scissors)	☐	☑
c. a description for the word he/she can't remember (such as, says "the brown one" for penny)	☑	☐
d. vague words for words he/she can't remember (such as, says "stuff, you know, watch-a-ma-call-it")?	☑	☐
5. Give a wrong answer and then self-correct (such as, says "basketball, no football")?	☐	☑
6. Have a long delay when he/she can't think of a word (such as, says "Give me the um ... ... video")?	☑	☐
7. Have difficulty remembering words during a conversation?	☑	☐
8. Repeat words and phrases when relating an experience ("We were, ... We were going shopping")?	☐	☑

(continues)

Figure 2.1. Sample completed Word-Finding Referral Checklist. *Note.* From *Word-Finding Referral Checklist,* by Diane J. German and Arthur E. German, 1992, Chicago: Word Finding Materials. Copyright 1992 by Diane J. German. Reprinted with permission.

Figure 2.1. ***Continued.***

Does the child usually	YES	NO
9. Make false starts and revisions when relating an experience ("We were ... Bob and I went to the game")?	☑	☐
10. Use gestures that indicate frustration (such as, hand waving, finger snapping) or mime the target word?	☑	☐
11. Use time fillers when trying to think of a word (such as, "um, ... er ... um ... computer")?	☑	☐
12. State, "I know that word, but I can't think of it" when he/she can't remember a word?	☑	☐

learner's word-finding response patterns. This includes information about the learner's

- speed and accuracy profile,
- responsiveness to phonemic cueing,
- nature of target word substitutions,
- ability to imitate multisyllabic words, and
- use of secondary characteristics when having word-finding difficulties (e.g., gestures, extra verbalizations).

The diagnostic model underlying the *Test of Word Finding–Second Edition* (TWF–2; German, 2000a) recommends the following questions be addressed to obtain this information. Answers to these questions will identify the word-finding error patterns that are typical of a particular learner.

WHAT IS THE LEARNER'S SPEED AND ACCURACY PROFILE?

Word-finding speed refers to the efficiency with which an individual retrieves words. *Word-finding accuracy* refers to the ability of an individual to retrieve words correctly on the first response. Learners with word-finding difficulties are typically inaccurate in their efforts to retrieve specific vocabulary. Although they may know the words they want to use, they respond incorrectly because they cannot retrieve the target words. When considering retrieval speed and accuracy together, learners who have word-finding difficulties with specific words tend to manifest the following time accuracy profiles (German, 1989, 1990, 2000a):

- Fast but inaccurate retrievers

- Slow and inaccurate retrievers
- Slow but accurate retrievers

IS THE LEARNER'S WORD FINDING AIDED BY PHONEMIC CUEING? *Phonemic cueing* is a diagnostic procedure in which the examiner provides the initial consonant–vowel combination (*yo* for *yolk*) or first syllable (*mi* for *microphone*) of the target word following a word-finding block. The phonemic cue is thought to make the word form search more effective by improving the link between the target word's semantic and phonological properties.

Therefore, if a learner is able to access the target word with the phonemic cue, it is assumed that his or her word-finding error was form-related, a failure to access the target word's phonological information (German, 2000a). This disruption is commonly know as the "tip of the tongue" error, and corresponding word-finding strategies are focused on making the phonological form of the target word more salient for the learner.

WHAT IS THE NATURE OF THE LEARNER'S RESPONSE SUBSTITUTIONS? Learners with word-finding difficulties typically produce unique target word substitutions when they have difficulty retrieving target words. An analysis of the learner's responses can provide information about the nature of his or her word-finding disruptions. Looking at the learner's response substitutions can guide the specialist's selection of word-finding strategies to facilitate a learner's word-finding skills. Individuals with word-finding difficulties often manifest the following response substitutions:

- Semantic substitutions are responses that are related in meaning to the target word, such a the following:
  - The category name for the word the learner cannot retrieve (e.g., substitutes *tool* for *hammer*)
  - The function of the word the learner cannot retrieve (e.g., substitutes *cutting* for *scissors*)
  - A word in the same category as the target word the learner cannot retrieve (e.g., substitutes *north* for *south*)
  - Description for the word the learner cannot retrieve (e.g., "the thing that has a cord and is hooked to the computer" for *mouse*)

- Phonological substitutions are responses that are related in sound form to the target word, such as the following:
  - A nonsense word that is similar in phonological pattern to the target word, such as the following substitutions for the word *octopus*:

    Phoneme shifts, as in *optucus*
    Phoneme substitutions, as in *octobus*
    Phoneme additions, as in *octgopus*
    Phoneme omissions, as in *ocpus*

  - A real word that shares the same phonological pattern as the target word (e.g., *emergency* for *emerging*)

- No response describes responses that do not contain content, such as the following:
  - "I don't know"
  - "I pass"
  - Omission (learner does not answer)

IS THE LEARNER ABLE TO CORRECTLY IMITATE THE ERRED TARGET WORD?

The imitation procedure focuses on the learner's ability to articulate the target word. By determining whether the learner can correctly imitate the erred target word, the specialist can observe whether a learner's failure to produce a known bisyllabic or multisyllabic target word is a problem of articulation. If a learner is able to imitate the target word syllable by syllable, it is assumed that he or she has sufficient articulatory ability to say the target word he or she failed to name. Otherwise, poor articulation would have been apparent when the learner imitated the word. It is therefore hypothesized that learners who can imitate an erred word they know probably failed to produce the word because of a word-finding difficulty.

In such cases, the learners' success on the imitation task occurred because the target word's phonological information was provided (German, 2000a). Hearing the model helps learners whose word-finding difficulties are due to problems in accessing all the phonological features of the target word. Word-finding strategies to reduce this error type, commonly known as "twist of the tongue" errors, are focused on making the word's syllabic structure explicit and the form of troublesome syllables more salient for the learners.

WHAT SECONDARY CHARACTERISTICS ARE PRESENT DURING A WORD-FINDING BLOCK?

Secondary characteristics in word-finding difficulties are behaviors that often accompany efforts to retrieve target words. Two types of secondary characteristics may be present during a word-finding block:

- *Gestures* are nonverbal responses that occur while an individual is having difficulty retrieving a specific word. Gestures of frustration include tapping, grimacing, eye blinking, and finger snapping. A learner might also mime the action associated with the target word referent (e.g., mime the action of cutting for *scissors* or mime exercising for *aerobics*).
- *Extra verbalizations* are additional comments produced when an individual is having difficulty retrieving a specific word. These comments can be *metacognitive,* where the learner comments on the word retrieval process itself (e.g., "I can't think of it") or *metalinguistic,* where the comments themselves provide cues to the naming process (e.g., "It starts with an *f*" for *film*).

IDENTIFYING THE LEARNER'S WORD-FINDING ERROR PATTERNS

By considering the information obtained from the five questions in the preceding section, the specialist can identify the learner's word-finding error patterns and use them to select appropriate word-retrieval strategies, plan self-advocacy instruction, and design word-finding accommodations. Matching the WFIP–2 word-finding intervention procedures to the learner's error patterns is the focus of Chapter 3.

Specialists can also use this information to relate errors to the four stages of word retrieval. Using the architectural stage model of lexical retrieval as a framework, German (2000a) suggested that children's word-finding errors, like adults' (Caramazza & Hillis, 1990; Hillis & Caramazza, 1995), may be due to disruptions at one of three points in the lexical process, leading to three descriptive error patterns:

- *Error Pattern 1: Lemma-Related Semantic Errors.* Lemma-related disruptions at Stage 2 result from a failure to access the target word's semantic or syntactic features (e.g., *boat* for *submarine*; German, 2000a; German & Newman, 2004).
- *Error Pattern 2: Word-Form Blocked Errors.* Word-form-related errors result from a failure at the juncture between Stages 2 and 3 to access

any of the target word-form information (e.g., no response or "I don't know"; German, 2000a; German & Newman, 2004).

- *Error Pattern 3: Word-Form Phonologic Errors.* Word-form segment-related disruptions at Stage 3 are demonstrated by partial access of the syllabic frame or segmental sound content associated with the lemma (e.g., *subrine* for *submarine*; German, 2000a; German & Newman, 2004).

Each of these word-finding error patterns is highlighted in the following section.

LINKING WORD-FINDING ERROR PATTERNS TO INTERVENTION

Using a learner's error patterns to guide selection of retrieval strategies results in individualized word-finding intervention. Therefore, three word-finding patterns are highlighted in this section and corresponding retrieval strategies are recommended.

ERROR PATTERN 1: LEMMA-RELATED SEMANTIC ERRORS

Failing to access the target word's lemma (i.e., its semantic and syntactic features) results in Error Pattern 1. This error pattern is marked by either a fast inaccurate response or a slow inaccurate response.

FAST, INACCURATE RESPONSES

Fast, inaccurate responses (commonly known as "slip of the tongue" errors) occur on the nouns (e.g., *cat* for *dog*), pronouns (e.g., *him* for *her*), or verbs (e.g., *skipping* for *running*) in a sentence. When learners manifest a fast, inaccurate response, they typically have failed to inhibit competing responses and thus retrieve the wrong names of known people, places, or objects (e.g., *calculator* for *computer*). Other characteristics include the following:

- Producing real-word substitutions that are related to the target word in either meaning (i.e., semantic neighbors such as *exponent* for *coefficient*) or sound pattern (i.e., phonological neighbors such as *emergency* for *emerging* or *octagon* for *octopus*)
- Self-correcting after producing an error

- Producing revisions or reformulations in discourse (e.g., "He is, she was late.")
- Typically not producing gestures

Intervention focused on reducing Error Pattern 1: Lemma-Related Semantic Errors (fast and inaccurate responses) should include all of the following:

1. Word-retrieval strategies that help learners slow the pace of their speaking
2. Word-finding self-advocacy instruction to improve self-mentoring and self-correction
3. Word-finding accommodations in the classroom that slow classroom discussion and encourage self-monitoring and self-correction

See Chapter 3 for more in-depth discussion of these WFIP–2 intervention components.

SLOW, INACCURATE RESPONSES

A slow, inaccurate response that is semantic in nature is thought to occur because of an inability to find the semantic (i.e., lemma) features of the target word. Typically, learners with this difficulty respond in the following ways:

- Produce real-word substitutions that are semantic neighbors to the target word (e.g., *robin* for *cardinal*)
- Do not self-correct
- Do not produce the target word when given the phonemic cue
- Are able to imitate the target word

Intervention focused on reducing Error Pattern 1: Lemma-Related Semantic Errors (slow, inaccurate responses) should include all of the following:

- Retrieval strategies that help learners anchor the semantic features of the target word include visual imagery and gesture mnemonics (see Lessons 6-4 and 6-5)
- Self-advocacy instruction focused on self-application of word-retrieval strategies (see all lessons in Chapters 6 through 10)
- Word-finding accommodations that include multiple-choice frames and resource materials (see Lessons 10-1 to 10-7)

ERROR PATTERN 2: WORD-FORM BLOCKED ERRORS

Error Pattern 2 results when the learner is able to access the semantic and syntactic features (i.e., the lemma) of the target word but fails to access the form of the target word. The outcome is a failure to access the corresponding syllabic frame and phonological content of the target word (known as a "lost address"). This error pattern is marked by slow inaccurate or slow accurate responses on the nouns (e.g., "Um ... I don't know" for *tambourine*), adjectives, or verbs (e.g., "Um ... skateboarding" as a delayed but correct response) within a sentence (commonly known as the "tip of the tongue" error type). Although learners know the words they cannot access, they typically manifest the following additional behaviors when trying to retrieve a word or respond to a question:

- A delay followed by an "I don't know" response (e.g., "Um ... I don't know")
- A delay followed by a semantic substitution response (e.g., "Um ... north" for *south*)
- Retrieval of the word when the learner is given a phonemic cue of the target word (e.g., the first syllable or consonant–vowel combination, *tam* for *tambourine*)
- Production of the correct word or name after an extended delay (e.g., "... uh ... uh ... clearance")
- A delay followed by a metalinguistic comment (e.g., "Um ... It starts with *tam* for *tambourine*") or a metacognitive comment (e.g., "I know it but cannot think of it.")
- Production of iconic gestures (e.g., mime of the target word action) or gestures of frustration (e.g., finger snapping, looking up)

Intervention focused on reducing Error Pattern 2: Word-Form Blocked Errors should include the following:

- Mnemonic word-finding strategies (see Lessons 7-1 through 7-3) that will make the target word form more salient
- Semantic alternate strategies (see Lessons 7-4 and 7-5) used to circumvent word-finding blocks
- Word-finding self-advocacy instruction (see retrieval strategy lessons in Chapter 7 and self-advocacy lessons in Chapter 9) to help with self-application of the retrieval strategies
- Word-finding accommodations (see Lessons 10-1 to 10-7) that reduce the retrieval load inherent in the learner's academic work

ERROR PATTERN 3: WORD-FORM PHONOLOGIC ERRORS

Error Pattern 3 results when the learner is able to access the target word's semantic and syntactic features but is only able to access part of the word's phonologic features (i.e., the syllabic frame or sound units). Errors at this level are typically phonemic substitutions that consist of phonemic approximations of the target word, such as the following:

- Phoneme exchanges (e.g., *carindal* for *cardinal*)
- Substitutions (e.g., *carbinal* for *cardinal*)
- Additions (e.g., *cardineral* for *cardinal*)
- Omissions (e.g., *carnal* for *cardinal*)

When learners display this error pattern, it is typically marked by a slow, inaccurate response when accessing bisyllabic or multisyllabic words—nouns (*octpus* for *octopus*), adjectives, or verbs (*skatebooding* for *skateboarding*)—within a sentence (commonly known as the "twist of the tongue" error). Although they know the meanings of these long words, learners with Error Pattern 3 typically manifest the following behaviors when trying to retrieve a word or respond to a question:

- Delay followed by a phonemic approximation of the target word (e.g., *amonlance* for *ambulance*) or no response (e.g., "Um ... I don't know")
- Delay followed by a semantic substitution (e.g., "Um ... fish thing" for *octopus*)
- Inability to retrieve with the phonemic cue
- Delay followed by a metacognitive comment (e.g., "Um ... I can't say those long words.")

Intervention focused on reducing Error Pattern 3: Word-Form Phonologic Errors should include the following:

- Segmenting strategies (see Lesson 8-1) that make the syllabic structure of the target word explicit
- Same-sounds syllable cues (see Lesson 8-2) that make the target word syllables more salient
- Rehearsal strategies (see all retrieval strategy lessons)
- A word-finding self-advocacy program (see all retrieval strategy lessons) that encourages self-application of the word-finding strategies
- Word-finding accommodations (see Lessons 10-1 to 10-7) that require multiple-choice frames in classroom questioning and resource materials that include the multisyllabic words in the curriculum

SUMMARY

When planning an intervention program for learners with word-finding difficulties, the specialist needs to have knowledge of a learner's word-finding skills in the following areas:

- Retrieval accuracy and speed
- Responsiveness to phonemic cueing
- Target word substitutions
- Ability to imitate
- Types of secondary characteristics produced

This information can be gleaned through collaborative observation in the classroom and formal diagnostic assessment.

Two standardized tests are available for formal diagnostic assessment: the *Test of Word Finding–Second Edition* (TWF–2; German, 2000a) and the *Test of Adolescent/Adult Word Finding* (German, 1990). These instruments provide information about a learner's word-finding speed and accuracy, responsiveness to phonemic cueing (TWF–2 only), response substitutions, and ability to imitate multisyllabic target words (TWF–2 only). An informal assessment of the learner's secondary characteristics (i.e., gestures and extra verbalizations) is also included in these instruments. Formal assessment of word-finding skills in discourse is available with the *Test of Word Finding in Discourse* (German, 1991).

SECTION 2

The Word-Finding Intervention Program

Implementing the WFIP-2: Components, Settings, and Forms

INSTRUCTIONAL COMPONENTS

When a learner has been identified as having word-finding difficulties, he or she is ready to begin the *Word-Finding Intervention Program–Second Edition* (WFIP–2). As indicated in earlier chapters, the WFIP–2 has three components: retrieval strategy instruction, word-finding self-advocacy instruction, and word-finding accommodations. Generally, specialists seeking to implement the WFIP–2 should follow the sequence described in this chapter.

COMPONENT 1: RETRIEVAL STRATEGY INSTRUCTION

Follow these steps to implement retrieval strategy instruction in the WFIP–2.

1. To begin, use the learner's word-finding error pattern for guidance in selecting the retrieval strategies that are appropriate for the learner (see discussion or error patterns in Chapter 2).
   a. Using the corresponding lesson plan (see the word-retrieval lesson plans in Chapters 6, 7, and 8), apply the preferred strategies, noting whether they facilitate the learner's retrieval.
   b. From these initial trials, identify those retrieval strategies that appear to best facilitate the learner's retrieval of words.
2. Identify vocabulary sets for use in the WFIP–2 lessons. Use Appendix A, which contains vocabulary lists and completed Syllable-Dividing and Same-Sounds Syllable Cue Study Forms, to demonstrate how to match retrieval strategies to selected vocabulary. See Chapter 4 for a discussion regarding procedures for matching retrieval strategies to target vocabulary.
3. Apply the WFIP–2 lesson plans that correspond to the retrieval strategies to improve the learner's word-finding skills with the target vocabulary.
4. Embed use of the retrieval strategies in various academic activities to teach learners how to aid their retrieval when they are having word-finding difficulties.

NOTE: The same lesson plans may be used many times; however, the selected vocabulary to which the retrieval strategies are applied will continue to change.

---

5. Teach self-application of retrieval strategies.

Although it is encouraged in all lessons, self-application of the selected strategies is the focus here. Using new vocabulary, the learner participates in retrieval strategy instruction. Charting the learner's self-application of strategies is encouraged. Jointly and strategically select settings to apply strategies, adding contexts as the learner achieves success in each setting.

COMPONENT 2: WORD-FINDING SELF-ADVOCACY INSTRUCTION

As you identify retrieval strategies, use the following steps to introduce the learner to the self-advocacy component of the WFIP–2:

1. Help the learner discover which retrieval strategies aid his or her retrieval.
2. Teach self-monitoring techniques to identify target behaviors.
3. Help the learner become aware of how different language settings, speaking situations, retrieval contexts, language contexts, times of day, and types of vocabulary influence his or her word-finding skills using the Word-Finding Self-Assessment Survey (see Appendix B).
4. Help the learner collaborate with teachers, parents, and supervisors about the word-finding accommodations needed to aid his or her word-finding skills in the school, home, and work environments.
5. Direct the learner to self-apply selected retrieval strategies in the language room and in the academic setting. Jointly create a written contract between you and the learner, specifying his or her commitment to self-apply the strategies in jointly identified settings by agreed-upon dates.

COMPONENT 3: WORD-FINDING ACCOMMODATIONS

After beginning the self-advocacy program, introduce the learner to the word-finding accommodations component of the WFIP–2. Implement it concurrently with the retrieval strategy and self-advocacy lessons, following these steps:

1. Begin the word-finding accommodations component by explaining to the learner the rationale for developing instructional modifications for students who have word-finding difficulties.
   a. Review with the learner his or her Word-Finding Self-Assessment Survey (see Appendix B). Discuss the learner's perception of his or her word-finding strengths and weaknesses as they relate to interpersonal communication, homework assignments, classroom assignments, and examinations.
   b. Complete the Classroom Observation Form (see Appendix C) for each of the learner's classrooms to identify the need for word-finding accommodations that will facilitate his or her learning.

2. Collaborate with teachers and parents to select and implement appropriate word-finding accommodations in the classroom and at home. Complete the Recommended Word-Finding Accommodations Form (see Appendix C).
3. After implementing the word-finding accommodations, use the learner's weekly language lesson time to discuss and analyze the appropriateness of those accommodations in the school and home settings.
4. Conduct ongoing review and revision of the word-finding accommodations chosen; note all the people involved (e.g., classroom teacher, parent, and learner).

Finally, develop Individualized Education Program (IEP) benchmarks (i.e., objectives) for the accommodations selected (see Chapter 5 for a discussion of benchmarks).

NOTE: Although the level of participation by each learner will vary depending on his or her age and ability to assess his or her own word-finding skills, children as young as 6 years can participate in conversations with the classroom teacher about word-finding accommodations.

INSTRUCTIONAL SETTINGS

Two distinct settings need to be considered when you implement the WFIP–2: the individual or group settings, and the language room or classroom settings.

INDIVIDUAL AND GROUP SETTINGS IN THE LANGUAGE ROOM

Lessons in the WFIP–2 are designed to be implemented in both individual and group formats. For example, initial strategy instruction lends itself to individual settings because it is focused on identification of appropriate retrieval strategies for a particular learner. However, a group format can also be used at this level. In a group setting, you would present the retrieval strategies selected for each learner to the entire group.

Strategy instruction lessons directed toward ongoing application and self-application of retrieval strategies are best implemented in a group format. Such use provides opportunities for practicing retrieving the target vocabulary in a discourse context provided by conversation among group members.

Self-advocacy instruction and planning word-finding accommodations can be implemented in either individual or group sessions. For example, completing and discussing the Word-finding Self-Assessment Survey can occur between you and the learner, or in a group format with learners responding in turn to questions on the survey. Similarly, identification of modifications needed in the classroom can emerge from a discussion among you, the teacher, and the learner, or from a group discussion where peers share their concerns and needs about instructional methods they may want modified.

IMPLEMENTING THE THREE INSTRUCTIONAL COMPONENTS IN THE CLASSROOM

RETRIEVAL STRATEGY INSTRUCTION IN THE CLASSROOM

You can facilitate the learner's oral language in cooperative group activities, oral language assignments, and written language tasks. In these contexts, facilitation might include the following:

- Linking same-sounds or familiar-word cues to target words, to anchor their retrieval
- Linking same-sound syllable cues to difficult syllables of multisyllabic words, to stabilize their retrieval
- Demonstrating syllable dividing to make the syllabic structure of multisyllabic words explicit
- Suggesting semantic alternates for target words the learner has difficulty retrieving
- Encouraging rehearsal of target words

WORD-FINDING ACCOMMODATIONS IN THE CLASSROOM

Although you will begin implementing the word-finding accommodation component in the context of the language lessons, the core of this component is actually implemented in the classroom. For example, to determine appropriate word-finding accommodations, you and the learner identify those accommodations that are needed at home and in the school language environments. Collaborate with the classroom teacher and the learner to determine the academic accommodations needed to encourage learning and facilitate communication in the learner's classroom. These accommodations should be documented in the learner's IEP. Final lessons involve the actual implementation of the accommodations planned for the learner in school.

SELF-ADVOCACY PROGRAMMING IN THE CLASSROOM

Initial lessons in self-advocacy instruction are implemented in the language lesson, which may or may not be in the classroom. However, the following lessons are implemented in the classroom:

- Self-monitoring of retrieval behaviors to be reduced
- Learner–teacher collaboration
- Self-application of retrieval strategies

WFIP–2 FORMS

The WFIP–2 provides a variety of forms for the learner and specialist to use in conjunction with various components of the intervention program. *You should not feel obligated to use all the WFIP–2 forms but should choose those that are most appropriate for the learner.* These forms are available in the appendixes of this manual and may be reproduced as needed. Following are descriptions of each form.

WORD-FINDING RETRIEVAL STRATEGY INSTRUCTION FORMS

Forms related to the retrieval strategy instruction component of the WFIP–2 are located in Appendix A of this manual. Specifically, the forms given are the Retrieval Strategy Lesson Plan and the Vocabulary and Retrieval Strategy Practice Form. Specialists and teachers may copy these forms for clinical and teaching purposes.

RETRIEVAL STRATEGY LESSON PLAN

The Retrieval Strategy Lesson Plan form is designed to assist you in planning and recording the WFIP–2 lessons implemented with each learner (see Appendix A). This form summarizes the following information:

1. The word-finding error patterns that are the focus of the retrieval strategy instruction
2. The retrieval strategies to be taught to facilitate the learners' word-finding skills
3. The corresponding WFIP–2 lesson plan for each retrieval strategy
4. The vocabulary and academic activity designated for a particular learner or group

Complete and update this form as needed for each learner using the WFIP–2. Use the following steps:

1. Enter the specialist and date information at the top of the form.
2. In Part 1: Assigning Lessons, in the columns under Learner's Name, enter the name of each learner enrolled in the WFIP–2.
3. Below each learner's name, indicate with a checkmark the retrieval strategies to be studied with that learner.
4. In Part 2: Selecting Content, enter the academic subject being studied (e.g., science, landforms) and the specific words being treated (e.g., *valley*).
5. Indicate the academic subject (e.g., reading, writing, math) that you plan to use to teach and reinforce the use of retrieval strategies being taught.

VOCABULARY AND RETRIEVAL STRATEGY PRACTICE FORM

The Vocabulary and Retrieval Strategy Practice Form is designed to help learners review and rehearse the vocabulary and retrieval strategies they have been taught in their WFIP–2 lessons. At the end of a lesson the specialist or the learner should do the following:

1. In Column 1, write the target words that have been identified as needing additional practice.
2. In Column 2, segment the target words into syllables.
3. Write the mnemonic retrieval strategy in Column 3 if the strategy is a same-sounds or familiar-word cue (i.e., *same-sounds cue, same-sounds meaning or syllable cue,* or *familiar-word cue,*) or in Column 4 if it is a synonym or category alternate.
4. Complete Column 5 by applying the retrieval strategy (in Column 3 or 4) to the target vocabulary word (from Column 1). Indicate responses with checkmarks in Column 5.
5. Complete Column 6 by verbalizing the target word in a brief sentence. Indicate responses with checkmarks in Column 6.

Instruct learners to use this form to guide their rehearsal of the vocabulary at home or at the beginning of each language session.

SELF-ADVOCACY INSTRUCTION FORM

WORD-FINDING SELF-ASSESSMENT SURVEY

The Word-Finding Self-Assessment Survey form (see Appendix B) is designed to be used in the self-advocacy component of the WFIP–2. Its purpose is to help learners identify influences that affect, both positively and negatively, their word-finding skills. Learners are asked to analyze the effects of the following variables on their word-finding skills using a scale of 1 to 3 where 1 indicates the *least difficulty* and 3 indicates the *most difficulty* in the corresponding context:

1. The speaking settings (e.g., reading class, dinner table, sports-related activities)
2. The language circumstances (i.e., one-on-one or in a group)
3. The retrieval contexts (i.e., retrieval of specific words in single-word or discourse contexts)
4. The language contexts (i.e., oral or written language)
5. The content area of the target word (e.g., people's names, science, math)
6. The lexical factors of the target word (e.g., the target word's frequency, length, syntax, phonological attributes)

The specialist and the learner should complete the Word-Finding Self-Assessment Survey together, following these steps:

1. Review the different language settings in which the learner is asked to talk. Have the learner rate his or her language difficulty in each setting.
2. Review the different language circumstances in which the learner is typically engaged. Ask the learner to rate his or her language difficulty in each setting.
3. Review the different retrieval contexts indicated on the survey where the learner is typically asked to respond orally. Ask the learner to rate his or her language difficulty in each context.
4. Review the different language contexts (i.e., oral or written language) in which the learner is typically asked to respond. Ask the learner to rate his or her language difficulty level in each context.
5. Review the different content areas in which the learner is typically asked to respond orally. Ask the learner to rate his or her language difficulty for the vocabulary in each subject.
6. Review the lexical factors of target words (i.e., frequency, syntax, length, and phonological complexity) that learners are typically asked to retrieve. Ask the learner to rate his or her language difficulty in using the corresponding vocabulary.

WORD-FINDING ACCOMMODATIONS FORMS

Word-finding accommodations forms assist specialists and teachers in identifying and recommending classroom word-finding accommodations.

The forms provided in Appendix C are the Classroom Observation Form and the Recommended Word-Finding Accommodations Form. Specialists and teachers may copy these forms for clinical or teaching purposes.

CLASSROOM OBSERVATION FORM

The Classroom Observation Form, shown in Appendix C, is provided to guide your discussions with teachers regarding implementation of word-finding accommodations in the learner's classrooms. With help from the classroom teacher, complete the form by following these steps:

1. Observe the learner's classroom and indicate on the form (depending on the column, mark ✗ or ✔) which tasks are expected of the learner in the areas of classroom discussion/oral classroom work, written classroom work, homework assignments, and evaluations. Also indicate the use of instructional technology in the classroom.
2. Collaborate with the classroom teacher to determine feasible word-finding accommodations in classroom activities that would facilitate the student's learning.

RECOMMENDED WORD-FINDING ACCOMMODATIONS FORM

The Recommended Word-Finding Accommodations Form (see Appendix C) is provided to guide specialists, teachers, and learners in determining the appropriate modifications to make in classroom discussions, oral classroom work, written classroom work, homework assignments, and evaluation. These recommended accommodations should be documented in the form of IEP objectives.

Complete the form with the learner and his or her classroom teachers. Note that the self-reflection required in this analysis may be difficult for younger learners. In such cases, feel free to select only those portions of the survey that the learner can complete. Use the following steps to complete the form:

1. Discuss the need to modify specific activities in the classroom to reduce the retrieval load inherent in these activities. Explain that the goal is to create activities that do not put high demands on the learner's word-retrieval skills.
2. Review classroom activities used in the various instructional areas listed on the Classroom Observation Form.
3. Discuss the appropriateness of these activities with learners who experience word-finding challenges.

4. Complete the Recommended Word-Finding Accommodations Form by checking the recommended modifications for instructional areas of concern.
5. Collaborate with the classroom teacher and the learner, if such an activity is age-appropriate for the learner, regarding the recommended accommodations.

WFIP–2 VOCABULARY FORMS

The WFIP–2 also includes selected vocabulary and offers two ways to incorporate those target words into the lessons. Appendix A contains the Syllable-Dividing and Same-Sound Syllable Cue Study Form (included both blank and completed, with selected vocabulary also listed by subject) and the Model Sentences for Selected WFIP–2 Vocabulary.

SYLLABLE-DIVIDING AND SAME-SOUNDS SYLLABLE CUE STUDY FORM

For Error Patterns 2 and 3 (see Chapter 2 for descriptions of the error patterns), the WFIP–2 lesson plans recommend that the learner use one of the mnemonic strategies—same-sounds cue, same-sounds meaning or syllable cue, or familiar-word cue—to anchor retrieval of target words or target word syllables. Appendix A provides the master form for the WFIP–2 Syllable-Dividing and Same-Sounds Syllable Cue Study Form, which is designed to be used as a worksheet to help learners apply the segmenting and retrieval strategies studied during the WFIP–2 lessons. Sample completed WFIP–2 Syllable-Dividing and Same-Sounds Syllable Cue Study Forms also are presented in Appendix A, showing how these forms could be used to teach a variety of vocabulary types.

In these examples, the WFIP–2 provides 13 vocabulary lists organized around themes typically relevant to school-age learners (e.g., sports themes such as baseball, tennis, swimming, golf, football, hockey, and soccer; academic themes such as math, social studies, and science). When it is appropriate for the learner, the specialist may use the vocabulary in Appendix A as the vocabulary for the WFIP–2 lessons.

MODEL SENTENCES FOR SELECTED WFIP–2 VOCABULARY

When using the WFIP–2, learners rehearse applying their retrieval strategies to target words in the context of a sentence and discourse. To aid in these lessons, Appendix A provides sentences for selected WFIP–2 vocabulary. When appropriate for the learner, you are encouraged to use the WFIP–2 sentences as the bases for creating meaningful narratives using the target vocabulary.

Word-Retrieval Strategy Instruction

The primary objective of teaching retrieval strategies is to aid learners in accessing specific words in single-word and discourse contexts. As a general rule, you should only apply the retrieval strategies to target words the learner comprehends. The WFIP–2 uses a set of nine procedures to achieve seven primary objectives, as shown in Figure 4.1. This chapter describes the objectives and their related procedures.

Enhance Lexical Access*

Procedure 1: Use retrieval strategies to enhance the learner's ability to access known target words.

Develop Individual Strategy Plans

Procedure 2: Identify retrieval strategies appropriate for the learner.
- Error Pattern 1: Lemma-Related Semantic Errors
  - Preferred retrieval strategies
  - Supplementary retrieval strategies
- Error Pattern 2: Word-Form Blocked Errors
  - Preferred retrieval strategies
  - Supplementary retrieval strategies
- Error Pattern 3: Word-Form Phonologic Errors
  - Preferred retrieval strategies

Procedure 3: Use relevant and thematic curriculum for word-finding intervention.

Procedure 4: Consider lexical factors of target words when matching the vocabulary to retrieval strategies.

Move from Single Word to Discourse

Procedure 5: Adjust application of strategies from retrieval of words in isolation to retrieval of those words in sentences and discourse.

Encourage Rehearsal

Procedure 6: Encourage ongoing rehearsal of vocabulary in isolation, sentences, and discourse.

Teach Self-Application

Procedure 7: Teach the learner to self-apply the retrieval strategies learned during the lessons.

Use Academic Activities in the Classroom

Procedure 8: Use academic activities in the classroom to teach and apply retrieval strategies.

Provide Generalization Activities

Procedure 9: Implement activities that encourage generalization of retrieval strategies to everyday classroom, home, and work situations.

*Incorporate appropriate technology across objectives and procedures.

Figure 4.1. Objectives and procedures for teaching word-retrieval strategies.

ENHANCE LEXICAL ACCESS

Procedure 1. Use retrieval strategies to enhance the learner's ability to access known target words.

Learners with word-finding difficulties struggle to retrieve words they know (see German, 2000a, for a discussion of subtypes of word-finding difficulties). The WFIP–2 provides retrieval strategies to help learners become automatic in accessing known target words. These retrieval strategies should be applied to words whose meanings the learner comprehends (i.e., the words' conceptual structure and lemma are stored), whose phonological schema (i.e., form or *lexeme*) the learner recognizes, and whose motor plan and capacity to articulate the learner possesses. For these words, instruction is focused on elaboration of the words' "retrieval strength" (Bjork & Bjork, 1992), thereby increasing the ease with which these known words can be accessed.

The WFIP–2 provides seven categories of retrieval strategies to help the learner gain access to known words. These strategies are memory tactics, or *mnemonics,* that aid retrieval of specific target words. Used before and during speech, each strategy has a different focus, as shown in Figure 4.2.

The three error patterns (see Chapter 2 for discussion of error patterns) also can be addressed using the WFIP–2 retrieval strategies (see Figure 4.3). These strategies form the basis for the WFIP–2 lesson plans in Section 3.

Mnemonic cueing retrieval strategies
- Same-sounds cue and same-sounds syllable cue
- Same-sounds meaning cue
- Familiar-word cue

Syllable-dividing retrieval strategies
- Target word segmenting
  - Visual syllable-dividing
  - Rhythm syllable-dividing

Alternate-word strategies
- Synonym and category substitution

Rehearsal
- Multiple repetitions
  - Isolation
  - Sentence
  - Discourse

Pausing
- Before noun phrase
- Before verb or noun in verb phrase

Self-monitoring and self-correcting strategy

Attribute-cueing retrieval strategies
- Graphemic cueing
- Imagery cueing
- Gesture cueing

Figure 4.2. Retrieval strategies used for enhancing lexical access of known words.

MNEMONIC-CUEING STRATEGIES

The first category of strategies is called "mnemonic cueing strategies" (German, 1993). Mnemonic cueing, based on knowledge of memory processes (Higbee, 1993), is a retrieval strategy in which the learner is taught to associate or link a cue word with the target word to aid retrieval of the target word. Researchers have indicated that the use of mnemonic

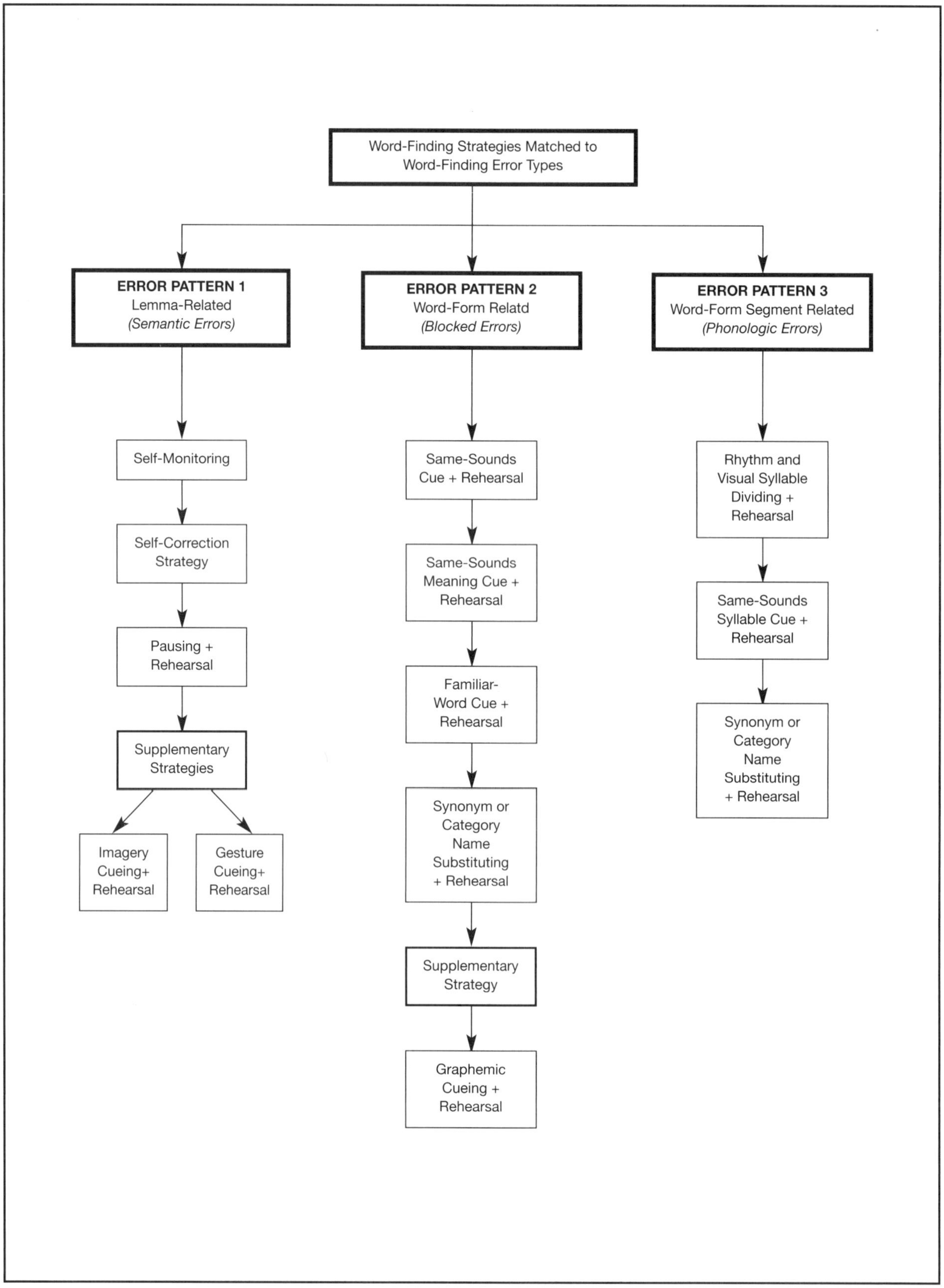

Word-Finding Strategies Matched to Word-Finding Error Types

- **ERROR PATTERN 1**
  Lemma-Related
  (Semantic Errors)
  - Self-Monitoring
  - Self-Correction Strategy
  - Pausing + Rehearsal
  - Supplementary Strategies
    - Imagery Cueing+ Rehearsal
    - Gesture Cueing+ Rehearsal
- **ERROR PATTERN 2**
  Word-Form Relatd
  (Blocked Errors)
  - Same-Sounds Cue + Rehearsal
  - Same-Sounds Meaning Cue + Rehearsal
  - Familiar-Word Cue + Rehearsal
  - Synonym or Category Name Substituting + Rehearsal
  - Supplementary Strategy
    - Graphemic Cueing + Rehearsal
- **ERROR PATTERN 3**
  Word-Form Segment Related
  (Phonologic Errors)
  - Rhythm and Visual Syllable Dividing + Rehearsal
  - Same-Sounds Syllable Cue + Rehearsal
  - Synonym or Category Name Substituting + Rehearsal

Figure 4.3. Word-finding strategies for each word-finding error pattern.

cues significantly decreases word-finding difficulties with target words (German, 2002) and improves general recall of everyday information (McNamara & Wong, 2003), episodic school experiences (Hudson & Fivush, 1991; Toglia, Shlechter, & Chevalier, 1992), and academic vocabulary (Mastropieri, Sweda, & Scruggs, 2000; Uberti, Scruggs, & Mastropieri, 2003).

Four types of mnemonic cues are provided in the WFIP–2:

- Same-sounds cue
- Same-sounds syllable cue
- Same-sounds meaning cue
- Familiar-word cue

Although similar to other memory strategies (e.g., "Key Word Method" in Uberti, Scruggs, & Mastropieri, 2003), the WFIP–2 mnemonic-cueing strategies differ in two important ways. First, application of mnemonic strategies in the WFIP–2 lessons are directed toward words whose meanings the learner already comprehends. For that reason the WFIP–2 mnemonic strategies do not focus on associating a function (e.g., *Christmas flower* for *poinsettia*) or an image (e.g., *red flower* for *poinsettia*) to the target word. Instead, the WFIP–2 mnemonic strategies are focused on helping speakers access the form or phonological schema of target words they already recognize. Further, other memory strategies may use form-related cues, but they are more broadly applied than the WFIP–2 retrieval strategies. Although these other memory strategies may be helpful for learners with general memory difficulties, learners with word-finding difficulties need a more targeted approach to their vocabulary instruction. For example, WFIP–2 lessons instruct you to match same-sounds cues to those syllables of a word that are troublesome for a particular learner. Associating a same-sounds cue to the problematic syllable of the target word results in an individualized strategic approach to improving a learner's retrieval of the target word. This is not to say that the WFIP–2 strategies supplant other memory techniques. Rather, the WFIP–2 retrieval strategies complement and refine other strategies, thus expanding your knowledge of effective instructional memory strategies for learners.

The following sections describe each of the WFIP–2 mnemonic strategies.

SAME-SOUNDS CUE AND SAME-SOUNDS SYLLABLE CUE

Same-sounds cues and *same-sounds syllable cues* are prompt words that use the form of the target word or syllable to cue its retrieval. The usefulness of cueing retrieval with words similar in sound to the target word or syllable (e.g., *coat* for *goat* or *daffy* for *daffodil,* an adaptation of what are referred to by Vitevitch [2002] and others as phonological neighbors of target words) has been verified in priming studies of adults. These investigations have reported that primes similar in sound form to the target word facilitate retrieval of that word during "tip of the tongue" blocks on picture naming tasks (Brown, 1991; Burke, MacKay, Worthley, & Wade, 1991; James & Burke, 2000; McNamara & Healy, 1988; Meyer & Bock, 1992). Child studies have also verified the usefulness of phonological priming to aid recall (McGregor & Windsor, 1996). German (2002) reported that students' word-finding skills improved on target words treated, in part, with the same-sounds cue and the same-sounds syllable cue over and beyond that of nontreated control words. Further, she reported that students' self-assessment of their ability to retrieve the treated words improved remarkably from pretreatment to posttreatment, whereas self-assessment of ease of retrieval of non-treated control words did not show improvement.

When using this strategy to improve word-finding skills, the learner is taught to associate or link a cue word to the target word or syllable. This cue word should be either an adapted phonological neighbor of the target word (i.e., shares some of the same sounds as the target word, such as *habit* for *habitat*) or a syllable or a homonym of the target word or syllable (e.g., *gym* for *Jim*). Before the speaking situation, the learner selects and practices thinking of a cue to prompt the target word or syllable (see Appendix A, Syllable-Dividing and Same-Sounds Syllable Cue Study Form). The learner is then instructed to think of the cue word while talking to aid his or her retrieval of specific words or word parts during a discourse.

The rehearsal strategy, described later in this chapter, is always used with a same-sounds cue (see Chapter 7, Lesson 7-1).

SAME-SOUNDS MEANING CUE

A same-sounds meaning cue is similar to the same-sounds cue in that it matches the phonological form of the target word, but it is also linked to the target word in meaning.

When using this strategy to improve word-finding skills, the learner is taught to associate, or link, a cue word that both sounds like the target word (e.g., *gym* for *Jim*) and is related to the target word in meaning (e.g., Jim is an athlete). The rehearsal strategy is always used with the same-sounds meaning cue (see Chapter 7, Lesson 7-2).

FAMILIAR-WORD CUE

The familiar-word cue is a prompt word that frequently co-occurs with the target word in a different context. Similar to, but more targeted than, collocation strategies (Woolard, 2004), the familiar-word cue strategy uses previously practiced word combinations to prime retrieval of a target word's form (e.g., *blue jeans* to retrieve the color blue).

When using this strategy to improve word-finding skills, the learner is taught to associate the target word with a word or phrase that is said with the target word in a different context. This association would be a word combination whose retrieval is already automatic for that learner, (e.g., *brown bear* to cue retrieval of *brown*). The rehearsal strategy, described later in this chapter, is always used with the familiar-word cue strategy (see Chapter 7, Lesson 7-3).

SYLLABLE-DIVIDING STRATEGIES

A second group of strategies, referred to as syllable-dividing strategies (German, 1993), uses target word segmenting. Researchers have indicated that focusing students on the metalinguistic properties of target words can aid their word-finding skills for these words (Catts, 1999; German & Schwanke, 2003; McGregor, 1994; VanKleeck, 1990; VanKleeck, Gillam, & McFadden, 1998; Wing, 1990). German (2002) reported that students' word-finding skills improved on target words treated, in part, with segmentation using the syllable-dividing strategy.

Syllable-dividing strategies are focused on the problematic word itself, directing the learner to analyze the target word (German, 1993; 2001). They provide metalinguistic reinforcement of the phonological structure of target words. These strategies are used before the speaking situation and in tandem with the same-sounds cue strategies to stabilize retrieval of multisyllabic words that the learner cannot retrieve or retrieves only partially (e.g., retrieves only the first syllable of the target word or a phonemic substitution).

Two types of syllable-dividing strategies are presented in this section: visual syllable dividing and rhythm syllable dividing (see Chapter 8, Lesson 8-1). Lesson 8-2, Same-Sounds Syllable Cue and Rehearsal, is used with these two syllable-dividing strategies.

VISUAL SYLLABLE DIVIDING

The visual syllable-dividing strategy is used to help the learner become automatic in retrieving multisyllabic words. This strategy is applied before the speaking situation and is used with learners who are familiar with syllabication concepts. The learner either writes each syllable in a grid representing the target word's syllabic structure (see Appendix A, Syllable-Dividing and Same-Sounds Syllable Cue Study Forms) or divides the target word into syllables by drawing a line between each syllable (e.g., ge/o/gra/phy). The learner then rehearses the target word, first syllable by syllable and then as a unit.

RHYTHM SYLLABLE DIVIDING

The rhythm syllable-dividing strategy is also used to help the learner become automatic in retrieving multisyllabic words. This strategy is applied before the speaking situation. When using this strategy to improve word-finding skills, the learner divides the target word into syllables by either marking each syllable with a rhythmic tap or clap or displaying fingers to indicate the number of syllables. Syllables also may be written in a grid for the student. The learner then rehearses the target word, first syllable by syllable and then as a unit.

ALTERNATE-WORD STRATEGY

The alternate-word strategy focuses on compensating for the retrieval block through synonym and category substitution (German, 1993, 2001; Harrell, Parenté, Bellingrath, & Lisicia, 1992). The goal is to aid the learner in making a smooth transition from attempts to retrieve the evasive word to an appropriate alternate. Used while talking, this strategy directs the speaker to use an alternate word for the target word that he or she is unable to retrieve.

When using this strategy, the speaker thinks ahead while talking, identifies the word that might cause difficulty, and then selects a synonym (e.g., *friendly* for *cordial*) or category name (e.g., *vegetable* for *artichoke*) for the evasive word.

To teach the alternate-word strategy, first identify synonyms or category names for target words, to increase the learner's word choices. Next, teach the learner to substitute these synonyms or category names for the target word he or she is unable to retrieve (see Chapter 7, Lessons 7-4 and 7-5). Then, following the block, have the learner use mnemonic-cueing and syllable-dividing strategies in tandem to anchor retrieval of troublesome words and avoid future word-finding disruptions.

REHEARSAL

Rehearsal strategies are employed to increase the automaticity of retrieving target words. These strategies require the learner to practice the retrieval of the target word through multiple repetitions, first in isolation and then in a sentence and discourse. Studies have indicated that an individual's retrieval processes are aided by rehearsal (Conca, 1989; Lesser, 1989; Ornstein, Naus, & Liberty, 1975). However, by itself, the rehearsal strategy does not appear to eliminate naming errors. German (2002) reported improvement in naming accuracy for words treated with mnemonic (i.e., same-sounds cues) strategies, whereas control words treated with rehearsal only (i.e., picture naming) did not improve significantly. When coupled with the mnemonic cueing and the syllable-dividing strategies, rehearsal aids retrieval of target words that the learner otherwise would not consistently retrieve accurately (German, 2002). Therefore, the rehearsal strategy is embedded in all the lesson plans for WFIP–2 word-finding strategies (see Chapters 6, 7, and 8, all lessons).

PAUSING

Pausing is a strategy that helps the speaker slow down the speaking process (German, 1993; Harrell et al., 1992). It involves cognitive modification to inhibit verbalization of erroneous words competing for selection. The learner is taught to strategically insert the pause before the noun or personal name in the noun phrase, or before the verb or adverb in the verb phrase. When strategically placed, the pause provides the learner with the time needed to screen out competing names or words and select the target word (see Chapter 6, Lesson 6-3).

SELF-MONITORING AND SELF-CORRECTING STRATEGY

The self-monitoring and self-correcting strategy is designed to help the learner self-monitor and self-correct his or her word-finding errors (Paul, 2001). Hallahan and Kauffman (2000) described self-monitoring as the practice of observing and recording one's own behavior, and Hanson (1996) indicated that the presence of this skill is a sign of increasing learner independence. Self-correction of word-finding errors is an outgrowth of self-monitoring and is important in maintaining accurate communication.

The WFIP–2's self-monitoring and self-correction lessons direct the learner to (a) listen to his or her speech while talking, (b) identify his or her word-finding errors, and (c) self-correct his or her word-finding errors before continuing the sentence. The self-monitoring and self-correcting strategy is taught in tandem with the pausing strategy (see Chapter 6, Lessons 6-1 and 6-2).

ATTRIBUTE-CUEING STRATEGIES

Attribute-cueing strategies are focused on specific attributes of the target word. They have been found helpful in prompting retrieval in both adults (Pease & Goodglass, 1978) and children (Johnson & Myklebust, 1967; McNamara & Wong, 2003; Rubin, Berstein, & Katz, 1989; Wiig & Semel, 1984; Wing, 1990).

The WFIP–2 provides lessons for attribute-cueing strategies focused on the spelling of the target word (i.e., graphemic cueing), the visual image of the word's referent (i.e., visual imagery), or the motor act associated with the target word (i.e., gesture cueing). These attribute strategies are classified as supplemental strategies because they are not direct links to the evasive sound form of the target word. However, they can be coupled with the other strategies for learners who may need additional mnemonic cueing. When learning each supplementary strategy, learners are first taught to use a presented cue and then to self-cue to aid retrieval.

GRAPHEMIC CUEING

Graphemic cueing is a retrieval strategy where the target word's form is primed with its spelling. First, the learner writes the target word, and then the learner is taught to revisualize the target word, spelling to self-cue his or her own retrieval of the target word. Graphemic cueing is most successful with learners who have grade-appropriate written language skills (see Chapter 7, Lesson 7-6).

IMAGERY CUEING

Although not focused on the sound form of the target word, this strategy is focused on priming or cueing the target word's meaning through visualization. Both adult and child studies have indicated that this type of strategy may be appropriate in the remediation of word-finding problems (Cermak, 1975; Johnson & Myklebust, 1967; Thompson, Hall, & Sison, 1986; Wing, 1990). The WFIP–2 provides a lesson to teach learners to revisualize the target word referent to cue retrieval. Exercises initially focus on the revisualization process itself and then move to using this process to prompt word retrieval (see Chapter 6, Lesson 6-4). Imagery cueing is most successful with learners who have visual memory strengths (Wiig & Semel, 1984).

GESTURE CUEING

Gesture cueing, used to prime the target word's meaning, focuses on the motor schema of the target word action. Similar strategies have been recommended for learners to aid their retrieval of verbs and both action–object and agent–action relations (Wiig & Becker-Caplan, 1984) and also have been identified as helpful for aphasic adults (Drummond & Rentschler, 1981). The WFIP–2 provides a lesson to teach learners to gesture the action associated with the target word to prompt its retrieval (see Chapter 6, Lesson 6-5). This strategy is applied only to relevant vocabulary whose associated action is easily represented through gesturing.

In all, the WFIP–2 strategies are applied first to the target word in isolation and then within the context of a sentence. Lesson goals begin with use of these strategies under your direction and then move to self-application of these strategies with vocabulary in the classroom, at home, or at work.

DEVELOP INDIVIDUAL STRATEGY PLANS

Procedure 2. Identify retrieval strategies appropriate for the learner.

When using the WFIP–2, it is important to identify a menu of strategies that will facilitate retrieval for a particular learner. Selection of strategies must consider the learner's error pattern and the lexical features of the target words to be accessed. (See Procedure 3 for a discussion of the effect of a target word's lexical factors on lexical access.)

The following retrieval strategies are matched to the three corresponding error patterns, as shown in Figure 4.3 by error pattern:

- Error Pattern 1: Lemma-Related Semantic Errors
- Error Pattern 2: Word-Form Blocked Errors
- Error Pattern 3: Word-Form Phonologic Errors

Note that the synonym and category substitution strategies are used with both Error Patterns 2 and 3. The retrieval strategies discussed earlier are summarized in this section and are presented in Figure 4.3 by error type.

Procedure 3. Use relevant and thematic curriculum for word-finding intervention.

The language curriculum for intervention should be based on relevant content with vocabulary drawn from the learner's classroom curriculum, daily routine, recreational life, or home environment. Instructional lessons should be thematic, with studied vocabulary grouped conceptually. Time spent on content or vocabulary not immediately relevant to the learner will not result in generalization of retrieval strategies across language situations. Rather, vocabulary practiced should consist of words drawn from the following:

- Words that the learner knows but has had difficulty retrieving
- Words you anticipate will be difficult for the learner to retrieve
- Vocabulary drawn from the learner's classroom curriculum
- Vocabulary from the learner's home or recreational experiences
- Vocabulary the learner uses in social situations
- Vocabulary from the learner's work environment

For example, a language lesson could be focused on applying mnemonic word-finding strategies to improve a learner's retrieval of art, reading, computer, science, or social studies vocabulary. Alternatively, a language lesson could be based on a learner's recreational interests. For the learner interested in sports, mnemonic strategies applied to vocabulary from football or basketball content could be the focus of the word-finding language lesson. Best results will be obtained by using words and contexts that have direct relevance and meaning for the learner.

Procedure 4. Consider lexical factors of target words when matching the vocabulary to retrieval strategies.

Use the following suggestions to guide you in your selection:

1. For high-frequency monosyllabic words from the learner's academic, social, or recreational vocabulary, use
   a. the pausing strategy to decrease fast, inaccurate substitutions,
   b. self-monitoring and self-correcting strategies to teach self-correction of fast and inaccurate responses,
   c. same-sounds mnemonic cues and familiar-word mnemonic cues to make the word's form more salient, and
   d. the rehearsal strategy to reinforce accurate retrieval of target words in sentences.

2. For long, phonologically complex (i.e., multisyllabic) words from the learner's academic, social, or recreational vocabulary, use
   a. syllable-dividing to make the syllabic structure of multisyllabic words explicit,
   b. same-sounds mnemonic cues to make the form of individual syllables salient, and
   c. synonym or category substituting for target words that can be meaningfully replaced in a discourse.

3. For rare words that are phonemically similar to few words (few phonological neighbors), use
   a. same-sounds mnemonic cues and familiar-word mnemonic cues to make the word's form more salient and
   b. the rehearsal strategy to reinforce accurate retrieval of target words in sentences.

MOVE FROM SINGLE WORD TO DISCOURSE

Procedure 5. Adjust application of strategies from retrieval of words in isolation to retrieval of words in sentences and discourse.

The goal for the learner with word-finding difficulties is to be able to apply the retrieval strategies when speaking in a variety of settings. Therefore, only in initial instruction, where word-finding strategies are introduced and applied for the first time, do activities focus on vocabulary in isolation. In subsequent lessons, the focus progresses to the development and practice of thematically related sentences that contain the target vocabulary. In final lessons for each set of words, scripts consisting of these sentences are practiced as examples of discourse with the targeted vocabulary. (See Appendix A for sample sentences using a variety of sports and selected academic vocabulary.)

ENCOURAGE REHEARSAL

Procedure 6. Encourage ongoing rehearsal of vocabulary in isolation, sentences, and discourse.

The literature on lexical memory supports rehearsal to maintain "retrieval strength" and to enhance "storage strength" of information (Bjork & Bjork, 1992). Vocabulary rehearsal should occur with both new and previously studied target vocabulary.

The WFIP–2 provides three types of rehearsal techniques:

- Rehearsal of target words in isolation
- Rehearsal of target words in sentences
- Rehearsal of target words in discourse

Rehearsal for target words in isolation is appropriate primarily in the beginning lessons and should always be connected to a particular word-finding strategy (e.g., mnemonic-cueing strategy, syllable-dividing strategy, or attribute-cueing strategy). Single-word rehearsal is meaningful when it is followed first by creating and rehearsing sentences with the target words and then by rehearsing brief narratives that contain the target vocabulary. Rehearsal is best when it occurs during the language lesson and at home. Learners should be encouraged to keep a list of target vocabulary in a notebook or in a computer file to use as a guide during their rehearsal sessions. Instruct students to rehearse a planned discourse with studied vocabulary before actually using that vocabulary in a particular conversation (e.g., rehearsal of basketball vocabulary before participating in a dialogue at a basketball game).

TEACH SELF-APPLICATION

Procedure 7. Teach the learner to self-apply the retrieval strategies learned during the lessons.

For retrieval strategies to be useful across language contexts, learners need to self-apply these strategies when they are having word-finding difficulties. To facilitate self-application, the WFIP–2 lessons employ cognitive modification techniques such as self-monitoring and self-instruction. The word-finding self-advocacy lessons in the WFIP–2 describe these cognitive modification strategies.

USE ACADEMIC ACTIVITIES IN THE CLASSROOM

Procedure 8. Use academic activities in the classroom to teach and apply retrieval strategies.

Retrieval strategy instruction in the context of academic activities aids the student's learning and facilitates his or her retrieval in a meaningful communication context. To encourage the teaching and application of retrieval strategies in academic contexts, collaborate with the teacher to use academic assignments to teach and apply the retrieval strategy. Activities could include using the following:

- Mnemonic-cueing and syllable-dividing strategies to develop the retrieval strength of technical terms in science, names and dates in social

studies and language arts, and vocabulary in math
- Pausing strategy to reduce fast inaccurate responses in class discussions in all content areas
- Syllable-dividing strategies plus rehearsal to aid silent and oral reading (if required) and spelling of multisyllabic words in science and math
- Semantic alternate strategies to circumvent word-finding blocks in oral and written language activities

PROVIDE GENERALIZATION ACTIVITIES

Procedure 9. Implement activities that encourage generalization of retrieval strategies to everyday classroom, home, and work situations.

When the learner indicates that he or she can self-apply the retrieval strategies studied in the WFIP–2 lessons and reinforced in academic activities, intervention should focus on helping the learner self-apply these strategies in academic situations inside and outside of school. Along with the classroom teacher and parents, observe the learner in various communication contexts. When necessary, remind the learner to self-apply the retrieval strategies appropriate for a given language situation.

SECTION 3

Goals, Objectives, and Lesson Plans

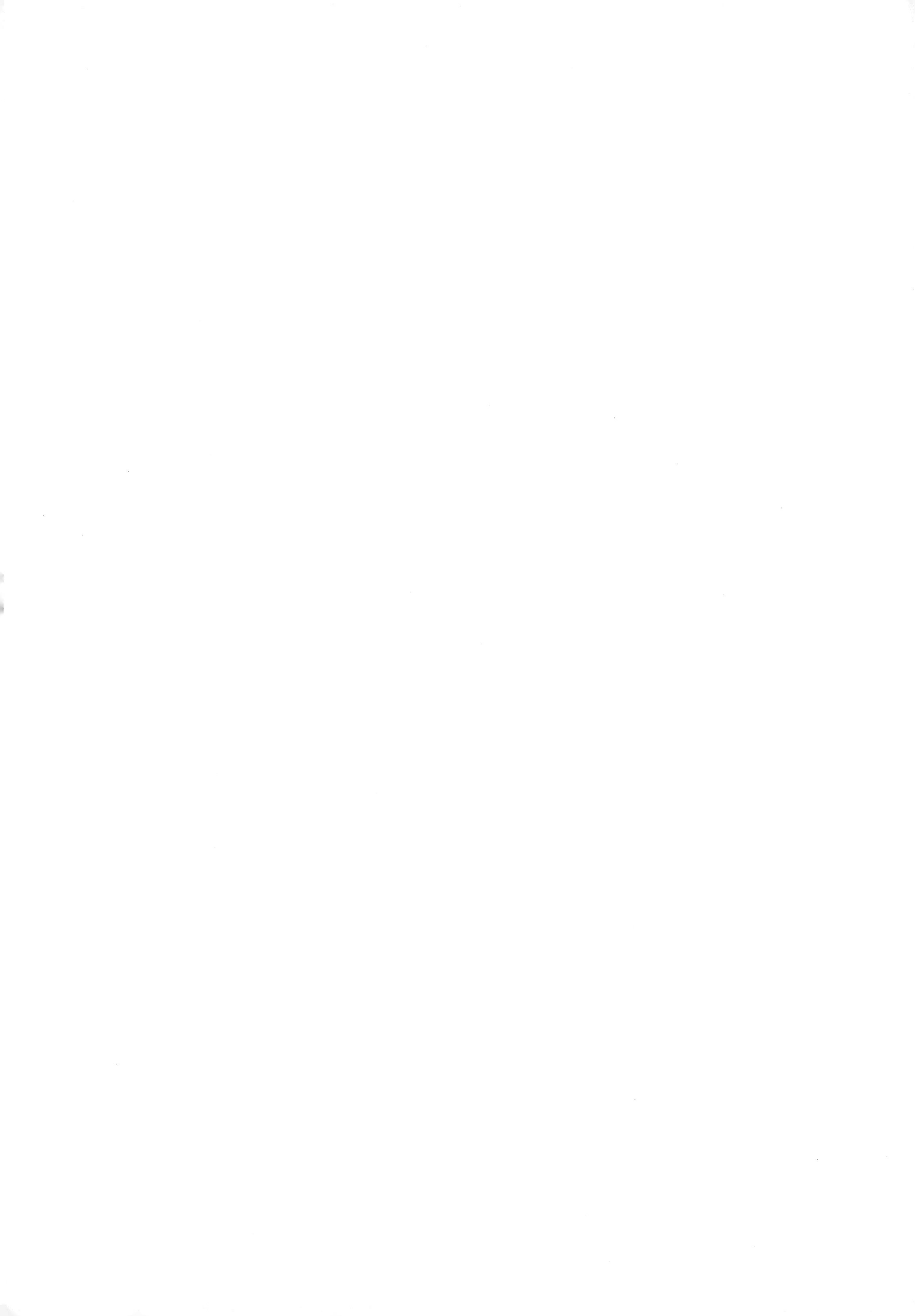

Developing Goals and Benchmarks and Using Lesson Plans

The first part of this chapter provides specific goals and benchmarks for use with the WFIP–2. *Although an extensive list of goals and benchmarks is provided, you do not need to use all the benchmarks indicated. Rather, select those goals and benchmarks that are most appropriate for your learners.* The second part of this chapter introduces the format of the WFIP–2 lesson plans and gives some guidelines for implementing the three kinds of lesson plans provided in the WFIP–2.

WRITING THE IEP OR IPP FOR STUDENTS WITH WORD-FINDING DIFFICULTIES

For specialists working with students in school settings, goals and benchmarks are presented in the context of the Individualized Education Program (IEP) mandated by the Individuals with Disabilities Education Act (IDEA) for learners deemed to have a disability. Because a word-finding difficulty is a communication or learning disability that is a condition eligible for special education services under IDEA, an IEP should be written for students receiving intervention in word finding. Similarly, an Individualized Program Plan (IPP) should be developed for any client receiving services in a clinical setting. Specialists who write IEPs or IPPs for their learners are encouraged to use the goals and benchmarks presented in this chapter (see the IEP/IPP Annual Goals and Benchmarks section).

Documentation of a learner's word-finding intervention benchmarks will help ensure that the learner obtains appropriate programming throughout his or her instruction. Goals and benchmarks clearly state the intention of each word-finding lesson. Keep in mind that you only need to use those goals and benchmarks that are appropriate for your learners.

Further, the format presented here should be considered only as a sample to illustrate the annual goals and short-term word-finding benchmarks. Ultimately, you will need to adapt these goals and benchmarks to the IEP/IPP format used in your work setting. The IEP/IPP should represent aspects that the multidisciplinary team deems appropriate in a program for improving word-finding skills. Select components of the IEP/IPP follow:

- A statement of the learner's present levels of performance
- Specific special education, related services, and ancillary treatments
- Annual long-term goals and instructional benchmarks
- Dates for initiation and duration of services
- Appropriate objective criteria and evaluation procedures

Following is a discussion of these IEP/IPP components as each relates to learners with word-finding difficulties.

A STATEMENT OF THE LEARNER'S PRESENT LEVELS OF PERFORMANCE

The law states that the IEP needs to indicate the present level of performance (PLOP). For a child with word-finding difficulties, the PLOP is derived from a deep assessment in word finding, including formal (both screening and deep evaluation) assessment, classroom observation, and parent or teacher feedback. In this PLOP statement, you would indicate the nature of the communication task or situation in which the student has word-finding difficulties. Retrieval difficulties can occur in oral questioning in the classroom (e.g., single word retrieval), when the learner is engaged in a conversation, or when the learner is asked to elaborate on or relate a story, event, or experience in or out of school (i.e., in discourse contexts). Indicate whether the student (a) has difficulties with communication tasks that require retrieval of single words, facts, phrases, or dates or (b) manifests word-finding difficulties in discourse contexts or in both single-word and discourse contexts. Information gleaned from both the informal and formal assessments in word finding can be used to report a learner's PLOP. Following is an example of a PLOP for Mark, a third-grade learner with word-finding difficulties.

MARK'S PLOP

In response to teachers' questions, Mark has exhibited difficulty retrieving multisyllabic names and words from stories read in class. Therefore, he needs to use segmenting and rehearsal strategies before class to become automatic in his retrieval of this vocabulary.

SPECIFIC SPECIAL EDUCATION, RELATED SERVICES, AND ANCILLARY TREATMENTS

As they relate to child word-finding intervention, the services involved and modifications to be made should be addressed in this IEP section.

SERVICES INVOLVED

The services that will be involved in the intervention must be stated clearly because the benchmarks of a comprehensive intervention program for a school-age student with word-finding difficulties cannot be met without the collaboration of the speech–language pathologist (SLP), special education teacher, and general classroom teacher. Therefore, everyone is encouraged to indicate his or her role in the intervention

program early in the planning process. Following is an example of the services that will be provided for Mark.

SLP SERVICES FOR MARK

The SLP will be providing Mark word-finding intervention that will focus on applying word-finding strategies to classroom vocabulary to help him become automatic in retrieval of multisyllabic words in the curriculum. The strategies used will be same-sounds cues and syllable dividing. The SLP will inform the classroom teacher when Mark has established automatic retrieval of vocabulary rehearsed.

MODIFICATIONS THAT WILL BE MADE

Typically, learners with word-finding difficulties need accommodations in their reading instruction, academic assessment, homework assignments, and classroom discourse to maintain grade-level achievement. Failure to create and implement accommodations early in a learner's schooling starts a lower achieving effect that compounds over the years and from which many students never recover. Chapter 10, Word-Finding Accommodations, describes accommodations typically needed by learners with word-finding difficulties. Following is an example of the accommodations that will be provided for Mark.

CLASSROOM ACCOMMODATIONS FOR MARK

The classroom and special education teachers will provide the SLP with lists of multisyllabic vocabulary so that Mark can be primed with needed strategies to establish automatic retrieval of this vocabulary before it is presented in the classroom. Until otherwise advised by the SLP, the classroom teacher will provide Mark with multiple-choice frames when calling on him instead of asking him to retrieve multisyllabic names or words.

ANNUAL LONG-TERM GOALS AND INSTRUCTIONAL BENCHMARKS (OBJECTIVES)

The annual long-term goals and benchmarks section of the word-finding IEP/IPP represents a progression of specific benchmarks[1] that, when

[1] *Benchmarks* and *short-term objectives* are often used interchangeably. Although we use the term *benchmarks* here, you will need to use whichever term is used in your setting.

met, move the learner toward meeting the annual goals. The goals and benchmarks indicated in this section focus on intervention techniques to improve retrieval of specific words in single-word and discourse language contexts. These goals and benchmarks are organized according to the WFIP–2 components: retrieval strategies, word-finding accommodations, and self-advocacy instruction. Nelson (1998) indicated that intervention benchmarks can be considered in a vertical sequence (first Objective 1, then Objective 2, etc.) during the initial acquisition stage and in a horizontal sequence later, when several benchmarks from the same or different areas are being considered together. Both sequences are appropriate for intervention in word finding. For example, initial intervention lessons may focus only on retrieval strategy instruction benchmarks, and subsequent lessons focus on self-advocacy benchmarks. Once the learner becomes knowledgeable of his or her retrieval strategies, lessons may focus on strategy application and self-advocacy goals concurrently.

ANNUAL LONG-TERM GOALS

The annual long-term goals section of the word-finding IEP/IPP addresses the long-range objectives of the intervention plan. It is a general estimate of what you hope to achieve within the school year or treatment period in each of the three areas of the word-finding intervention program. Following the WFIP–2 model for learners with word-finding difficulties, consider goals for three instructional components: retrieval strategy instruction, word-finding accommodations, and word-finding self-advocacy. Consider the following examples of Mark's long-term word-finding goals, which are described using two different measurement criteria: a percentage and a rubric.

MARK'S LONG-TERM GOALS

Retrieval Strategy Long-Term Goals

- By applying retrieval strategies to multisyllabic names and vocabulary studied in science class, Mark will increase his ability to retrieve science vocabulary by 80% when he is called on in class.
- By applying retrieval strategies to multisyllabic names and vocabulary studied in science class, Mark's ability to retrieve science vocabulary when he is called on in class will move from Emerging to Sometimes along the following rubric: Just beginning ► Emerging ► Sometimes ► Always.

Word-Finding Accommodations Long-Term Goals

- The classroom or special education teacher will provide the SLP with lists of multisyllabic science vocabulary before classroom presentation for all units so that Mark can be taught to apply word-finding strategies to 100% of the relevant science vocabulary studied in class.

- The classroom or special education teacher will provide the SLP with lists of multisyllabic science vocabulary in advance of classroom presentation for all units so that Mark's ability to apply word-finding strategies will progress from Sometimes to Always along the following rubric: Just beginning ► Emerging ► Sometimes ► Always.

Word-Finding Self-Advocacy Long-Term Goals

- Mark's ability to ask for the multisyllabic science vocabulary for each unit will increase from 0% to 50%.

- Mark's ability to ask for the multisyllabic science vocabulary for each unit will progress from Just beginning to Emerging along the following rubric: Just beginning ► Emerging ► Sometimes ► Always.

INSTRUCTIONAL BENCHMARKS FOR RETRIEVAL STRATEGIES

The specific instructional objectives on a student's IEP/IPP stem directly from assessment and focus on the retrieval strategies described in Chapter 4. The answers to diagnostic questions guide your selection of word-finding strategies for each learner. After selecting strategies, write benchmarks (i.e., objectives) that apply those word-finding strategies to important, relevant vocabulary in the learner's life. For example, the same-sounds cue retrieval strategy would be used for a learner whose word-finding assessment indicates that he or she typically gives a "No Response" during a word-finding block but does respond to the phonemic cue. This strategy makes a target word's form more salient for the learner.

Similarly, to stabilize retrieval of multisyllabic words, the syllable dividing strategy would be used for the learner who produces phonemic substitutions (i.e., omits sounds, substitutes sounds, or exchanges sounds) during word-finding blocks. The same-sounds syllable cue strategy (see Lesson 8-2) is also appropriate to use to aid retrieval of multisyllabic words. However, in this context, same-sounds syllable cues are linked to the troublesome syllable of the multisyllabic word (e.g., link

mom to the middle syllable of the target word *ther**mom**eter*) to aid future retrieval of that target word).

APPROPRIATE BENCHMARKS AND EVALUATION PROCEDURES

Progress toward a long-term (i.e., annual) goal can be measured by accomplishment of the short-term objectives, or *benchmarks.* The criteria for attainment should be individualized and should vary for each learner.

IEP/IPP ANNUAL GOALS AND BENCHMARKS

Figures 5.1 through 5.3 present annual goal statements and benchmarks for the three WFIP–2 components. Activities for these benchmarks are indicated in the corresponding WFIP–2 lesson plans later in this manual.

The lesson plans in Chapters 6 through 10 specify the goals and benchmarks for the three different components of the word-finding program. Though these chapters address different word-finding components, the format of each lesson plan is the same. This format is outlined in the following section.

USING WFIP–2 LESSON PLANS

This section presents the structure of WFIP–2 lesson plans and gives instructions for implementing lesson plans for each of the three WFIP–2 components: word-finding retrieval strategy instruction, word-finding self-advocacy instruction, and word-finding accommodations.

The WFIP–2 lesson plans are designed to be flexible and selective. *You do not need to implement every lesson in the WFIP–2. Choose only those lessons that present strategies appropriate for the learner receiving intervention.* Guidelines presented in this section, as well as in Chapter 4, should be followed in selecting the most appropriate lessons for each learner.

PARTS OF A LESSON PLAN

The WFIP–2 lesson plans consist of the following parts:

- Lesson number and title
- Retrieval context
- Error pattern targeted (only in retrieval strategy lessons and self-accommodations lessons)

ANNUAL GOALS AND BENCHMARKS FOR WORD-FINDING RETRIEVAL STRATEGIES

Instructional Area: Retrieval Strategy Instruction (Select strategies appropriate for the learner.)

Annual Goal Statement 1: Reduce Error Pattern 1: Lemma-Related Semantic Errors that produce fast, inaccurate responses (commonly known as "slip of the tongue" errors).

Benchmarks for Retrieval Strategy Instruction

1. The learner will use the pausing strategy to inhibit the retrieval of competing words.
2. The learner will use self-monitoring strategies to avoid producing fast, inaccurate responses.
3. The learner will use self-correction strategies to correct fast, inaccurate responses.
4. The learner will use the same-sounds meaning cue to reduce retrieval of competing words.
5. The learner will self-apply retrieval strategies in activities other than the language lesson.

Annual Goal Statement 2: Reduce the occurrence of Error Pattern 2: Word-Form Blocked Errors that produce slow, inaccurate or slow, accurate responses (commonly known as "tip of the tongue" errors).

Benchmarks for Retrieval Strategy Instruction

1. The learner will use the same-sounds cue to improve word retrieval of evasive target words.
2. The learner will use same-sounds meaning cue to improve word retrieval of evasive target words.
3. The learner will use the familiar-word cue to improve word retrieval of evasive target words.
4. The learner will use synonym and category substituting to circumvent word-finding blocks.
5. The learner will use rehearsal techniques to increase automaticity of target words.
6. The learner will self-apply retrieval strategies in activities other than the language lesson.

Annual Goal Statement 3: Reduce Error Pattern 3: Word-Form Phonologic Errors that result in phonemic substitution for multisyllabic words (commonly known as "twist of the tongue" errors).

Benchmarks for Retrieval Strategy Instruction

1. The learner will use syllable-dividing to improve word retrieval of multisyllabic words.
2. The learner will use same-sounds syllable cue to improve word retrieval of difficult syllables.
3. The learner will use rehearsal techniques to increase automaticity of target words.
4. The learner will use synonym and category substituting to circumvent word-finding errors on multisyllabic words.
5. The learner will self-apply retrieval strategies in activities other than the language lesson.

Figure 5.1. Annual goals and benchmarks for word-finding retrieval strategies.

- Benchmarks (i.e., retrieval strategy benchmarks, self-advocacy benchmarks, or accommodations benchmarks)
- Participants
- Time
- Setting
- Materials
- Recommended technology
- Activities
- Generalization activities

ANNUAL GOALS AND BENCHMARKS FOR WORD-FINDING SELF-ADVOCACY INDTRUCTION

Instructional Area: Word-finding self-advocacy instruction

Annual Goal Statement: The learner will demonstrate the ability to self-advocate by self-applying his or her retrieval strategies.

Benchmarks for Self-Advocacy Instruction

1. The learner will demonstrate awareness of his or her word-finding profile.
2. The learner will apply self-monitoring and self-correction techniques to identify and self-correct her or his word-finding errors.
3. The learner will self-apply his or her retrieval strategies.

Annual Goal Statement: The learner will demonstrate awareness of his or her retrieval strengths and weaknesses by completing the Word-Finding Self-Assessment Survey.

Benchmark for Self-Advocacy Instruction

1. The learner will identify speaking situations, language circumstances, retrieval contexts, nature of target words, and times of day that facilitate or impair his or her word retrieval.

Annual Goal Statement: The learner will self-advocate regarding his or her word-finding skills.

Benchmarks for Self-Advocacy Instruction

1. The learner will demonstrate awareness of the benchmarks of his or her lessons.
2. The learner will collaborate with teachers, relatives, or supervisors to determine the accommodations needed to reinforce his or her word-finding skills, both inside and outside school.
3. The learner will practice the retrieval strategies selected to aid his or her word-finding skills.
4. The learner will self-apply his or her retrieval strategies.

Figure 5.2. Annual goals and benchmarks for word-finding self-advocacy.

- Word-finding self-advocacy goals
- Word-finding accommodation activities (only in retrieval strategy lesson plans)
- Academic context applications (only in retrieval strategy and self-advocacy lesson plans)

Descriptions of each lesson plan part follow.

- **Lesson number and title.** At the top of each lesson plan, a unique number and title identify the lesson. In Chapters 6, 7, and 8, the lesson title corresponds to the specific retrieval strategy the learner will be taught to use when he or she is having difficulty retrieving a target word.

- **Retrieval context.** All lessons provided in the WFIP–2 are directed toward improving lexical access of specific words in both single-word and discourse contexts.

ANNUAL GOALS AND BENCHMARKS FOR WORD-FINDING ACCOMMODATIONS

Instructional Area: Word-finding accommodations

Annual Goal Statement: The learner will collaborate with his or her teachers to reduce activities and interactions that put high demands on his or her word-finding skills by modifying the language environment as demonstrated by the term *benchmarks.*

Benchmarks for Word-Finding Accommodations

1. The learner will collaborate with his or her teachers to identify the accommodations needed in oral discourse that will help him or her express his or her knowledge both inside and outside school.
2. The learner will collaborate with his or her teachers to identify electronic sources (e.g., hardware, Web sites, software) that can aid him or her in the classroom, when doing homework, and when taking exams.
3. The learner will collaborate with his or her teachers to identify the accommodations needed when completing classroom work, doing homework, taking examinations, and participating in home or job activities.
4. The learner will collaborate with school personnel, family members, and friends to modify those activities that put high demands on his or her word-retrieval skills.

Figure 5.3. Annual goals and benchmarks for word-finding accommodations.

- **Error Pattern.** The term *error pattern* refers to the type of word-finding disruption targeted by the lesson (e.g., Error Pattern 1: Lemma-Related Semantic Errors; Error Pattern 2: Word-Form Blocked Errors; or Error Pattern 3: Word-Form Phonologic Errors). Note that the retrieval strategy lessons are divided into three chapters (Chapters 6, 7, and 8) according to the specific error pattern they address. Specialists should match retrieval strategies to the error patterns most common for the individual learner. Word-finding accommodations lessons address all three error patterns.

- **Benchmark (objective).** The term *benchmark* refers to the strategy or concept being taught and the outcome expected. For retrieval strategy lessons, this part of the lesson is called the "word-finding intervention benchmark (objective)." For word-finding self-advocacy lessons, it is called the "self-advocacy benchmark (objective)," and for word-finding accommodations lessons, it is called the "accommodation benchmark (objective)." Word-finding accommodation benchmarks indicate the specific academic assessment and instruction to be differentiated and the actual accommodation to be recommended.

- **Participants.** The number and roles of specific participants recommended for each word-finding lesson are indicated in this part of the lesson. The number varies depending on whether the WFIP–2 lessons are implemented in the language room, special education classroom, or

general education classroom. Participants could include the specialist and the learner or learners in an individual or small group format. The classroom teacher and other members of the class may be included when lessons are taught, applied, and reinforced in the context of academic activities or class discussions.

- **Time.** The estimated time to complete each lesson is indicated in this part of the lesson. However, because the actual time required for each lesson will vary depending on the learner, the setting, and the format chosen, the time listed in the lesson plan is only a suggestion.

- **Setting.** The choice of setting will vary as a function of (a) the specialist's and learner's schedules, (b) whether the WFIP–2 is being used in a school or center, and (c) where the learner is in his or her ability to apply the WFIP–2 components. Therefore, recommendations should be viewed only as suggestions to guide you in setting up the WFIP–2. Possible settings include the language room in the school or clinic, a small language group in the general education or special education class, or a dual-focus vocabulary lesson in a classroom. Once learners have had some experience with the lessons or are focused on self-application of the component concepts, lessons can be implemented in cooperative group situations or large discussion groups, in general education or special education classes, or in the context of academic activities. Dialogue between the specialist and the teacher can occur in the general and or special education classroom. If you decide to observe the learner in the classroom, then the appropriate setting would be the classroom.

- **Materials.** The materials needed for each lesson may include specialists' forms, learner activity forms, word lists (see discussion of vocabulary selection in Chapter 4), and model sentences. Most of the necessary materials can be found in the appendixes of this manual. Retrieval strategy forms, vocabulary lists, and sample sentences containing selected vocabulary are presented in Appendix A. The Word-Finding Self-Assessment Survey is described in the following text and also in Appendix B. The two forms needed for the accommodations lessons are described in the following text and are presented in Appendix C:

    - *Classroom Observation Form.* This form is designed to guide observations of the learner's classroom to identify areas of the curriculum where there is a high demand on the learner's word-retrieval skills (see Appendix C).
    - *Recommended Word-Finding Accommodations Form.* Selected accommodations for the learner's classroom in each of the curriculum areas are indicated on this form (see Appendix C). The form is designed to

guide discussions with classroom teachers to help identify those curriculum accommodations appropriate for a particular student.
- *Word-Finding Self-Assessment Survey.* This form is used to help learners identify those influences that affect, both positively and negatively, their word-finding skills (see Appendix B).

Additional materials to support a game format also may be suggested in this part of the lesson. Some lessons call for materials that the teacher or specialist must provide, such as lists of teachers, subjects, and course schedules.

- **Recommended technology.** This part of the lesson plan lists Web sites and technologies that assist with the lesson. Technology can be used to support automatic application of retrieval strategies. For example, Web sites providing similar-sounding words are good sources for identifying cues for retrieval strategies. Similarly, software providing word choices can support retrieval in written-language tasks. Therefore, Web sites and software related to retrieval strategy instruction are recommended in each retrieval strategy lesson plan (see Chapters 6, 7, and 8). Word-finding accommodations lessons also encourage use of technology. As accommodations are created in the learner's classes, appropriate technology supports should be integrated into the instructional program.

- **Activities.** The specific intervention activities are the central focus of each lesson. In retrieval strategy lessons, activities are separated into intervention levels:.

- *Level 1: Awareness.* Make the learner aware of the focus of the retrieval strategy being studied.
- *Level 2: Instruction and Rehearsal.* Identify and teach the specific retrieval strategies appropriate for the learner, and then guide practice in applying retrieval strategies to chosen vocabulary, first in isolation, then in sentences, and finally in discourse scripts.
- *Level 3: Self-Application.* Always encourage the learner to self-apply the retrieval strategies taught.

NOTE: The time spent at each intervention level is difficult to predict because it is dependent on various specialist and learner variables. Therefore, use your professional judgment to determine when a learner is ready to progress to the next level.

Initial word-finding accommodations lessons focus on helping learners self-evaluate their learning environment to identify needed classroom modifications. The Word-Finding Self-Assessment Survey is designed to aid in this process. The Classroom Observation Form, which you complete, indicates the type of tasks required of the learner in the classroom. In the final word-finding accommodations lessons, the Recommended Word-Finding Accommodations Form is used as a focus for teacher–learner–specialist conferences, where decisions are made on which aspects of the curriculum will need specific modifications to accommodate for the learner's word-finding difficulties. All word-finding accommodations lessons are directed toward three basic activities:

1. Self-analysis of the learner's word-finding skills across language and contexts
2. Observation of the learner's classroom to identify instruction and assessment activities that put a high demand on the learner's word-finding skills in oral or written tasks (completion of the Classroom Observation Form)
3. Collaboration with the classroom teacher to select and implement accommodations needed in each academic area (completion of the Recommended Word-Finding Accommodations Form)

- **Generalization activities.** To ensure mastery and generalization of the strategies and concepts being taught, each WFIP–2 lesson includes activities designed to help establish generalization by applying the strategy in settings outside the language lesson. In the word-finding self-advocacy lessons, these generalization activities require learners to monitor their own word-finding skills between language lessons in order to identify those experiences that interfere with or facilitate their retrieval. In word-finding accommodation lessons, the generalization activities focus on the learner's continuous monitoring to identify new curriculum activities that need modification because of high demands on the learner's word-finding skills.

- **Word-finding self-advocacy goals.** Self-advocacy goals for a particular lesson are indicated in this part of the lesson. These goals focus on (a) providing learners with a better understanding of their word-finding difficulties by helping them become aware of the benchmarks of their intervention lessons and (b) learning to self-apply the retrieval strategies that best facilitate their word-finding skills. For word-finding accommodation lessons, self-advocacy goals include sensitizing learners to those aspects of their learning, social, or work environment that may need to be modified; teaching learners to self-monitor their learning environment; and instructing learners how to negotiate with teachers for the accommodations needed in their curriculum.

• **Word-finding accommodation activity.** The word-finding accommodation activities for the lesson are indicated here. Generally, the activities focus on modifying the learner's language environment in school to reduce the retrieval load inherent in his or her classroom work. Classroom accommodations might include aiding the learner's oral participation in the classroom by either cueing the learner or providing multiple-choice questions. See Chapter 10 for classroom accommodation recommendations.

• **Using academic (and home) contexts.** Learners are encouraged to apply their lessons in academic and home settings. Self-advocacy lessons use this part of the lesson to solicit participation from teachers and family members. Retrieval strategy lessons may use this part of the lesson to acquire lists of multisyllabic words relevant for each curricular unit. Retrieval strategies then can be applied to vocabulary that is important in the classroom. For example, a learner having difficulty retrieving the word *habitat* in science or retrieving the word *numerator* in math class would be aided by applying the retrieval strategies he or she studied in the WFIP–2. In these situations, you could encourage the learner to do one of the following:

1. Apply the same-sounds cue strategy in science class to aid retrieval of the target word *habitat* (e.g., *habit* for *habitat*)
2. Apply the segmenting strategy and rehearsal (i.e., the syllable-dividing strategy) in math class to provide metalinguistic support for the target word *numerator.*

WFIP–2 lesson plans are organized according to the word-finding component that they address: retrieval strategy instruction, self-advocacy instruction, or word-finding accommodations. Depending on the component, some lessons may have additional parts. The following sections discuss the WFIP–2 lessons by component.

WORD-FINDING RETRIEVAL STRATEGY LESSONS

Chapters 6, 7, and 8 present the WFIP–2 lesson plans for intervention. Using these WFIP–2 retrieval strategy lesson plans, you can create a menu of strategies that are appropriate for the learner's error pattern. Retrieval strategy lessons are identified as either *preferred* or *supplementary.* Preferred retrieval strategies should be taught to all learners demonstrating the error pattern indicated. Supplementary strategies

should only be used if they match the student's learning strengths and are judged to aid his or her retrieval.

The lesson designed for a particular WFIP–2 retrieval strategy does not change in the intervention program. The same lesson is to be used unlimited times. However, the vocabulary, which is the curriculum of the lesson, continuously changes. As the learner's retrieval of vocabulary improves, selected retrieval strategies are applied to new vocabulary. Further, the WFIP–2 lessons may be modified as learners use the program. The following are appropriate modifications:

1. Elimination of the awareness activities for a retrieval strategy after the learner has had experience with the lesson
2. Reduction in the number of target words used in each lesson as a function of the difficulty level of the vocabulary
3. Elimination or modification of the choice of game format
4. Reduction in the number or variation in the choice of support forms and worksheets used with the learner

The WFIP–2 retrieval strategy lessons are presented in Chapters 6, 7, and 8 and are displayed in Figure 5.4 by error pattern.

WORD-FINDING SELF-ADVOCACY LESSONS

Chapter 9 presents word-finding self-advocacy lessons, which help learners use their retrieval strategies to self-advocate for appropriate learning experiences. Lesson 9-1 focuses on teaching self-monitoring strategies, whereas later lessons are directed toward completing a self-assessment analysis of one's word-finding skills across various contexts. Following are discussions concerning the appropriate age to begin self-advocacy instruction and how the self-advocacy lesson objectives integrate with retrieval strategy lesson objectives.

WHAT AGE TO BEGIN SELF-ADVOCACY INSTRUCTION

To be successful in meeting word-finding self-advocacy objectives, learners need to be able to carry out certain metacognitive and metalinguistic processes. These include self-reflection and self-assessment of one's language usage, and self-application of retrieval strategies and classroom accommodations. To make the best decisions about your learners' ability to carry out such metacognitive and metalingusitic processes, you will need to be aware of individual differences among learners' abilities to carry out self-advocacy tasks.

Error Pattern 1: Lemma-Related Semantic Errors
Preferred word-retrieval strategies:
- Lesson 6-1: Self-Monitoring
- Lesson 6-2: Self-Correcting
- Lesson 6-3: Pausing
- Lesson 7-2: Same-Sounds Meaning Cue and Rehearsal

Supplementary word-retrieval strategies:
- Lesson 6-4: Imagery Cueing and Rehearsal
- Lesson 6-5: Gesture Cueing and Rehearsal

Error Pattern 2: Word-Form Blocked Errors
Preferred word-retrieval strategies:
- Lesson 7-1: Same-Sounds Cue and Rehearsal
- Lesson 7-2: Same-Sounds Meaning Cue and Rehearsal
- Lesson 7-3: Familiar-Word Cue and Rehearsal
- Lesson 7-4: Synonym Substituting and Rehearsal
- Lesson 7-5: Category Substituting and Rehearsal

Supplementary word-retrieval strategies:
- Lesson 7-6: Graphemic Cueing

Error Pattern 3: Word-Form Phonologic Errors
Preferred word-retrieval strategies:
- Lesson 8-1: Syllable-Dividing and Rehearsal
- Lesson 8-2: Same-Sounds Syllable Cue and Rehearsal
- Lesson 7-4: Synonym Substituting and Rehearsal
- Lesson 7-5: Category Substituting and Rehearsal

Figure 5.4. Word-retrieval strategy lesson plans by error pattern.

Note that German (2002), using an interview paradigm, reported that elementary students, first and third graders, were able to self-reflect on their word-finding improvement. After engaging in a 13-week word-finding intervention program, these learners were able to report improvement on experimental treated target words in contrast to little improvement on untreated control words. Yet, for certain learners the word-finding self-advocacy objectives (i.e., metacognitive tasks) may be difficult because those learners have not developed these skills or they have cognitive difficulties that make it hard for them to process this information. In these cases, focus on retrieval strategy awareness activities and teacher-directed word-finding accommodations and save the word-finding self-advocacy objectives for later. However, for learners with developed metacognitive skills, the word-finding self-advocacy tasks will not be difficult and the lessons for this component should be implemented along with retrieval strategy instruction and word-finding accommodations.

WORD-FINDING SELF-ADVOCACY BENCHMARKS (OBJECTIVES)

Benchmarks for the word-finding self-advocacy component are initially taught as separate word-finding self-advocacy lessons and are integrated later into each of the other lessons. During word-finding self-advocacy instruction, the following cognitive modification techniques will be learned:

1. Self-monitoring to identify one's own word-finding error patterns (see Lesson 6-1)
2. Self-assessment of word-finding strengths (see Lessons 9-1 to 9-6)
   a. To identify speaking settings (e.g., classroom, playground, home) that facilitate word retrieval versus experiences that make word finding more difficult
   b. To identify language situations (e.g., group discussion, one-on-one) that facilitate word finding versus language situations that make word retrieval more difficult
   c. To identify those retrieval contexts (e.g., single-word, discourse) that facilitate word retrieval versus those contexts that make word finding more difficult
   d. To identify those language contexts (e.g., oral, written) that facilitate word retrieval versus those language contexts where word finding is more difficult
   e. To identify the subjects of words that are retrieved with the least and greatest difficulty
   f. To identify the lexical factors of words (e.g., frequency of usage, length, syntax, phonological attributes) that contribute to or interfere with ease of retrieval

Word-finding self-advocacy benchmarks are also integrated into the word-finding retrieval strategy lessons presented in Chapters 6, 7, and 8. These benchmarks focus on helping learners self-apply their retrieval strategies and request appropriate word-finding accommodations. These word-finding self-advocacy benchmarks help learners

1. become aware of the benchmarks of their retrieval strategy lessons,
2. become aware of the retrieval strategies that aid their word finding,
3. self-apply their retrieval strategies, and
4. learn to collaborate with their teachers, parents, or supervisors relative to the accommodations needed to aid their learning in school, at home, and in a work environment.

WORD-FINDING ACCOMMODATION LESSONS

Chapter 10 presents both the word-finding accommodations lessons themselves and some guidelines for selecting and implementing accommodations. Note that it is best to complete word-finding accommodations lessons after self-advocacy lessons have been completed.

TEACHING WORD-FINDING ACCOMMODATION LESSONS

The word-finding accommodation lessons should be used concurrently with the retrieval strategy instruction and the word-finding self-advocacy lessons. The initial accommodations lessons require collaboration with the learner's classroom teachers and, if necessary, observation of the learner in his or her various classrooms. If you decide to observe the learner in the classroom, it is appropriate to schedule the observations in place of the learner's scheduled language sessions.

Recommended Lesson Sequence

1. *Lesson 10-1 (approximately 2 sessions).* Review rationale and awareness for the word-finding accommodations component.
   - Session 1: Meet with the learner to discuss the rationale for requesting differentiated assessment and instruction to accommodate for his or her word-finding difficulties. Explain that together you are going to identify those components of his or her school, social, home, or work language environment that need to be modified. (The extent to which the learner participates in developing this program will depend on his or her awareness of the retrieval demands in his or her environment.) Explain that ultimately you hope the learner will direct his or her own word-finding accommodations.
   - Session 2: Together with the learner, review the Word-Finding Self-Assessment Survey (see Appendix B). This self-assessment provides information on the learner's perceptions of his or her retrieval strengths and weaknesses in various language settings, situations, and retrieval contexts.
2. *Lesson 10-2 (1 session).* Analyze survey results and select academic settings to observe. Discuss with the learner the results of the Word-Finding Self-Assessment Survey. Decide which teachers to contact and identify classrooms that need to be visited or observed.
3. *Lessons 10-3 through 10-6 (approximately 1 to 4 sessions).* Collabora-

tively evaluate the learner's classrooms. Arrange to visit the classrooms you think may need to be modified for the learner with word-finding difficulties. (For younger learners, this may mean meeting with only one or two teachers; for older learners, it may mean meeting with several teachers from different classrooms.) The purpose of these observations is to obtain information relative to the oral and written retrieval demands placed on the learner during the school day. Complete the Classroom Observation Form in Appendix C for the selected classrooms. Following your observations, meet with the teachers in those classrooms you observed. The goal is to come to a consensus on acceptable accommodations during oral discourse, written or oral exams, and assignments that will enable the learner to express his or her knowledge without being penalized for his or her retrieval difficulties. When you meet with the student's teachers, begin with a list of specific accommodations you think would be most beneficial to the student. With the teacher, complete the Recommended Word-Finding Accommodation Form for the learner.

4. *Lesson 10-7 (1 session).* Make recommendations for modification of language environments. Discuss with the learner the accommodations you and the classroom teacher or supervisor would like to implement. Together, review the Recommended Word-Finding Accommodation Form in Appendix C.

NOTE: The level of learner involvement in this decision-making process will vary with each learner. For example, with primary learners, you may want to be more general, assuring the learner that you and the teacher are going to work together to aid the learner's word-finding skills in the classroom. However, with intermediate and secondary-level learners, you will want them to participate in all decisions relative to these accommodations.

---

5. *Future lessons.* Monitor the use of suggested accommodations by asking the learner about his or her classroom activities and also by reviewing the accommodations with the classroom teacher on a regular basis (e.g., weekly.).

When the word-finding accommodations lessons have been completed, you may want to establish a schedule for (a) monitoring the effectiveness of the selected modifications and (b) determining whether a different set of accommodations is needed.

CURRICULUM AREAS CONSIDERED FOR ACCOMMODATION

For learners, the curriculum areas considered for accommodation include the following:

- Oral classroom participation
- Classroom work and assignments
- Homework assignments
- Class examinations

See Figure 5.3 for annual goals and benchmarks for word-finding accommodations.

The remaining chapters in this manual present the lessons and accommodations central to the WFIP–2. Chapters 6, 7, and 8 include retrieval strategy lessons; Chapter 9 gives word-finding self-advocacy lessons; and Chapter 10 presents both examples of word-finding accommodations and the lessons for identifying and implementing those accommodations.

Retrieval Strategy Lessons for Error Pattern 1

This chapter presents lesson plans for preferred and supplementary retrieval strategies for Error Pattern 1: Lemma-Related Semantic Errors. This word-finding disruption is thought to represent a failure to access the correct semantic features of the target word (e.g., *boat* for *submarine*; German, 2000a). When learners demonstrate this error pattern they manifest one of the following:

- Fast, inaccurate responses, (a verbalization of interfering words competing for selection, commonly known as a "slip of the tongue" error)
- Slow, inaccurate responses (a verbalization of semantic substitutions not corrected by the phonemic cue)

Retrieval strategies that encourage self-monitoring and self-correction (see Lessons 6-1 and 6-2) and reduce the learner's speaking rate (see Lesson 6-3) are recommended to reduce the fast, inaccurate responses typical of this error pattern. Strategies that focus on the target word's visual image (see Lesson 6-4) or on its associated motor act (see Lesson 6-5) may also serve to cue accurate retrieval of the target word's semantic features (i.e., lemma). Successful application of these retrieval strategies does require rehearsal activities. Lessons for these retrieval strategies follow.

LESSON 6-1

PREFERRED RETRIEVAL STRATEGY—SELF-MONITORING

Apply this strategy while the learner is talking. Use this lesson to help the learner master the self-monitoring technique.

RETRIEVAL CONTEXT: Retrieval of specific words in sentences or discourse

ERROR PATTERN: Error Pattern 1: Lemma-Related Semantic Errors

RETRIEVAL STRATEGY BENCHMARK (OBJECTIVE): To learn self-monitoring techniques to identify word-finding errors

PARTICIPANTS: Learner or learners, specialist, and teacher

TIME: 10 to 15 minutes

SETTING: Small language group in language room, general education classroom, or special education classroom, or entire class in general education classroom

MATERIALS: Paper and pencil

TECHNOLOGY OR ELECTRONIC MATERIALS: Video camera or audio recorder and tapes

ACTIVITIES

1. Explain to the learner that he or she can observe his or her own language, noting when and where word-finding errors occur.

2. To demonstrate self-monitoring, choose a behavior (e.g., raising your arm) that you will use during a conversation. Direct the learner to verbally note (e.g., count, or say "now") each time you use that behavior or action while engaged in a discourse with the learner.

3. Next, choose a word-finding behavior, such as saying time fillers like "um" or "er." Tape or videotape the learner in a conversation with you or in a language group. Watch or listen to the recording and direct the learner to verbally note (e.g., count, or say "now") each time he or she says a time filler while engaged in a discourse with you.

4. Last, choose a word-finding error and ask the learner to monitor his or her production of that language behavior. Watch or listen to the recording and direct the learner to verbally note (e.g., count, or say "now") each time he or she makes the word-finding error while engaged in a discourse with you.

GENERALIZATION ACTIVITIES

1. Identify a word-finding behavior that the learner typically demonstrates when he or she is having difficulty retrieving a target word. Ask the learner to monitor his or her use of this target behavior at home or school.

2. Ask the learner to report his or her self-observations at the next language session.

LESSON 6-2

PREFERRED RETRIEVAL STRATEGY—SELF-CORRECTING

Apply this strategy while the learner is talking. Use this lesson to teach self-correction of word-finding errors.

RETRIEVAL CONTEXT: Retrieval of specific words in sentences or discourse

ERROR PATTERN: Error Pattern 1: Lemma-Related Semantic Errors

RETRIEVAL STRATEGY BENCHMARK (OBJECTIVE): To self-correct fast, inaccurate responses while talking using the self-correction strategy

PARTICIPANTS: Learner or learners, specialist, and teacher

TIME: 10 to 15 minutes

SETTING: Initially, Level 1: Awareness and Level 2: Instruction activities are best taught in a small language group in the language room, general education classroom, or special education classroom. Later, Level 3: Self-Application activities can be taught in cooperative groups, during class discussion, or in the context of an academic activity.

LEARNER'S MATERIALS:

- WFIP–2 Retrieval Strategy Lesson Plan
- Paper and pencil

TECHNOLOGY OR ELECTRONIC MATERIALS: Audio and video recorder and tapes

INTERVENTION LEVEL 1: AWARENESS OF RETRIEVAL STRATEGY

Preparation: Provide audio or video recorder and tapes.

1. Explain to the learner that to ensure accurate communication, it is important to listen to one's speech while talking and to self-correct word-finding errors.
2. Audiotape or videotape the learner when talking in the classroom or in a language group.
3. Listen to or watch the recorded tape with the learner.
4. Ask the learner to stop the tape each time he or she makes an error. Discuss the need to listen to your own speech when talking.

INTERVENTION LEVEL 2: INSTRUCTION OF RETRIEVAL STRATEGY AND REHEARSAL

Preparation: Provide audio or video recorder and tapes.

1. Listen to or watch again the tape of the learner when talking in the classroom or in a language group.
2. Have the learner stop the tape each time he or she makes an error.
3. Demonstrate to the learner how to self-correct his or her word-finding errors by inserting the phrase "No, I mean ..." or the correct word itself in the sentence.

INTERVENTION LEVEL 3: SELF-APPLICATION OF RETRIEVAL STRATEGY AND REHEARSAL

During future language lessons, monitor and review as needed how to self-correct word-finding errors when talking.

GENERALIZATION ACTIVITIES

Ask the learner to self-monitor his or her speech in the classroom and report at the next language lesson when self-correction of word-finding errors occurred.

WORD-FINDING SELF-ADVOCACY GOALS

1. The learner will recognize his or her word-finding errors when speaking.

2. The learner will self-correct his or her word-finding errors by inserting the correct target word or the phrase “I mean ...” followed by the correct word.

CLASSROOM ACCOMMODATION ACTIVITY

Preparation: Collaborate with the teacher to monitor whether the learner self-corrects his or her word-finding errors when talking.

The teacher should direct the learner to self-correct word-finding errors observed in and out of the classroom.

USING ACADEMIC CONTEXTS

Collaborate with the teacher to identify those academic subjects (e.g., science, math, language arts, social studies) where learners need to apply the self-correction strategy when talking to ensure they are communicating correctly and, thus, demonstrating their knowledge.

LESSON 6-3

PREFERRED RETRIEVAL STRATEGY—PAUSING

Apply this strategy while the learner is talking. Use the lesson to improve word-finding accuracy.

RETRIEVAL CONTEXT: Retrieval of specific words in sentences and discourse

ERROR PATTERN: Error Pattern 1: Lemma-Related Semantic Errors

RETRIEVAL STRATEGY BENCHMARK (OBJECTIVE): To apply strategic pausing to inhibit retrieval of interfering words and reduce semantic substitutions

PARTICIPANTS: Learner or learners and specialist

TIME: 20 to 30 minutes

SETTING: Initially, Level 1: Awareness and Level 2: Instruction activities are best taught in a small language group in the language room, general education classroom, or special education classroom. Later, Level 3: Self-Application activities can be taught in cooperative groups, during class discussion, or in the context of an academic activity.

LEARNER'S MATERIALS (SEE APPENDIX A):

- WFIP–2 Retrieval Strategy Lesson Plan
- WFIP–2 Vocabulary and Retrieval Strategy Practice Form
- WFIP–2 Vocabulary
- Other word lists developed from learner's word-retrieval errors or drawn from the learner's classroom curriculum or home, recreational, or work environment
- Model Sentences for Selected WFIP–2 Vocabulary
- Age-appropriate board game with spinner, if needed

TECHNOLOGY AND ELECTRONIC MATERIALS:

- Audio and video recorder and tapes

- For readers, electronic word lists and sentences to demonstrate strategic placement of pauses in sentences

---

INTERVENTION LEVEL 1: AWARENESS OF ERROR PATTERN AND RETRIEVAL STRATEGY

Preparation: Provide word lists and paper and pencil or word processor.

1. Start with error pattern awareness. Familiarize the learner with Error Pattern 1 using the following steps:

   a. Explain to the learner that often when individuals are having difficulty retrieving a word or name, they misspeak and say the wrong word or name. As an example, ask learners if their grandparents or other members of their family ever call them by their sister's or brother's name.

   b. Present to the learner other examples of target word substitutions that would suggest that a person is having difficulty retrieving a word or name.

   c. Tape a brief monologue where you intentionally produce wrong names or substitutions in the context of sentences. Listen to the audiotape together, asking the learner to raise his or her hand when a word-finding error occurs.

   d. Tape a brief dialogue with the learner requiring him or her to retrieve names of friends, family members, and objects or events. Listen to the audiotape with the learner. Raise your hand each time the learner produces a word-finding substitution. Then ask the learner to listen to the discourse again and raise a hand each time he or she uses

or starts to use a target word substitution. Continue until the learner is aware of his or her target word substitutions.

2. To teach strategy awareness, familiarize the learner with the pausing strategy using the following steps:

   a. Explain to the learner that instead of producing a substitution, he or she should pause before a target name or word.

   b. Indicate that the pause needs to occur at the beginning (pause before noun or adjective of the noun phrase) or at the end of a sentence (before verb, object, or adverb of the verb phrase).

   c. Demonstrate the use of the pausing strategy. Select and verbalize three different sentences from the taped discourse, pausing before retrieving the target name or word in each of the sentences. Continue this activity until the learner is familiar with the pausing strategy.

INTERVENTION LEVEL 2: INSTRUCTION OF RETRIEVAL STRATEGY AND REHEARSAL

Preparation: Provide word lists and game spinner, if needed.

1. *Target word selection.* Select five target names or words that are relevant and that the learner understands.

2. *Pausing in sentences.* Have the learner verbalize three different sentences for the target name or word, applying the pausing strategy before saying the noun in the noun phrase or the verb in the verb phrase of the sentence. The learner may develop original sentences or use those provided in Appendix A. *If a game format is used, have the learner spin*

the spinner to determine the number of sentences to generate for the target word.

3. *Pausing in discourse.* Have the learner generate a brief discourse using the target names or words. Ask the learner to apply the pausing strategy to avoid saying the wrong name or a target word substitution when speaking. Model a discourse for the learner. *If a game format is used, have the learner spin the spinner to determine the number of target words to include in each discourse.*

4. *Pausing strategy reminder.* If the learner produces a wrong name or target word substitution during his or her discourse in Steps 2 and 3, remind the learner to apply the pausing strategy to inhibit interfering words when talking.

INTERVENTION LEVEL 3: SELF-APPLICATION OF RETRIEVAL STRATEGY AND REHEARSAL

1. Explain to the learner that the pausing strategy needs to be self-applied in conversations or when talking in the classroom, with friends, or at home.

2. Choose five additional target names or words that the learner understands and encourage the learner to self-apply the pausing strategy, repeating Steps 1 through 4 of Intervention Level 2.

3. Create a contract with the learner that directs him or her to apply retrieval strategies in specific settings or an agreed number of times within selected contexts.

GENERALIZATION ACTIVITY

Preparation: Provide the learner with the WFIP–2 Vocabulary and Retrieval Strategy Practice Form.

The learner enters in his or her WFIP–2 Vocabulary and Retrieval Strategy Practice Form the names or words he or she needs to rehearse. Then the learner applies the pausing strategy when retrieving the target name or word in a sentence.

WORD-FINDING SELF-ADVOCACY GOALS

1. The learner is able to recognize that when he or she interchanges names of classmates or produces inappropriate target word substitutions, he or she is manifesting a word-finding error.

2. The learner understands that instead of producing the incorrect name or an inappropriate target word substitution, he or she should pause (i.e., use the pausing strategy) until he or she is able to retrieve the name or word. The learner will also be aware that during pausing, he or she is to apply the retrieval strategies being studied.

WORD-FINDING ACCOMMODATION ACTIVITY

Preparation: Collaborate with the teacher to identify word lists and review the pausing strategy.

1. Request that the teacher direct the learner to raise his or her hand only after he or she has silently rehearsed a response.

2. To help the learner inhibit verbalization of erroneous words, recommend the teacher subtly signal (e.g., raise hand to

collar or lift index finger to mouth) to the learner to pause before answering questions in class (see Chapter 10 for other suggestions on how to modify the learner's language environment).

USING ACADEMIC CONTEXTS

Collaborate with the teacher to identify those academic subjects (e.g., science, math, language arts, social studies) where the learner should apply the pausing strategy (see Chapter 10 for suggestions on how to use technology to reduce substitutions in written language).

LESSON 6-4

SUPPLEMENTARY RETRIEVAL STRATEGY—IMAGERY CUEING AND REHEARSAL

Practice this strategy prior to the speaking situation and apply it while the learner is talking. Use this lesson to improve word-finding accuracy and speed.

RETRIEVAL CONTEXT: Retrieval of specific words in sentences and discourse

ERROR PATTERN: Error Pattern 1: Lemma-Related Semantic Errors (an inability to find the semantic features of the target word; learner does not retrieve the word with the phonemic cue)

RETRIEVAL STRATEGY BENCHMARK (OBJECTIVE): To mentally picture the target word referent to cue target words that are difficult to retrieve (Note: This lesson should be used only with target vocabulary whose referents can be easily pictured.)

PARTICIPANTS: Learner or learners and specialist

TIME: 20 to 30 minutes

SETTING: Initially, Level 1: Awareness and Level 2: Instruction activities are best taught in a small language group in the language room, general education classroom, or special education classroom. Later, Level 3: Self-Application activities can be taught in cooperative groups, during class discussion, or in the context of an academic activity.

LEARNER'S MATERIALS (SEE APPENDIX A):

- WFIP–2 Retrieval Strategy Lesson Plan
- WFIP–2 Vocabulary and Retrieval Strategy Practice Form
- WFIP–2 Vocabulary
- Other word lists developed from learner's word-retrieval errors or drawn from the learner's classroom curriculum or home, recreational, or work environment.

- Model Sentences for Select WFIP–2 Vocabulary
- Age-appropriate board game with spinner, if needed

TECHNOLOGY OR ELECTRONIC MATERIALS: For readers, electronic word lists and sentences and Web sites with icons corresponding to referents of target words; hand-held voice recorders to remind the learner when and how to apply retrieval strategies

INTERVENTION LEVEL 1: AWARENESS OF RETRIEVAL STRATEGY

Preparation: Provide word processor and electronic file of words, or lists and paper and pencil.

1. To teach awareness of referents, or visual images, for target words, explain to the learner that the referents of many words can be pictured. Show pictures of familiar words, such as *apple, orange, fork, book,* and *cup.*

2. Explain to the learner that for those types of target words, remembering how the referents look can help one remember the word.

   a. Show pictures of the words *apple, orange, fork, book,* and *cup.* Ask the learner to look at the pictures and then, with eyes closed, picture each object in his or her mind. (Other words whose referents are easily visualized may be used for this exercise.)

   b. Ask the learner to close his or her eyes and say the names while visualizing each target word referent (i.e., the pictures in his or her mind).

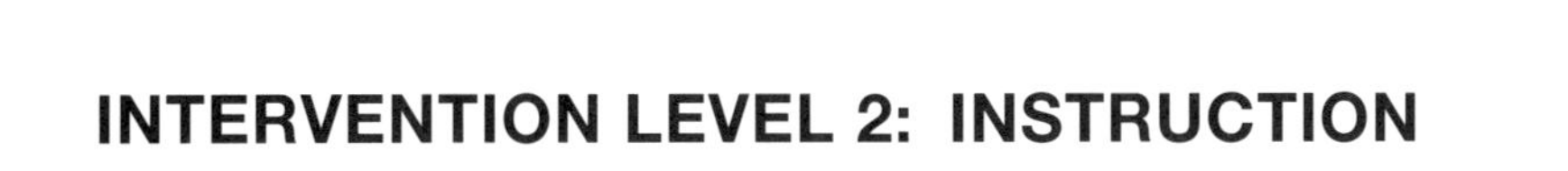

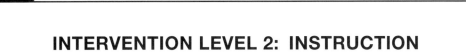

INTERVENTION LEVEL 2: INSTRUCTION OF RETRIEVAL STRATEGY AND REHEARSAL

Preparation: Provide word lists and game spinner.

1. *Target word selection.* From the learner's materials list, select five known and relevant words whose referent can be easily visualized.

2. *Target word and visualizing referent.* Name each word and have the learner visualize the target word referent in his or her mind.

3. *Target word practice.* Have the learner say each target word three times while picturing the target word referent in his or her mind. *If a game format is used, have the learner spin the spinner to determine the number of times to rehearse the target word.*

4. *Target word rehearsal in a sentence.* Have the learner say each target word in a sentence three times while picturing the target word referent in his or her mind. The learner may develop original sentences or, if appropriate, use those provided in Appendix A. *If a game format is used, have the learner spin the spinner to determine the number of sentences to rehearse.*

5. *Target word rehearsal in discourse.* Have the learner use each target word in a discourse while picturing the target word referent in his or her mind. *If a game format is used, have the learner spin the spinner to determine the number of target words to use in each discourse. Have the learner record his or her points after each spin. The learner with the most points at the end of the lesson wins the game.*

6. *Visual imagery cueing reminder.* If the learner has difficulty retrieving the target words in Steps 4 and 5, encourage him

or her to visualize the target word referent to prime retrieval of each target word.

INTERVENTION LEVEL 3: SELF-APPLICATION OF THE RETRIEVAL STRATEGY AND REHEARSAL

Choose five additional known target words whose referents can be pictured and ask the learner to self-apply the retrieval strategy as he or she repeats Steps 2 through 5.

GENERALIZATION ACTIVITY

Preparation: Provide the learner with the WFIP–2 Vocabulary and Retrieval Strategy Practice Form.

The learner enters the words he or she has had difficulty retrieving into the WFIP–2 Vocabulary and Retrieval Strategy Practice Form. The learner practices, visualizing the referent of each target word while saying each word three times alone and in a sentence.

WORD-FINDING SELF-ADVOCACY GOALS

1. The learner will recognize that when he or she has difficulty retrieving a specific word, he or she can be aided by visualizing the target word referent.

2. The learner will be able to predict that he or she is going to have difficulty retrieving a word and try to self-cue by visualizing the target word referent.

CLASSROOM ACCOMMODATION ACTIVITY

Preparation: Collaborate with the teacher to identify word lists and review the imagery cueing strategy.

Until the learner becomes automatic in retrieving target words, suggest that the teacher frame questions to the learner in a "find the answer" or multiple-choice format to facilitate his or her class participation. For example, say, "The commander in chief of our country is the ... secretary of state, president, or senator?" or "Find the answer in your book." (See Chapter 10 for other suggestions on how to design accommodations for the learner's language environment.)

USING ACADEMIC CONTEXTS

1. Collaborate with the teacher to identify vocabulary and apply the imagery cueing strategy to academic vocabulary that can be visualized.

2. When a learner indicates difficulty retrieving previously treated academic vocabulary, suggest that the teacher ask the learner to picture the target word referent in his or her mind to aid retrieval.

LESSON 6-5

SUPPLEMENTARY RETRIEVAL STRATEGY—GESTURE CUEING AND REHEARSAL

Practice this strategy prior to the speaking situation and apply it while the learner is talking. Use this lesson to improve word-finding accuracy and speed.

RETRIEVAL CONTEXT: Retrieval of specific words in sentences and discourse

ERROR PATTERN: Error Pattern 1: Lemma-Related Semantic Errors (an inability to find the semantic [i.e., lemma] features of the target word; learner does not retrieve the word with the phonemic cue)

RETRIEVAL STRATEGY BENCHMARK (OBJECTIVE): To subtly gesture the action associated with the target word referent to aid retrieval of the word (to be used only with target vocabulary whose associated action can be gestured)

PARTICIPANTS: Learner or learners and specialist

TIME: 20 to 30 minutes

SETTING: Initially, Level 1: Awareness and Level 2: Instruction activities are best taught in a small language group in a language room, general education classroom, or special education classroom. Later, Level 3: Self-Application activities can be taught in a cooperative group, during a class discussion, or in the context of an academic activity

LEARNER'S MATERIALS (SEE APPENDIX A):

- WFIP–2 Retrieval Strategy Lesson Plan
- WFIP–2 Vocabulary and Retrieval Strategy Practice Form
- WFIP–2 Vocabulary
- Other word lists (whose associated action can be gestured) developed from learner's word retrieval errors or drawn from the learner's classroom curriculum or home, recreational, or work environment

- Model Sentences for Select WFIP–2 Vocabulary
- Age-appropriate board game with spinner, if needed

TECHNOLOGY OR ELECTRONIC MATERIALS: For readers, electronic word lists and sentences; hand-held voice recorders to remind the learner when and how to apply retrieval strategies

INTERVENTION LEVEL 1: AWARENESS OF RETRIEVAL STRATEGY

Preparation: Provide electronic file and word processor, or word lists and paper and pencil.

1. To teach awareness of gestures representing the action associated with some target word referents, explain to the learner that for some words, the action associated with the word can be gestured. Show pictures of familiar words that are associated with actions that can be gestured, such as *scissors, pencil sharpener,* or *key.*

2. Explain to the learner that for these target words, remembering how their associated action can be gestured can help word retrieval.

   a. Demonstrate the action associated with various objects as you name them. For example, show pictures of the words *scissors, pencil sharpener, key, fork,* and *cup.* Ask the learner to listen to the words and watch you subtly gesture the action for each word. *Always demonstrate the gesture with the least exaggerated movement so as not to distract the listener when self-gesturing to cue retrieval.*

   b. Ask the learner to subtly gesture the action associated with three common verbs (e.g., *eating, brushing teeth,* and *writing*) while he or she says each word.

INTERVENTION LEVEL 2: INSTRUCTION OF RETRIEVAL STRATEGY AND REHEARSAL

Preparation: Provide word lists and board game.

1. *Target word selection.* Select five known and relevant target words whose associated action can be easily gestured.

2. *Target word and gesture strategy.* Name each of the five words and have the learner subtly gesture the action associated with each target word as it is named.

3. *Target word practice.* Have the learner gesture the action associated with the target word while he or she says it three times. *If a game format is used, have the learner spin the spinner and move around the game board after subtly gesturing the action associated with each word before saying it three times.*

4. *Target word rehearsal in a sentence.* Have the learner subtly gesture the action associated with each target word while verbalizing the words in three different sentences. The learner may develop original sentences or use those provided in Appendix A. *If a game format is used, have the learner spin the spinner and move around the game board after saying each word in a sentence three times.*

5. *Target word rehearsal in discourse.* Have the learner verbalize each target word in a discourse. Model a discourse for the learner if needed. *If a game format is used, have the learner spin the spinner, move around the game board, and verbalize a short discourse. The learner who circles the board a specified number of times wins the game.*

6. *Gesture cueing reminder.* If the learner has difficulty retrieving any of the target words in Steps 4 and 5, encourage him

or her to gesture the action associated with the target word to prime retrieval of that word.

INTERVENTION LEVEL 3: SELF-APPLICATION OF THE RETRIEVAL STRATEGY AND REHEARSAL

Choose five additional relevant target words that the learner understands and encourage the learner to self-apply the retrieval strategy as he or she repeats Steps 2 through 5.

GENERALIZATION ACTIVITY

Preparation: Provide the learner with the WFIP–2 Vocabulary and Retrieval Strategy Practice Form.

The learner enters the words he or she has had difficulty retrieving into the WFIP–2 Vocabulary and Retrieval Strategy Practice Form. The learner practices, at home or in class, saying each target word three times alone and in a sentence while subtly gesturing the action associated with each word.

WORD-FINDING SELF-ADVOCACY GOALS

1. The learner will recognize that when he or she has difficulty retrieving a specific word, he or she can be aided by gesturing the action associated with that word.

2. The learner will be able to predict that he or she is going to have difficulty retrieving a word and self-cue by gesturing the action associated with the target word.

CLASSROOM ACCOMMODATION ACTIVITY

Preparation: Collaborate with the teacher to identify word lists and review the gesture cueing strategy.

If the learner is not able to retrieve a target word, suggest that the teacher frame questions to the learner in a multiple-choice or "find the answer" format to facilitate his or her class participation. For example, in language arts class ask the student, "In baseball the players wait in the ... stands, dugout, or bleachers?" or "Find the answer in your book." (See Chapter 10 for other suggestions on how to design accommodations for the learner's language environment.)

USING ACADEMIC CONTEXTS

1. Collaborate with the teacher to identify academic vocabulary whose action can be gestured.

2. When a learner indicates difficulty retrieving a previously treated word, suggest that the teacher ask the learner to subtly gesture the action associated with the target word.

3. If the gesture self-cueing does not aid the learner's retrieval of the target word, ask the teacher to accept the learner's mime of the target word's action.

Retrieval Strategy Lessons for Error Pattern 2

This chapter presents preferred and supplementary retrieval strategies for learners who display Error Pattern 2: Word-Form Blocked Errors, a failure to access any of the target words' form information. This pattern is commonly known as a "tip of the tongue" error. When learners demonstrate this error pattern, they produce slow, inaccurate responses, *but are able to retrieve the target word when a phonemic cue (first syllable or consonant–vowel combination) is provided.* They either produce a no-response type that does not add content (e.g., "I don't know," "I pass," or no response) or a semantic substitution, which is corrected with the phonemic cue. See Chapter 3 for a discussion of this error pattern.

Retrieval strategies that link words similar in sound or words frequently associated with the target word can reduce these word-form-related errors. These strategies make the target word form more salient. Their use has been reported to be helpful in reducing slow, inaccurate

responses in children (German, 2002). Retrieval strategies that help learners circumvent word-finding blocks (e.g., synonym and category substituting) also aid learners during connected discourse. Further, for learners who have good written-language skills, strategies that focus on the target words' spelling can also help make the phonological schema of the target word more salient.

LESSON 7-1

PREFERRED RETRIEVAL STRATEGY—SAME-SOUNDS CUE AND REHEARSAL

Practice this strategy prior to the speaking situation and have the learner apply it while talking. Use this strategy to improve word-finding accuracy and speed.

RETRIEVAL CONTEXT: Retrieval of specific words in sentences and discourse

ERROR PATTERN: Error Pattern 2: Word-Form Blocked Errors (commonly known as "tip of the tongue" errors; learner retrieves target word with phonemic cue)

RETRIEVAL STRATEGY BENCHMARK (OBJECTIVE): To link a same-sounds cue (i.e., an adapted phonological neighbor) to the target word to make the word's form more salient

PARTICIPANTS: Learner or learners and specialist

TIME: 20 to 30 minutes

SETTING: Initially, activities for Level 1: Awareness and Level 2: Instruction are best taught in a small language group in the language room, general education classroom, or special education classroom. Later, Level 3: Self-Application activities can be taught in cooperative groups, during class discussion, or in the context of an academic activity.

LEARNER'S MATERIALS (SEE APPENDIX A):

- WFIP–2 Retrieval Strategy Lesson Plan
- WFIP–2 Syllable-Dividing and Same-Sounds Syllable Cue Study Forms
- WFIP–2 Vocabulary and Retrieval Strategy Practice Form
- WFIP–2 Vocabulary
- Other word lists developed from learner's word retrieval errors or drawn from the learner's classroom curriculum or home, recreational, or work environment

- Model Sentences for Selected WFIP–2 Vocabulary
- Age-appropriate board game with spinner, if needed

TECHNOLOGY OR ELECTRONIC MATERIALS: Electronic dictionaries and word lists available on the Internet are good sources for identifying same-sounds cues for target words and syllables. The following are three helpful Web sites:

- http://www.rhymezone.com
- http://www.onelook.com
- http://www.rhymer.com

If these Web sites are no longer available, search the Internet using the descriptors *rhymes, homophones, dictionary,* and *mnemonics* to identify additional Web sites to assist you in teaching the retrieval strategy in this lesson.

INTERVENTION LEVEL 1: AWARENESS OF RETRIEVAL STRATEGY

Preparation: Provide word lists and paper and pencil or word processor.

1. Teach the concept of linking cue words to target words to aid the retrieval of the target words.

   a. Explain to the learner that when you use the same-sounds cue you associate or link a prompt word that shares sounds with the target word (adapted phonological neighbor).

   b. To serve as an example of how one can use this strategy, share Emily's story with the learner.

EMILY'S STORY

Emily was a second-grade student who, late in the school year, still could not remember the names of her science and math teachers, Mrs. Tucker and Mrs. Freed, respectively. To help Emily remember her teachers' names, she was taught to use the same-sounds cue retrieval strategy. She linked the cue word *tuck* as in "tuck in your clothes" to the teacher's name Mrs. Tucker, and she linked the cue word *freedom* to the teacher's name, Mrs. Freed. Emily practiced thinking of her cue word *tuck* before saying "Mrs. Tucker" out loud three times. She practiced thinking of her cue word *freedom* before saying "Mrs. Freed" out loud three times. After applying the same-sounds cue strategy, Emily was able to address her teachers by their names the next day in class.

c. Ask the learner to think of a same-sounds cue to remember your name. Have the learner practice thinking of the same-sounds cue and saying your name out loud three times. *Stress to learner that he or she is not to verbalize the cue word out loud. Rather, the learner should only think of the same-sounds cue while saying the target word out loud.*

INTERVENTION LEVEL 2: INSTRUCTION OF RETRIEVAL STRATEGY AND REHEARSAL

Preparation: Provide electronic file and word processor or word lists and paper and pencil.

1. *Target word selection.* Select five target words that are relevant and that the learner understands. (See Appendix A for various academic and recreation vocabulary lists.)

2. *Same-sounds cue practice.* Have the learner link each of the target words with a cue word that sounds like the target word. Use the Syllable-Dividing and Same-Sounds Syllable Cue Study Form (see Appendix A) to display how the cue word is

linked to the target word. For monosyllabic and multisyllabic words, write the target word syllable or syllables in the boxes in Step 2 on the form, and then write the same-sounds cue in the space in Step 3.

3. *Target word rehearsal in isolation.* Have the learner think of, not say, the same-sounds cues for the target words while verbalizing each word three times. *If a game format is used, have the learner spin the spinner, move around the game board, and with each turn, think of the same-sounds cue when saying the target word three times.*

4. *Target word rehearsal in a sentence.* Have the learner think of, not say, the same-sounds cue for each target word while verbalizing that target word in three different sentences. The learner may develop his or her own sentences or, if appropriate, use the model sentences provided in Appendix A. *If a game format is used, have the learner spin the spinner and move around the game board. With each turn, have the learner think of the same-sounds cue before saying the target word out loud in three different sentences.*

5. *Target word rehearsal in discourse.* While verbalizing a short discourse using five target words, have the learner think of (not say aloud) the same-sounds cue before saying each target word. If needed, model a discourse for the learner by telling a story or relating an event using the five target words. *If a game format is used, have the learner spin the spinner, move around the game board, and with each turn, verbalize five sentences to create a short discourse using the five target words. The learner who circles the board a specified number of times wins the game.*

6. *Same-sounds cue reminder.* If the learner has difficulty retrieving a target word in Steps 4 and 5, remind the learner of the same-sounds cue for that target word.

INTERVENTION LEVEL 3: SELF-APPLICATION OF RETRIEVAL STRATEGY AND REHEARSAL

Choose five additional relevant target words that the learner understands and encourage the learner to self-apply the same-sounds cue retrieval strategy as he or she repeats Steps 2 through 5.

GENERALIZATION ACTIVITY

Preparation: Provide the learner with the WFIP–2 Vocabulary and Retrieval Strategy Practice Form.

On the WFIP–2 Vocabulary and Retrieval Strategy Practice Form, the learner writes the words he or she has had difficulty retrieving, along with the same-sounds cues for those target words. The learner practices these words, at home or in class, thinking of the same-sounds cue while rehearsing each word out loud and in a sentence three times.

WORD-FINDING SELF-ADVOCACY GOALS

1. The learner will recognize that when he or she has difficulty retrieving a specific word, he or she can be aided by using same-sounds cues and rehearsal.
2. The learner will be able to predict potentially troublesome vocabulary, names, and other words and apply the same-sounds cue strategy and rehearsal.

CLASSROOM ACCOMMODATION ACTIVITY

Preparation: Collaborate with the classroom teacher to identify word lists and review the same-sounds cue strategy.

When a learner is not able to retrieve a target word like *cumulus* in science class, suggest that the teacher either cue the learner with the first syllable of the target word (e.g., *cum* for *cumulus*) or frame questions to the learner in a multiple-choice or "find the answer" format to facilitate his or her class participation. For example, to check knowledge of clouds in science the teacher should ask, "What is the name of the clouds that are fluffy on top and flat on the bottom ... stratus, cumulus, or cirrus?" or "Find the answer in your book." (See Chapter 10 for other suggestions on how to modify the learner's language environment.)

USING ACADEMIC CONTEXTS

1. Collaborate with the teacher to identify vocabulary and apply the same-sounds cue strategy to aid the learner's oral retrieval of selected terms in math, science, social studies, and language arts.

2. Following retrieval strategy instruction, suggest that the teacher encourage the learner to self-apply the same-sounds cue retrieval strategy when learning new vocabulary.

LESSON 7-2

PREFERRED RETRIEVAL STRATEGY— SAME-SOUNDS MEANING CUE AND REHEARSAL

Practice this strategy prior to the speaking situation and apply it while the learner is talking. Use this strategy to improve word-finding accuracy and speed.

RETRIEVAL CONTEXT: Retrieval of specific words in sentences and discourse

ERROR PATTERN: Error Pattern 1: Lemma-Related Semantic Errors (commonly known as "slip of the tongue" errors) and Error Pattern 2: Word-Form Blocked Errors (commonly known as "tip of the tongue" errors; learner retrieves target word with the phonemic cue)

RETRIEVAL STRATEGY BENCHMARK (OBJECTIVE): To link the same-sounds meaning cue (i.e., a word that shares sounds and meaning with the target word, making the link between the target word meaning and form more salient)

PARTICIPANTS: Learner or learners and specialist

TIME: 20 to 30 minutes

SETTING: Initially, activities for Level 1: Awareness and Level 2: Instruction are best taught in a small language group in the language room, general education classroom, or special education classroom. Later, Level 3: Self-Application activities can be taught in cooperative groups, during class discussion, or in the context of an academic activity.

LEARNER'S MATERIALS (SEE APPENDIX A):

- WFIP–2 Retrieval Strategy Lesson Plan
- WFIP–2 Syllable-Dividing and Same-Sounds Syllable Cue Study Forms
- WFIP–2 Vocabulary and Retrieval Strategy Practice Form
- WFIP–2 Vocabulary
- Other word lists developed from learner's word-retrieval errors or drawn from the learner's classroom curriculum or home, recreational,

or work environment
- Model Sentences for Selected WFIP–2 Vocabulary
- Age-appropriate board game with spinner, if needed

TECHNOLOGY OR ELECTRONIC MATERIALS: Electronic dictionaries and word lists available on the Internet are good sources for identifying same-sounds cues for target words and syllables. The following are three helpful Web sites:
- http://www.rhymezone.com
- http://www.dictionary.com
- http://www.rhymer.com

If these Web sites are no longer available, search the Internet using the descriptors *rhymes, homophones, dictionary,* and *mnemonics* to identify additional Web sites to assist you in teaching the retrieval strategy in this lesson.

INTERVENTION LEVEL 1: AWARENESS OF RETRIEVAL STRATEGY

Preparation: Provide word lists and paper and pencil or word processor.

1. Teach the concept of linking cue words to target words to aid word retrieval.

   a. Explain to the learner that when you use the same-sounds meaning cue, you associate a cue word that *both shares sounds with the target word (such a cue word is called an adapted phonological neighbor) and is also related in meaning to the target word.*

b. To serve as an example of how one can use this strategy, share Brian's story with the learner.

BRIAN'S STORY

Brian was a kindergartener who had difficulty naming his body parts. The specialist taught him to link the same-sounds meaning cue *older* to remember the body part *shoulder. Older* was a same-sounds meaning cue for *shoulder* because it shared some of the same sounds as the target word, and Brian's older brother had big shoulders. Brian first practiced thinking of his cue word *older* while saying the target word *shoulder* in isolation and in three sentences, after which he was able to name his shoulder in class.

---

c. Ask the learner to think of a same-sounds meaning cue to remember your name or another teacher's name. Have the learner identify and practice thinking of the same-sounds meaning cue while saying the target name out loud. *Stress to learner that he or she is not to verbalize the same-sounds meaning cue out loud. Rather the learner is to only think of the cue word and say the target word out loud.*

INTERVENTION LEVEL 2: INSTRUCTION OF RETRIEVAL STRATEGY AND REHEARSAL

Preparation: Provide word lists and, if needed, a board game.

1. *Target word selection.* Select five target words that are relevant and that the learner understands. See Appendix A for various academic and recreation vocabulary lists.

2. *Same-sounds meaning cue practice.* Have the learner link each of the target words with a cue word that sounds like the target word and is related to the target word in meaning. Use the Syllable-Dividing and Same-Sounds Syllable Cue

Study Form to display how the cue word is linked to the target word. For monosyllabic and multisyllabic words, write the target word syllable or syllables in the boxes in Step 2 on the form, and then write the same-sounds meaning cue in the space in Step 3.

3. *Target word rehearsal in isolation.* Have the learner think of, not say, the same-sounds meaning cue while verbalizing each target word three times out loud.

4. *Target word rehearsal in a sentence.* Have the learner think of, not say, the same-sounds meaning cue for the target word while verbalizing that target word in three different sentences. The learner may develop his or her own sentences or, if appropriate, use the model sentences provided in Appendix A.

5. *Target word rehearsal in discourse.* Have the learner think of, not say, the same-sounds meaning cue before each target word while verbalizing a short discourse using the five target words the learner is studying. If necessary, model a discourse for the learner by telling a story or relating an event using the target words. *If a game format is used, with each turn have the learner verbalize five sentences to create a short discourse using the five target words. Have the learner use a spinner to determine the number of spaces to move around the game board. The learner who circles the board a specified number of times wins the game.*

6. *Same-sounds meaning cue reminder.* If the learner has difficulty retrieving a target word in Steps 4 and 5, remind the learner of the same-sounds meaning cue for that target word.

INTERVENTION LEVEL 3: SELF-APPLICATION OF RETRIEVAL STRATEGY AND REHEARSAL

1. Explain to the learner that, prior to conversations with friends or discussions in class, the same-sounds meaning cue strategy needs to be self-applied to target names and words.

2. Choose five additional relevant target words that the learner understands, and encourage the learner to self-apply the same-sounds meaning cue retrieval strategy as he or she repeats Steps 2 through 5 for these additional words.

GENERALIZATION ACTIVITY

Preparation: Provide the learner with the WFIP–2 Vocabulary and Retrieval Strategy Practice Form.

On the Vocabulary and Retrieval Strategy Practice Form, the learner writes the words he or she has had difficulty retrieving along with their same-sounds meaning cues. The learner practices these words, at home or in class, thinking of the same-sounds meaning cue while rehearsing each word out loud and in a sentence three times.

WORD-FINDING SELF-ADVOCACY GOALS

1. The learner will recognize that when he or she has difficulty retrieving a specific word, he or she can be aided by using the same-sounds meaning cue and rehearsal strategy.

2. The learner will be able to predict potentially troublesome vocabulary, names, and other words and apply the same-sounds meaning cue and rehearsal strategy.

CLASSROOM ACCOMMODATION ACTIVITY

Preparation: Collaborate with the classroom teacher to identify word lists.

When a learner is not able to retrieve a target word, suggest that the teacher either cue the learner with the first syllable of the target word (e.g., *at* for *atlas*) or frame questions to the learner in a multiple-choice or "find the answer" format to facilitate his or her class participation. For example, say, "A book of maps is called a ... globe, legend, or an atlas?" or "Find the answer in your book." (See Chapter 10 for other suggestions on how to modify the learner's language environment.)

USING ACADEMIC CONTEXTS

1. Collaborate with the teacher to identify vocabulary and apply the same-sounds meaning cue strategy to aid the learner's oral retrieval of selected terms in math, science, social studies, and language arts.

2. Following retrieval strategy instruction, suggest that the teacher encourage the learner to self-apply the same-sounds meaning cue retrieval strategy when learning new vocabulary.

LESSON 7-3

PREFERRED RETRIEVAL STRATEGY—FAMILIAR-WORD CUE AND REHEARSAL

Practice this retrieval strategy prior to the speaking situation and apply it while the learner is talking. Use this strategy to improve word-finding accuracy and speed.

RETRIEVAL CONTEXT: Retrieval of specific words in sentences and discourse

ERROR PATTERN: Error Pattern 2: Word-Form Blocked Errors (commonly known as "tip of the tongue" errors; learner retrieves the target word with phonemic cue)

RETRIEVAL STRATEGY BENCHMARK (OBJECTIVE): To link the familiar-word cue (i.e., a cue word that frequently co-occurs with the target word in a different context) to the target word

PARTICIPANTS: Learner or learners and specialist

TIME: 20 to 30 minutes

SETTING: Initially, activities for Level 1: Awareness and Level 2: Instruction are best taught in a small language group in the language room, general education classroom, or special education classroom. Later, Level 3: Self-Application activities can be taught in cooperative groups, during class discussion, or in the context of an academic activity.

LEARNER'S MATERIALS (SEE APPENDIX A):

- WFIP–2 Retrieval Strategy Lesson Plan
- WFIP–2 Syllable-Dividing and Same-Sounds Syllable Cue Study Forms
- Vocabulary and Retrieval Strategy Practice Form
- WFIP–2 Vocabulary
- Other word lists developed from learner's word-retrieval errors or drawn from the learner's classroom curriculum or home, recreational, or work environment

- Model Sentences for Select WFIP–2 Vocabulary
- Age-appropriate board game with spinner, if needed

TECHNOLOGY OR ELECTRONIC MATERIALS: Electronic dictionaries and word lists available on the Internet are good sources for identifying familiar word cues for target words. The following are four helpful Web sites:

- http://www.rhymezone.com
- http://www.dictionary.com
- http://www.onelook.com
- http://www.longmanwebdict.com

If these Web sites are no longer available, search the Internet using the descriptors *collocational dictionaries, rhymes, homophones, dictionary,* and *mnemonics* to identify additional Web sites to assist you in teaching the retrieval strategy in this lesson.

INTERVENTION LEVEL 1: AWARENESS OF RETRIEVAL STRATEGY

Preparation: Provide word lists and paper and pencil or word processor.

1. Teach the concept of linking cue words to target words to aid word retrieval.

   a. Explain to the learner that when you use the familiar-word cue, you link a cue word that is frequently said with the target word (i.e., it co-occurs) in a different context. For example, if you wanted to remember *pizza,* you could think of the familiar-word cue *cheese.* For *helmet* you could think of the cue word *football,* and for *candles* you could think of the cue word *birthday.*

   b. To serve as an example of how one can use this strategy, share Thomas's story with the learner.

THOMAS'S STORY

Thomas was a kindergarten student who had difficulty naming his colors, even though he could always point to each color when he heard the color's name. To help him remember color names, he was taught to use the familiar-word cue retrieval strategy. He linked the familiar-word cues *red light* to the color *red* and *blue jeans* to the color *blue.* He practiced thinking of his familiar-word cue *red light* while saying *red* out loud, and he practiced thinking of his familiar-word cue *blue jeans* while saying *blue* out loud. The next day in class, Thomas was able to name those two color words consistently.

c. Ask the learner to think of a familiar-word cue to teach someone how to remember the color *green.* If he or she has difficulty thinking of a familiar-word cue, model how thinking of the familiar word cue *green bean* can help a learner remember the color *green.*

INTERVENTION LEVEL 2: INSTRUCTION OF RETRIEVAL STRATEGY AND REHEARSAL

Preparation: Provide word lists and, if needed, a board game.

1. *Target word selection.* Select five target words that are relevant and that the learner understands. (See Appendix A for various academic and recreation vocabulary lists.)

2. *Familiar-word cue practice.* Have the learner link the target words to familiar-word cues. For words that do not have frequently co-occurring words, have the learner use a same-sounds cue (see Lesson 7-1). Use the Syllable-Dividing and Same-Sounds Syllable Cue Study Form to display how the cue word is linked to the target word. For both monosyllabic and multisyllabic words, write the target word syllable or syllables in the boxes in Step 2 on the form and then write the familiar-word cue in the space in Step 3 on the form.

3. *Target word rehearsal in isolation.* Have the learner think of, not say, the familiar-word cue for the target word while verbalizing each target word three times.

4. *Target word rehearsal in a sentence.* Have the learner think of, not say, the familiar-word cue for the target word while verbalizing each target word in three different sentences. The learner may develop his or her own sentences or, if appropriate, use the model sentences provided in Appendix A. *If a game format is used, have the learner spin the spinner to move around the game board. With each turn, have the learner think of the familiar-word cue before saying the target words out loud in three different sentences.*

5. *Target word rehearsal in discourse.* Have the learner think of the familiar-word cue while verbalizing the five target words in a short discourse. If needed, model a discourse for the learner by telling a story or relating event using the target words. *If a game format is used, have the learner spin the spinner to move around the game board. With each turn, have the learner verbalize five sentences to create a short discourse using the five target words. The learner who circles the board a specified number of times wins the game.*

6. *Familiar-word cue reminder.* If the learner has difficulty retrieving a target word in Steps 4 and 5, remind the learner of the familiar-word cue for that target word.

INTERVENTION LEVEL 3: SELF-APPLICATION OF RETRIEVAL STRATEGY AND REHEARSAL

Choose five additional relevant target words that the learner understands and encourage the learner to self-apply the retrieval strategy as he or she repeats Steps 2 through 5 with the additional words.

GENERALIZATION ACTIVITY

Preparation: Provide the learner with the WFIP–2 Vocabulary and Retrieval Strategy Practice Form.

When using the WFIP–2 Vocabulary and Retrieval Strategy Practice Form in Appendix A, you may want to create an electronic file of this form or produce hard copies on which the learner can write. On the form, the learner writes the words he or she has had difficulty retrieving, along with the familiar-word cue. The learner rehearses these words, at home or in class, thinking of the familiar-word cue while saying each word alone and in a sentence three times.

WORD-FINDING SELF-ADVOCACY GOALS

1. The learner will recognize that when he or she has difficulty retrieving a specific word, he or she can be aided by using the familiar-word cue and rehearsal.

2. The learner will be able to predict potentially troublesome vocabulary, names, and so on, and apply the familiar-word cue and rehearsal strategy.

CLASSROOM ACCOMMODATION ACTIVITY

Preparation: Collaborate with the classroom teacher to identify word lists and review the familiar-word cue strategy.

When a learner is not able to retrieve a target word in social studies, suggest that the teacher either cue the learner with the first syllable of the target word (e.g., *con* for *continent*) or frame questions to the learner in a multiple-choice or “find the answer” format to facilitate his or her class participation. For example, say, "A large area of land is called a ... continent, boundary, or equator?" or "Find the answer in your book." (See Chapter 10 for other suggestions on how to modify the learner's language environment.)

USING ACADEMIC CONTEXTS

1. Collaborate with the teacher to identify vocabulary and apply the familiar-word cue strategy to aid the learner's oral retrieval of selected terms in math, science, social studies, and language arts.

2. Following instruction of the familiar-word cue retrieval strategy, suggest that the teacher encourage the learner to self-apply the retrieval strategy when practicing new vocabulary.

LESSON 7-4

PREFERRED RETRIEVAL STRATEGY— SYNONYM SUBSTITUTING AND REHEARSAL

Apply this strategy while the learner is talking. Use this strategy to circumvent a word-finding block.

RETRIEVAL CONTEXT: Retrieval of specific words in sentences and discourse

ERROR PATTERN: Error Pattern 2: Word-Form Blocked Errors (commonly known as "tip of the tongue" errors) or Error Pattern 3: Word-Form Phonologic Errors (commonly known as "twist of the tongue" errors)

RETRIEVAL STRATEGY (OBJECTIVE): To substitute synonyms for evasive or multisyllabic words that are difficult to retrieve

PARTICIPANTS: Learner or learners and specialist

TIME: 20 to 30 minutes

SETTING: Initially, activities for Level 1: Awareness and Level 2: Instruction are best taught in a small language group in the language room, general education classroom, or special education classroom. Later, Level 3: Self-Application activities can be taught in cooperative groups, during class discussion, or in the context of an academic activity.

LEARNER'S MATERIALS (SEE APPENDIX A):

- WFIP–2 Retrieval Strategy Lesson Plan
- WFIP–2 Vocabulary and Retrieval Strategy Practice Form
- WFIP–2 Vocabulary
- Other word lists developed from learner's word-retrieval errors or drawn from the learner's classroom curriculum or home, recreational, or work environment
- Model Sentences for Select WFIP–2 Vocabulary
- Age-appropriate board game with spinner, if needed

TECHNOLOGY OR ELECTRONIC MATERIALS: Electronic dictionaries and word lists available on the Internet are good sources for identifying synonyms. The following are two helpful Web sites:

- http://www.rhymezone.com
- http://www.dictionary.com

If these Web sites are no longer available, search the Internet using the descriptors *mnemonics, dictionary, rhymes,* and *synonyms* to identify additional Web sites to assist you in using the retrieval strategy in this lesson.

INTERVENTION LEVEL 1: AWARENESS OF RETRIEVAL STRATEGY

Preparation: Provide word processor or paper and pencil, and electronic or hard copy of word lists.

1. Review the definition of a synonym with the learner. Explain to the learner that for some words, a speaker could substitute a synonym and still retain the intended meaning of the sentence. As examples, present the following target words to the learner (orally, printed, or pictured): *a cook, happy,* and *movie.* Review these words with the learner, explaining that each of these words can be matched with another word that has the same or similar meaning. Demonstrate by giving the synonyms for these target words: *chef* for *cook, glad* for *happy,* and *show* for *movie.*

2. Emphasize to the learner that when talking it is better to substitute a synonym for a target word than to experience a word-finding block. Say two sentences for each sample target word in Step 1. Develop a sentence using the target word, and then repeat the sentence substituting the synonym for the target word in the sentence.

INTERVENTION LEVEL 2: INSTRUCTION OF RETRIEVAL STRATEGY AND REHEARSAL

Preparation: Provide word lists and target word cards.

1. *Target word selection.* From the vocabulary list, select target words that are easily paired with synonyms. Use an electronic thesaurus or Web site to identify synonyms for target words.

2. *Target word and synonym rehearsal.* Name each of the selected words and have the learner repeat each word followed by its synonym.

3. *Target word and synonym game.* Have the learner draw a card and verbalize target words and synonyms printed on the card. Continue through the cards until each learner has had an opportunity to practice all the target words.

4. *Target word and synonym substitution in a sentence.* Have the learner draw a card and say two sentences, one sentence with the target word and one sentence substituting the synonym for the target word.

5. *Target word and synonym in different sentences.* Have the learner draw a card and say three sentences for the target word. Then have the learner say the same three sentences, substituting the synonym for the target word.

6. *Target word and synonym in discourse.* Have the learner draw three cards and verbalize the three target words in a discourse script. Model a discourse for the learner.

7. *Synonym substitution reminder.* If the learner has difficulty retrieving a target word in Step 6, encourage him or her to substitute a synonym for the evasive target word.

INTERVENTION LEVEL 3: SELF-APPLICATION OF RETRIEVAL STRATEGY AND REHEARSAL

1. Explain to the learner that the synonym substituting strategy should be self-applied when talking in the classroom, with friends, or at home, to circumvent potential word-finding blocks.

2. Choose additional target words that the learner knows and encourage the learner to self-apply the retrieval strategy as he or she repeats Steps 2 through 6 with the additional target words.

GENERALIZATION ACTIVITY

Preparation: Provide the learner with the WFIP–2 Vocabulary and Retrieval Strategy Practice Form.

On the Vocabulary and Retrieval Strategy Practice Form, the learner writes the words he or she has had difficulty retrieving, along with their synonyms. The learner practices, at home or in class, saying sentences once with the target word and once with the synonym substitute. The sentences with each target word should be rehearsed three times.

WORD-FINDING SELF-ADVOCACY GOALS

1. The learner will recognize that when he or she anticipates that a specific word will be difficult to retrieve, he or she can substitute a synonym for the target word.

2. The learner will be able to predict that he or she is going to have difficulty retrieving a word and substitute a synonym for the target word rather than produce a word-finding error.

WORD-FINDING ACCOMMODATIONS

Preparation: Collaborate with the teacher to identify word lists and review the synonym substituting strategy.

1. When a learner indicates difficulty retrieving a specific word either in discourse or in responding to a question, encourage the teacher to accept a synonym in place of the target word.

2. If the learner is not able to substitute a synonym for the target word, suggest that the teacher either cue the learner with the first syllable of the target word (e.g., *air* for *area*) or frame questions to the learner in a multiple-choice or "find the answer" format to facilitate his or her class participation. For example, in math class the teacher could ask the learner, "The surface of objects is called the ... angle, circumference, or area?" (See Chapter 10 for other suggestions on how to modify the learner's language environment.)

USING ACADEMIC CONTEXTS

1. Collaborate with the teacher to identify vocabulary and apply the synonym substituting strategy to maintain the learner's oral fluency in math, science, social studies, and language arts, as well as to facilitate his or her written language expression.

2. If the learner is not able to retrieve a treated word, the teacher should ask for and accept a word that is similar in meaning to the target word.

LESSON 7-5

PREFERRED RETRIEVAL STRATEGY—CATEGORY SUBSTITUTING AND REHEARSAL

Apply this strategy while the learner is talking. Use this strategy to circumvent a word-finding block.

RETRIEVAL CONTEXT: Retrieval of specific words in sentences and discourse

ERROR PATTERN: Error Pattern 2: Word-Form Blocked Errors (commonly known as "tip of the tongue" errors) or Error Pattern 3: Word-Form Phonologic Errors (commonly known as "twist of the tongue" errors)

RETRIEVAL STRATEGY BENCHMARK (OBJECTIVE): To substitute category words for evasive or multisyllabic words that are difficult to retrieve

PARTICIPANTS: Learner or learners and specialist

TIME: 20 to 30 minutes

SETTING: Initially, activities for Level 1: Awareness and Level 2: Instruction are best taught in a small language group in the language room, general education classroom, or special education classroom. Later, Level 3: Self-Application activities can be taught in cooperative groups, during class discussion, or in the context of an academic activity.

LEARNER'S MATERIALS (SEE APPENDIX A):

- WFIP–2 Retrieval Strategy Lesson Plan
- WFIP–2 Vocabulary and Retrieval Strategy Practice Form
- WFIP–2 Vocabulary
- Other word lists developed from learner's word-retrieval errors or drawn from the learner's classroom curriculum or home, recreational, or work environment
- Model Sentences for Select WFIP–2 Vocabulary
- Age-appropriate board game with spinner, if needed

TECHNOLOGY OR ELECTRONIC MATERIALS: For readers, provide electronic word lists and sentences. Electronic dictionaries and word lists available on the Internet are good sources for identifying category names for target words. The following are two helpful Web sites:

- http://www.rhymezone.com (definitions)
- http://www.mydictionary.com

If neither of these Web sites are available, search the Internet using the descriptors *mnemonics, dictionary, rhymes,* and *category* to identify additional Web sites to assist you in using the retrieval strategy in this lesson.

INTERVENTION LEVEL 1: AWARENESS OF RETRIEVAL STRATEGY

Preparation: Provide word processor or paper and pencil, and learner's word lists.

1. Review with the learner the concept of categorization and the definition of a category word.

   a. Present (orally, written, or pictured) the following target words to the learner: *apple, hammer,* and *football.*

   b. Review this vocabulary list with the learner, explaining that each of these words can be matched with another word that names its category.

   c. Demonstrate by giving the category name for the target words: *fruit* for *apple, tool* for *hammer,* and *sport* for *football.*

2. Emphasize to the learner that, when talking, it is better to substitute the category name of a target word then to have a word-finding block. To demonstrate, say two sentences for each sample target word in Step 1. Develop a sentence using the target word, and then repeat the sentence substituting the category name for the target word. Emphasize to the learner that it is appropriate to substitute a category name for a word that is difficult to retrieve.

INTERVENTION LEVEL 2: INSTRUCTION OF RETRIEVAL STRATEGY AND REHEARSAL

Preparation: Provide word lists and target word cards.

1. *Target word selection.* Select from the vocabulary list those target words that can be easily substituted with their category word. If needed, use one of the electronic dictionaries indicated in the learner's materials section of this lesson to identify category names for target words.

2. *Target word and category word rehearsal.* Name each of the words and have the learner repeat each word followed by its category name.

3. *Target word and category word game.* Have the learner draw a card and verbalize first the target word on the card and then its category name. Continue through the cards until each learner has had an opportunity to practice each target word.

4. *Target word and category word substitution in a sentence.* Have the learner draw a card and say two sentences, one with the target word on the card and one substituting the category word on the card for the target word.

5. *Target word and category word substitution in different sentences.* Have the learner draw a card and say three different sentences for the target word. Then have the learner say the same three sentences, substituting the category name for

the target word. The learner may develop his or her own sentences or, if appropriate, use those provided in Appendix A.

6. *Target word and category word in discourse.* Have the learner draw three cards and verbalize the three target words in a discourse script.

7. *Category word substituting reminder.* If the learner has difficulty retrieving a target word in Steps 4 and 5, encourage him or her to substitute a category name for the evasive target word.

INTERVENTION LEVEL 3: SELF-APPLICATION OF RETRIEVAL STRATEGY AND REHEARSAL

1. Explain to the learner that the category substituting strategy should be self-applied to circumvent potential word-finding blocks when talking in the classroom, with friends, or at home.

2. Choose additional words that the learner knows and encourage the learner to self-apply the category substituting strategy as he or she repeats Steps 2 through 6 from Level 2: Instruction (earlier in this lesson).

GENERALIZATION ACTIVITY

Preparation: Provide the learner with the WFIP–2 Vocabulary and Retrieval Strategy Practice Form.

On the WFIP–2 Vocabulary and Retrieval Strategy Practice Form, the learner writes the words he or she has had difficulty retrieving, along with their category names. The learner practices, at home or in class, saying sentences, one with the target word and one with the category word substitute. The sentences with each target word should be rehearsed three times.

WORD-FINDING SELF-ADVOCACY GOALS

1. The learner will recognize that when he or she has difficulty retrieving a specific word, he or she can substitute the category name for the target word.

2. The learner will be able to predict that he or she is going to have difficulty retrieving a target word and substitute the category name for that word, rather than produce a word-finding error.

WORD-FINDING ACCOMMODATIONS

Preparation: Collaborate with the teacher to identify word lists and to review the category substituting strategy.

1. When a learner indicates difficulty retrieving a specific word either in discourse or in responding to a question, encourage the teacher to accept the learner's use of a category name in place of the target word.

2. If the learner is not able to substitute a category word for the target word, suggest that the teacher cue the learner with the first syllable of the target word (e.g., *sub* for *subtraction*) or frame questions to the learner in a multiple-choice or "find the answer" format to facilitate his or her class participation. For example, in math class a teacher could say, "When you take away, it is called ... subtraction, addition, or multiplication?" (See Chapter 10 for other suggestions on how to modify the learner's language environment.)

USING ACADEMIC CONTEXTS

1. Collaborate with the teacher to identify vocabulary and apply the category substituting strategy to maintain the learner's oral fluency in math, science, social studies, and language arts, as well as to facilitate his or her written-language expression.

2. If the learner is not able to retrieve a target word, encourage the teacher to ask the learner to think of the category name for that word.

LESSON 7-6

SUPPLEMENTARY RETRIEVAL STRATEGY—GRAPHEMIC CUEING

Practice this strategy prior to the speaking situation and apply it while the learner is talking. Use this lesson only with learners who have grade-appropriate spelling skills. The purpose of this lesson is to improve word-finding accuracy and speed.

RETRIEVAL CONTEXT: Retrieval of specific words in sentences and discourse

ERROR PATTERN: Error Pattern 2: Word-Form Blocked Errors (commonly known as "tip of the tongue" errors; learner retrieves target word with the phonemic cue)

RETRIEVAL STRATEGY BENCHMARK (OBJECTIVE): To use target word spellings to cue retrieval of words difficult to retrieve

PARTICIPANTS: Learner or learners and specialist

TIME: 20 to 30 minutes

SETTING: Initially, activities for Level 1: Awareness and Level 2: Instruction are best taught in a small language group in the language room, general education classroom, or special education classroom. Later, Level 3: Self-Application activities can be taught in cooperative groups, during class discussion, or in the context of an academic activity.

LEARNER'S MATERIALS (SEE APPENDIX A):

- WFIP–2 Retrieval Strategy Lesson Plan
- WFIP–2 Vocabulary and Retrieval Strategy Practice Form
- WFIP–2 Vocabulary
- Other word lists developed from learner's word-retrieval errors or drawn from the learner's classroom curriculum or home, recreational, or work environment
- Model Sentences for Selected WFIP–2 Vocabulary
- Age-appropriate board game with spinner, if needed

TECHNOLOGY OR ELECTRONIC MATERIALS: Electronic dictionaries and word lists available on the Internet are good sources for identifying target word spellings. The following are two helpful Web sites:

- http://www.dictionary.com
- http://www.onelook.com

If these Web sites are no longer available, search the Internet using the descriptors *dictionary* and *spellings* to identify additional Web sites to assist you in using the retrieval strategy in this lesson.

INTERVENTION LEVEL 1: AWARENESS OF RETRIEVAL STRATEGY

Preparation: Provide electronic or learner's word lists and a word processor or paper and pencil.

NOTE: Use this strategy only with learners who have grade-appropriate spelling skills.

1. Remind learners that each word has a specific spelling. Write the words *apple, orange, fork, book,* and *cup.* Show each word to the learner and spell each word aloud, pointing to each letter as you spell the word.

2. Explain to the learner that visualizing or writing how a target word is spelled can help future retrieval of that word when speaking and writing.

   a. Write the words *apple, orange, fork, book,* and *cup.* Have the learner look at each word, then, with his or her eyes closed, visualize spelling while saying each target word.

b. Have the learner visualize and then write the target word while verbalizing the word three times. For example, say to the learner, "Picture how the word *apple* is spelled in your head. Write the word *apple,* and then say 'apple.'")

INTERVENTION LEVEL 2: INSTRUCTION OF RETRIEVAL STRATEGY AND REHEARSAL

Preparation: Provide electronic file or learner's word lists and game spinner.

1. *Target word selection.* Select five target words that are relevant and that the learner understands.

2. *Target word and spelling practice.* Have the learner write or type each of the words and then say each word three times as he or she looks at it.

3. *Target word and spelling visualization (eyes closed).* Ask the learner to close his or her eyes and listen. As you say each of the target words, ask the learner to visualize each word's spelling and say the word aloud.

4. *Target word and spelling rehearsal.* Have the learner say each target word three times while visualizing its spelling.

5. *Target word rehearsal in a sentence.* Have the learner say each word in a sentence three times, while visualizing its spelling. The learner may develop his or her own sentences or, if appropriate, use those provided in Appendix A. *If a game format is used, have the learner spin the spinner to determine the number of sentences to rehearse.*

6. *Target word rehearsal in discourse.* Have the learner use the words in a discourse, visualizing the words' spellings while

saying each target word. Model a discourse for the learner. *If a game format is used, have the learner spin the spinner to determine the number of target words to use in each discourse. For example, if the learner spins* 3, *have him or her develop a discourse around three target words. Have the learner record the number of points obtained after each spin. The learner with the most points at the end of the lesson wins the game.*

7. *Graphemic cueing reminder.* If the learner has difficulty retrieving the target word in Steps 5 and 6, encourage him or her to visualize the target word's spelling to cue retrieval of the target word.

INTERVENTION LEVEL 3: SELF-APPLICATION OF RETRIEVAL STRATEGY AND REHEARSAL

1. Explain to the learner that the graphemic cueing strategy needs to be self-applied when he or she has difficulty remember names and words when speaking in the classroom, with friends, or at home.

2. Choose five additional relevant target words that the learner understands and encourage the learner to self-apply the retrieval strategy as he or she repeats Steps 2 through 6 with the additional words.

GENERALIZATION ACTIVITY

Preparation: Provide the learner with the WFIP–2 Vocabulary and Retrieval Strategy Practice Form.

On the WFIP–2 Vocabulary and Retrieval Strategy Practice Form, the learner writes the words he or she has had difficulty

retrieving. The learner practices, at home or in class, visualizing the spelling of each target word while saying each word alone and in sentences.

WORD-FINDING SELF-ADVOCACY GOALS

1. The learner will recognize that when he or she has difficulty retrieving a specific word, he or she can be aided by visualizing the spelling of the target word.

2. The learner will be able to predict that he or she is going to have difficulty retrieving a word and try to self-cue by visualizing the spelling of the target word.

CLASSROOM ACCOMMODATION ACTIVITY

Preparation: Collaborate with the teacher to identify vocabulary lists for each unit.

If the learner is not able to retrieve a target word, suggest that the teacher either cue the learner with the first syllable of the target word (e.g., *pla* for *plateau*) or frame questions to the learner in a multiple-choice or "find the answer" format to facilitate his or her class participation. For example, in social studies class a teacher could ask the student, "The flat part on the top of a hill is called a ... prairie, pond, or plateau?" (See Chapter 10 for other suggestions on how to modify the learner's language environment.)

USING ACADEMIC CONTEXTS

1. Collaborate with the teacher to identify vocabulary and apply the graphemic cueing strategy (i.e., target word spelling)

to academic vocabulary to aid the learner's word finding in oral and written discourse.

2. When a learner indicates difficulty retrieving a specific word, either in discourse or in responding to a question, suggest that the teacher ask the learner to picture the word's spelling in his or her mind to aid retrieval.

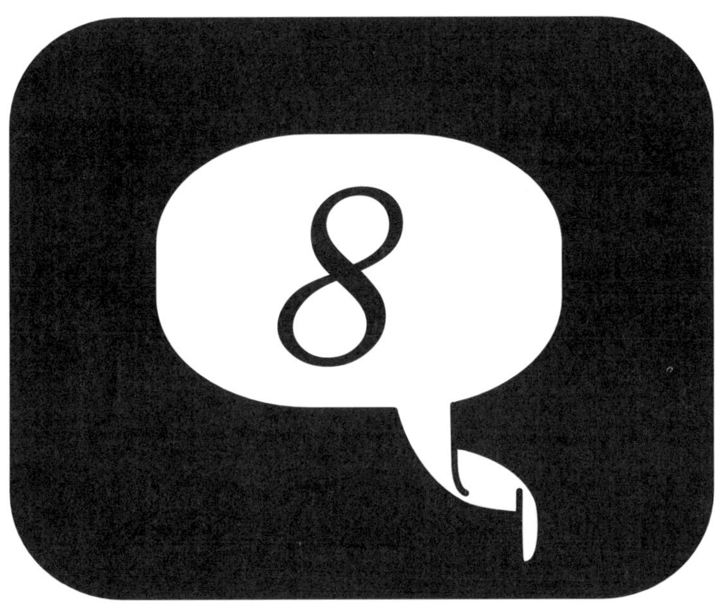

Retrieval Strategy Lessons for Error Pattern 3

This chapter presents preferred and supplementary retrieval strategies for Error Pattern 3: Word-Form Phonologic errors. Typically this error pattern is demonstrated by a phonemic substitution, indicating partial access of the syllabic frame or segmental sound units associated with the target word (e.g., *subrine* for *submarine; commonly referred to as a "twist of the tongue" error). Typically resulting in slow and inaccurate responses, these phonemic substitutions are not corrected with the phonemic cue.*

Pairing retrieval strategies that make the syllabic structure of the target word explicit (e.g., syllable dividing) with strategies that make individual syllables more salient (e.g., same-sounds syllable cues) is helpful to learners when they manifest form-segment-related errors on multisyllabic words (German, 2002). See Chapter 4 for a discussion of this strategic approach.

Further, retrieval strategies that help learners circumvent word-finding disruptions on multisyllabic words (e.g., synonym and category substituting) also aid learners during discourse (see Lessons 7-4 and 7-5).

LESSON 8-1

PREFERRED RETRIEVAL STRATEGY— SYLLABLE DIVIDING + REHEARSAL

Practice this strategy prior to the speaking situation. Use it to improve word-finding accuracy and speed of retrieving multisyllabic words.

RETRIEVAL CONTEXT: Retrieval of specific words in sentences and discourse.

ERROR PATTERN: Error Pattern 3: Word-Form Phonologic Errors (commonly known as "twist of the tongue" errors; the learner does not access the target word with the phonemic cue)

RETRIEVAL STRATEGY BENCHMARK (OBJECTIVE): To use syllable dividing and rehearsal to improve retrieval of multisyllabic words (Note: Use this strategy only if the learner understands how to divide words into syllables.)

PARTICIPANTS: Learner or learners and specialist

TIME: 20 to 30 minutes

SETTING: Initially, activities for Level 1: Awareness and Level 2: Instruction are best taught in a small language group in the language room, general education classroom, or special education classroom. Later, Level 3: Self-Application activities can be taught in cooperative groups, during class discussion, or in the context of an academic activity.

LEARNER'S MATERIALS (SEE APPENDIX A):

- WFIP–2 Retrieval Strategy Lesson Plan
- WFIP–2 Syllable-Dividing and Same-Sounds Syllable Cue Study Forms
- WFIP–2 Vocabulary and Retrieval Strategy Practice Form
- WFIP–2 Vocabulary
- Other multisyllabic word lists developed from learner's word-retrieval errors or drawn from the learner's classroom curriculum or home, recreational, or work environment

- Model Sentences for Selected WFIP–2 Vocabulary
- Age-appropriate board game with spinner, if needed

TECHNOLOGY OR ELECTRONIC MATERIALS: Electronic dictionaries on the Internet are good sources for identifying correct syllabication of multisyllabic target words. The following are three helpful Web sites:

- http://www.rhymezone.com
- http://www.dictionary.com
- http://www.rhymer.com

If these Web sites are no longer available, search the Internet using the descriptors *syllabication, syllables, English pronunciation,* and *dictionary* to identify additional Web sites to assist you in using the retrieval strategy in this lesson.

INTERVENTION LEVEL 1: AWARENESS OF RETRIEVAL STRATEGY

Preparation: Provide word lists and paper and pencil or word processor.

1. Teach awareness of retrieval difficulties with multisyllabic target words.

   a. Contrast shorter monosyllabic words (e.g., *cup*) with longer multisyllabic words (e.g., *temperature*) for the learner.

   b. Indicate to the learner that he or she often has difficulty retrieving the longer words, which are multisyllabic words.

   c. Have the learner name pictures of monosyllabic and multisyllabic words (e.g., *worm* and *caterpillar*). With the learner, contrast the ease with which he or she can say

shorter monosyllabic words versus longer multisyllabic words.

2. Demonstrate to the learner the purpose and use of the syllable dividing and rehearsal strategy. (Note that syllabication of target words should be based on pronunciation.) Explain to the learner that the syllable dividing and rehearsal strategy can improve retrieval of long words.

   a. Using the Syllable-Dividing and Same-Sounds Syllable Cue Study Form, segment the following multisyllabic words into syllables by writing each syllable in the corresponding box on the form or drawing a line between each syllable as you write the word: *com/pu/ter, te/le/phone,* and *te/le/vis/ion.*

   b. Mark each syllable with a rhythmic tap, or a raise a finger for each syllable as it is said.

INTERVENTION LEVEL 2: INSTRUCTION OF RETRIEVAL STRATEGY + REHEARSAL

Preparation: Provide word lists, pencil and paper, and a spinner.

---

1. *Target word selection.* From the materials listed for this lesson, select five multisyllabic target words that are relevant and that the learner understands.

2. *Syllable-dividing strategy.* Using the Syllable-Dividing and Same-Sounds Syllable Cue Study Form, segment the multisyllabic words into syllables by writing each syllable in a box on Step 2 of the form, or by writing each word and drawing a line between each syllable. Have the learner mark each

syllable with a rhythmic tap or raise a finger for each syllable as it is said.

3. *Multisyllabic word rehearsal.* Have the learner say each multisyllabic word three times while segmenting the word into syllables. *If a game format is used, have the learner spin the spinner for each multisyllabic word to determine how many times he or she should rehearse the target word.*

4. *Multisyllabic word rehearsal in sentences.* Have the learner verbalize the target word in three sentences. The learner may develop his or her own sentences or, if appropriate, use those provided in the Model Sentences for Selected WFIP–2 Vocabulary (see Appendix A). *If a game format is used, have the learner spin the spinner to determine how many sentences he or she should verbalize with the target word.*

5. *Multisyllabic word rehearsal in discourse.* Have the learner generate a discourse using the five target words. If needed, model a discourse for the learner. Continue until each learner has had an opportunity to practice his or her target words in a brief discourse. *If a game format is used, have the learner spin the spinner to determine how many target words to include in his or her brief discourse.*

6. *Syllable-dividing strategy reminder.* If the learner has difficulty retrieving the target word in Step 5, encourage him or her to rehearse these target words, both segmented and as a unit, three times.

INTERVENTION LEVEL 3: SELF-APPLICATION OF RETRIEVAL STRATEGY + REHEARSAL

1. Explain to the learner that the syllable-dividing strategy needs to be self-applied when he or she has difficulty re-

trieving multisyllabic names or words in the classroom, with friends, or at home.

2. Choose five additional multisyllabic target words that are relevant and that the learner understands and encourage the learner to self-apply the retrieval strategy as he or she repeats Steps 2 through 5 of Level 2: Instruction (earlier in this lesson) with those additional target words.

GENERALIZATION ACTIVITY

Preparation: Provide the learner with the WFIP–2 Vocabulary and Retrieval Strategy Practice Form.

The WFIP–2 Vocabulary and Retrieval Strategy Practice Form is presented in Appendix A. You are encouraged to create an electronic file of this form or produce hard copies. On the Vocabulary and Retrieval Strategy Practice Form, the learner writes the words he or she has had difficulty retrieving. The learner rehearses, at home or in class, saying sentences with the target words. If he or she has difficulty retrieving the target words, the learner should segment the words into syllables using the syllable-dividing strategy.

WORD-FINDING SELF-ADVOCACY GOALS

1. The learner will recognize that he or she has difficulty retrieving multisyllabic words.
2. The learner will use the syllable-dividing and rehearsal strategy to improve retrieval of multisyllabic words.
3. The learner will predict when he or she is going to have difficulty retrieving multisyllabic words.

4. The learner will ask for the correct pronunciation of the word to prepare to apply the syllable-dividing strategy.

CLASSROOM ACCOMMODATION ACTIVITY

Preparation: Collaborate with the teacher to identify multisyllabic word lists and review the syllable-dividing rehearsal strategy.

1. Prior to each academic unit studied, teachers should provide learners and specialists with a list of important multisyllabic words.

2. In class, suggest that the teacher frame questions to the learner in a multiple-choice format when a learner has difficulty retrieving a multisyllabic word. (See Chapter 10 for other suggestions on how to modify the learner's language environment.)

USING ACADEMIC CONTEXTS

Collaborate with the teacher to identify multisyllabic vocabulary and apply the syllable-dividing and rehearsal strategy to aid the learner's retrieval of multisyllabic words in science, math, language arts, and social studies.

LESSON 8-2

PREFERRED RETRIEVAL STRATEGY— SAME-SOUNDS SYLLABLE CUE AND REHEARSAL

Practice this strategy prior to the speaking situation, and apply it while the learner is talking. Use this strategy to improve word-finding accuracy and speed of multisyllabic words.

RETRIEVAL CONTEXT: Retrieval of specific words in sentences and discourse

ERROR PATTERN: Error Pattern 3: Word-Form Phonologic Errors (commonly known as "twist of the tongue" errors; the learner does not access the target word with the phonemic cue)

RETRIEVAL STRATEGY BENCHMARK (OBJECTIVE): To link the same-sounds syllable cue (i.e., similar-sounding words) to difficult-to-retrieve syllables to improve retrieval of multisyllabic words

PARTICIPANTS: Learner or learners and specialist

TIME: 20 to 30 minutes

SETTING: Initially, activities for Level 1: Awareness and Level 2: Instruction are best taught in a small language group in the language room, general education classroom, or special education classroom. Later, Level 3: Self-Application activities can be taught in cooperative groups, during class discussion, or in the context of an academic activity.

LEARNER'S MATERIALS (SEE APPENDIX A):

- WFIP–2 Retrieval Strategy Lesson Plan
- WFIP–2 Syllable-Dividing and Same-Sounds Syllable Cue Study Forms
- WFIP–2 Vocabulary and Retrieval Strategy Practice Form
- WFIP–2 Vocabulary
- Other multisyllabic word lists developed from learner's word-retrieval errors or drawn from the learner's classroom curriculum or home, recreational, or work environment

- Model Sentences for Selected WFIP–2 Vocabulary
- Age-appropriate board game with spinner, if needed

TECHNOLOGY OR ELECTRONIC MATERIALS: Electronic dictionaries and word lists available on the Internet are good sources for identifying same-sounds cues for syllables. The following are three helpful Web sites:

- http://www.rhymezone.com
- http://www.onelook.com
- http://www.rhymer.com

If these Web sites are no longer available, search the Internet using the descriptors *rhymes, homophones, dictionary,* and *mnemonics* to identify additional Web sites to assist you in teaching the retrieval strategy in this lesson.

INTERVENTION LEVEL 1: AWARENESS OF RETRIEVAL STRATEGY

Preparation: Provide word lists and paper and pencil or word processor.

1. Teach the concept of linking words to syllables that share the same sounds.

   a. Explain to the learner that when you use the same-sounds syllable cue with multisyllabic words, you associate or link a prompt word that has some of the same sounds as the target syllable.

   b. To serve as an example of how to use this strategy, share Matt's story with the learner.

MATT'S STORY

Matt, a second-grade student, often had difficulty remembering all the syllables of long words. As an example, Matt had difficulty retrieving the word *thermometer.*

He would incorrectly say "theroneter." To help Matt remember how to say *thermometer* correctly, his speech and language clinician helped him divide the word *thermometer* into the syllables *ther/mom/me/ter.* Next she taught him to link the cue word *mom* to the second syllable because that was the most difficult syllable for Matt to retrieve. Matt then practiced saying the target word *thermometer* three times, thinking each time of his cue word *mom* before saying "thermometer" out loud. After that language lesson, Matt was able to say "thermometer" correctly in class.

INTERVENTION LEVEL 2: INSTRUCTION AND APPLICATION OF RETRIEVAL STRATEGY AND REHEARSAL

Preparation: Provide a copy of the WFIP–2 Syllable-Dividing and Same-Sounds Syllable Cue Study Form, word lists, and, if needed, a board game.

1. *Same-sounds syllable cue instruction.* Ask the learner to think of a long (i.e., multisyllabic) word that he or she has difficulty saying. Using the Syllable-Dividing and Same-Sounds Syllable Cue Study Form, divide the target word in syllables. To link a same-sounds cue to the syllable that is most difficult for the learner to say, enter the same-sounds syllable cue in the callout corresponding to the evasive syllable (see Step 3 on the form). Have the learner practice thinking of the same-sounds syllable cue while saying the multisyllabic word out loud three times. *Stress to the learners that he or she is not supposed to verbalize the same-sounds syllable cue out loud. Rather, the learner should only think of the same-sounds syllable cue and say the target word out loud.*

2. *Target word selection.* Select five multisyllabic target words that are relevant and that the learner understands (see Appendix A for selected vocabulary).

3. *Same-sounds syllable cue practice.* First, using the WFIP–2 Syllable-Dividing and Same-Sounds Syllable Cue Study Form, segment the multisyllabic words into syllables by writing each syllable in a box on the form (see Step 2 on the form). Second, have the learner link a cue word that sounds like the evasive syllable by writing it in the callout corresponding to the troublesome syllable (see Step 3 on the form).

4. *Target word rehearsal in isolation.* Have the learner think of, not say, the same-sounds syllable cue as he or she verbalizes each word three times. *If a game format is used, have the learner spin the spinner, move around the game board, and with each turn, think of the same-sounds syllable cue while saying the target word three times.*

5. *Target word rehearsal in a sentence.* Have the learner think of, not say, the same-sounds syllable cue as he or she verbalizes each target word in three different sentences. The learner may develop his or her own sentences or use those provided in Appendix A. *If a game format is used, have the learner spin the spinner and move around the game board. With each turn, have the learner think of the same-sounds syllable cue before saying the target word out loud in three different sentences.*

6. *Target word rehearsal in discourse.* Using the five target words, have the learner think of the appropriate same-sounds syllable cue while verbalizing each word in a short discourse. If needed, model a discourse for the learner by telling a story or relating an event using the target words. *If a game format is used, have the learner spin the spinner, move around the game board, and with each turn, verbalize five sentences to create a short discourse using the five target words. The learner who circles the board a specified number of times wins the game.*

7. *Same-sounds syllable cue reminder.* If the learner has difficulty retrieving a target word in Steps 5 and 6, remind the learner of his or her same-sounds syllable cue for that target word.

INTERVENTION LEVEL 3: SELF-APPLICATION OF RETRIEVAL STRATEGY AND REHEARSAL

1. Explain that the same-sounds syllable cue strategy needs to be self-applied when the learner has difficulty retrieving multisyllabic names or words in the classroom, with friends, or at home.

2. Choose five additional relevant target words that the learner understands and encourage the learner to self-apply the retrieval strategy as he or she repeats Steps 2 through 6 of Level 2: Instruction (earlier in this lesson).

GENERALIZATION ACTIVITY

Preparation: Provide the learner with the WFIP–2 Vocabulary and Retrieval Strategy Practice Form.

On the WFIP–2 Vocabulary and Retrieval Strategy Practice Form, the learner writes the words he or she has had difficulty retrieving, along with their same-sounds syllable cues. The learner practices these words, at home or in class, thinking of the same cue while rehearsing each target word out loud and in a sentence three times.

WORD-FINDING SELF-ADVOCACY GOALS

1. The learner will recognize that when he or she has difficulty retrieving a multisyllabic word, he or she can be aided by using the same-sounds syllable cue and rehearsal.

2. The learner will be able to predict potentially troublesome multisyllabic words, names, and other words and apply the same-sounds syllable cue strategy and rehearsal.

CLASSROOM ACCOMMODATION ACTIVITY

Preparation: Collaborate with the classroom teacher to identify multisyllabic word lists and review application of the same-sounds syllable cue strategy.

When a learner is not able to retrieve a mutisyllabic word, suggest that the teacher frame questions to the learner in a "find the answer" or multiple-choice format to facilitate his or her class participation. For example, in math class a teacher could ask the student, "Train tracks are an example of ... an angle, parallel lines, or the area?" (See Chapter 10 for other suggestions on how to modify the learner's language environment.)

USING ACADEMIC CONTEXTS

1. Collaborate with the teacher to identify vocabulary and apply the same-sounds syllable cue strategy to aid the learner's oral retrieval of selected multisyllabic words in math, science, social studies, and language arts.

2. Following retrieval strategy instruction, suggest that the teacher encourage the learner to self-apply the same-sounds syllable cue retrieval strategy when learning new vocabulary.

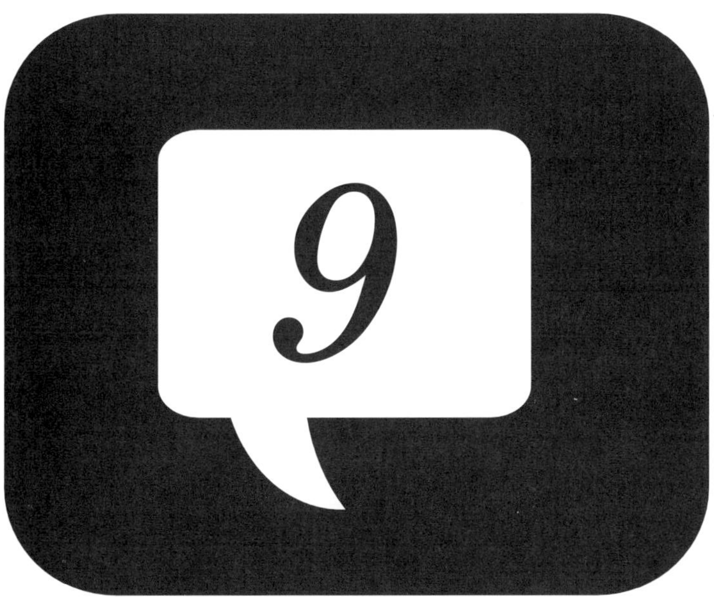

Word-Finding Self-Advocacy Lessons

The purpose of the WFIP–2 word-finding self-advocacy lessons is to empower learners to use their retrieval strategies and to self-advocate for appropriate learning experiences. Emphasis is placed on self-application of retrieval strategies and self-selection of classroom accommodations that will improve learning in school.

Specifically, the goals of these lessons are

1. to help learners become aware of their word-finding error patterns through self-monitoring,
2. to empower learners to take responsibility for improving their word-finding skills through self-application of retrieval strategy instruction, and
3. to teach learners to advocate for language accommodations to facilitate their communication.

Meeting the first two goals is important if learners are to be motivated to self-apply retrieval strategies. The third goal is important if students are to negotiate the word-finding accommodations needed in their language environment to further their learning.

The following are the WFIP–2 word-finding self-advocacy lesson plans. Once these lessons have been completed, word-finding self-advocacy objectives should be addressed in the context of other instructional lessons.

Note that all the self-advocacy lesson plans should be completed before beginning the lessons for word-finding accommodations.

LESSON 9-1

SELF-ASSESSMENT OF WORD-FINDING SKILLS—LANGUAGE SETTINGS

Use this lesson to guide the learner's word-finding self-assessment.

RETRIEVAL CONTEXT: Retrieval of specific words in sentences and discourse

SELF-ADVOCACY BENCHMARK (OBJECTIVE): To identify language settings (e.g., school, home) where the learner experiences the most and the least difficulty with word finding

PARTICIPANTS: Learner or learners, specialist, and teacher or teachers

TIME: 10 to 15 minutes

SETTING: Small language group in language room, general education classroom, or special education classroom, or entire class in general education classroom

MATERIALS: Word-Finding Self-Assessment Survey (see Appendix B)

ACTIVITIES

NOTE: Lessons 9-1 through 9-5 may be combined as time allows.

1. Explain to the learner that word finding may be easier in some language settings and more difficult in others.

2. Use the Word-Finding Self-Assessment Survey to identify different language settings where word-finding skills may

vary. Point out these language settings to the learner and discuss common elements among the language settings.

3. Have the learner complete the portion of the Word-Finding Self-Assessment Survey that focuses on word-finding skills in different language settings.

GENERALIZATION ACTIVITIES

1. Ask the learner to use the self-monitoring technique taught in Lesson 6-1 to monitor his or her own word-finding skills in the various language settings discussed. Focus on identifying those language settings that facilitate or interfere with the learner's word-finding skills.

2. Ask the learner to report his or her observations at the next language session.

USING ACADEMIC AND HOME CONTEXTS

Ask teachers and family members to note whether the learner's word-finding skills vary depending on the language setting. If so, these observations should be shared with the learner along with modifications that can be made in these different language settings to reduce heavy demands on the learner's word-finding skills.

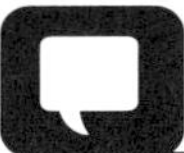

LESSON 9-2

SELF-ASSESSMENT OF WORD-FINDING SKILLS—LANGUAGE CIRCUMSTANCES

Use this lesson to guide the learner's word-finding self-assessment.

RETRIEVAL CONTEXT: Retrieval of specific words in sentences and discourse

SELF-ADVOCACY BENCHMARK (OBJECTIVE): To identify which language circumstances (e.g., one-on-one, group) present the learner with the most and the least word-finding difficulty

PARTICIPANTS: Learner or learners, specialist, and teacher or teachers

TIME: 10 to 15 minutes

SETTING: Small language group in language room, general education classroom, or special education classroom, or entire class in general education classroom

MATERIALS: Word-Finding Self-Assessment Survey (see Appendix B)

ACTIVITIES

NOTE: Lessons 9-2 through 9-5 may be combined as time allows.

1. Explain to the learner that word finding may be easier in some language circumstances (e.g., one-on-one, group participation) and more difficult in others.

2. Use the Word-Finding Self-Assessment Survey to identify whether one-on-one or group participation puts more demands on the learner's word-finding skills.

3. Complete the portion of the Word-Finding Self-Assessment Survey that focuses on word-finding skills under different language circumstances.

GENERALIZATION ACTIVITIES

1. Using self-monitoring techniques taught in Lesson 6-1, ask the learner to monitor his or her own word-finding skills in a group versus when talking to one person. Ask the learner to focus on identifying which circumstance facilitates or interferes with his or her word-finding skills.

2. Ask the learner to report his or her observations at the next language session.

USING ACADEMIC AND HOME CONTEXTS

Ask teachers and family members to note if the learner's word-finding skills vary depending on whether he or she is talking in a group or in a one-on-one situation. The learner should use these observations to guide his or her self-monitoring.

LESSON 9-3

SELF-ASSESSMENT OF WORD-FINDING SKILLS—RETRIEVAL CONTEXTS

Use this lesson to guide the learner's word-finding self-assessment.

RETRIEVAL CONTEXT: Retrieval of specific words in sentences and discourse

SELF-ADVOCACY BENCHMARK (OBJECTIVE): To identify retrieval contexts (e.g., single word or discourse) that create the most and least difficulty in retrieval

PARTICIPANTS: Learner or learners, specialist, and teacher or teachers

TIME: 10 to 15 minutes

SETTING: Small language group in language room, general education classroom, or special education classroom, or entire class in general education classroom

MATERIALS: Word-Finding Self-Assessment Survey (see Appendix B)

ACTIVITIES

NOTE: Lessons 9-3 through 9-5 may be combined as time allows.

1. Explain to the learner that he or she may have more or less difficulty with word retrieval depending on whether he or she is asked to retrieve a specific word, give an explanation or a description, or relate an experience.

2. Use the Word-Finding Self-Assessment Survey to identify different retrieval contexts where word-finding skills may vary. Point out these contexts to the learner and discuss common elements among the contexts.

3. Complete the portion of the Word-Finding Self-Assessment Survey that focuses on word-finding skills in different retrieval contexts.

GENERALIZATION ACTIVITIES

1. Using self-monitoring techniques taught in Lesson 6-1, ask the learner to monitor his or her own word-finding skills in school and at home. The focus of this lesson is on identifying whether the learner has more word-finding difficulty when asked questions that require retrieval of specific names or words versus when engaged in a discourse, conversation, or narrative.

2. Ask the learner to report his or her observations at the next language session.

USING ACADEMIC AND HOME CONTEXTS

Ask teachers and family members to note if the learner's word-finding skills vary depending on whether the learner needs to retrieve a specific word or fact or to engage in a discourse. The learner should use this information to guide his or her self-monitoring.

LESSON 9-4

SELF-ASSESSMENT OF WORD-FINDING SKILLS—ACADEMIC SUBJECT OF TARGET WORD

Use this lesson to guide the learner's word-finding self-assessment.

RETRIEVAL CONTEXT: Retrieval of specific words in sentences and discourse

SELF-ADVOCACY BENCHMARK (OBJECTIVE): To identify academic subjects related to vocabulary that is difficult to retrieve or vocabulary that is easy to retrieve

PARTICIPANTS: Learner or learners, specialist, and teacher or teachers

TIME: 10 to 15 minutes

SETTING: Small language group in language room, general education classroom, or special education classroom, or entire class in general education classroom

MATERIALS: Word-Finding Self-Assessment Survey (see Appendix B)

ACTIVITIES

NOTE: Lessons 9-4 through 9-5 may be combined as time allows.

1. Explain to the learner that vocabulary from some subjects (e.g., academic, recreational, political) may be more difficult to retrieve than other vocabulary.

2. Use the Word-Finding Self-Assessment Survey to identify words from different subjects that may be harder or easier

for the learner to retrieve. Point out and discuss these academic subjects with the learner.

3. Complete the portion of the Word-Finding Self-Assessment Survey that focuses on changes in word-finding skills based on the subject of the target word the learner is attempting to retrieve.

GENERALIZATION ACTIVITIES

1. Using self-monitoring techniques taught in Lesson 6-1, ask the learner to monitor his or her own word-finding skills when attempting to retrieve vocabulary from different academic subjects. Ask the learner to identify those academic subjects in which vocabulary is the most challenging to retrieve.

2. Ask the learner to report his or her observations at the next language session.

USING ACADEMIC AND HOME CONTEXTS

Ask teachers and family members to note whether the learner's word-finding skills vary depending on the academic subject area being discussed. The learner should use this information to guide his or her self-monitoring.

LESSON 9-5

SELF-ASSESSMENT OF WORD-FINDING SKILLS— LEXICAL FACTORS OF THE TARGET WORD

Use this lesson to guide the learner's word-finding self-assessment.

RETRIEVAL CONTEXT: Retrieval of specific words in sentences and discourse

SELF-ADVOCACY BENCHMARK (OBJECTIVE): To identify whether a target word's frequency of occurrence, syntax, length, or phonological complexity affects a learner's word-finding skills

PARTICIPANTS: Learner or learners, specialist, and teacher or teachers

TIME: 10 to 15 minutes

SETTING: Small language group in language room, general education classroom, or special education classroom, or entire class in general education classroom

MATERIALS: Word-Finding Self-Assessment Survey (see Appendix B)

ACTIVITIES

NOTE: Lessons 9-5 through 9-6 may be combined as time allows.

1. Explain to the learner that certain types of words may be more difficult to retrieve because of their frequency of usage, length, syntax, or phonological complexity (i.e., the number of syllables, letter sounds).

2. Use the Word-Finding Self-Assessment Survey to identify and discuss different types of words that may be more difficult or easier for the learner to retrieve based on the lexical factors indicated.

3. Complete the portion of the Word-Finding Self-Assessment Survey that examines the effect of lexical factors on a word's ease of retrieval.

GENERALIZATION ACTIVITIES

1. Using self-monitoring techniques taught in Lesson 6-1, ask the learner to monitor his or her word-finding skills when attempting to retrieve words of varying lexical factors. Focus on identifying the word characteristics that facilitate or interfere with the learner's word-finding skills.

2. Ask the learner to report his or her observations at the next language session.

USING ACADEMIC AND HOME CONTEXTS

Ask teachers and family members to note whether the learner's word-finding skills vary depending on the syntactical category, length, or the phonological complexity of the target word. The learner should use these observations to guide his or her self-monitoring.

LESSON 9-6

SELF-ASSESSMENT OF WORD-FINDING SKILLS—SUMMARY LESSON

Use this lesson to guide the learner's word-finding self-assessment.

RETRIEVAL CONTEXT: Retrieval of specific words in sentences and discourse

SELF-ADVOCACY BENCHMARK (OBJECTIVE): To complete and summarize the self-assessment analysis

PARTICIPANTS: Learner or learners, specialist, and teacher or teachers

TIME: 10 to 15 minutes

SETTING: Small language group in language room, general education classroom, or special education classroom, or entire class in general education classroom

MATERIALS: Word-Finding Self-Assessment Survey (see Appendix B)

ACTIVITIES

1. Discuss and summarize for the learner the results from the Word-Finding Self-Assessment Survey.

2. Discuss with the learner the possible modifications that can be made to reduce retrieval demands inherent in those areas on the survey that were identified as the most troublesome. For example if the learner indicated that he or she finds it difficult to retrieve answers to questions asked in class, tell the learner to ask the teacher for choices or for a

phonemic cue. (See Chapter 10 for other suggestions on how to modify the learner's language environment.)

GENERALIZATION ACTIVITY

Using self-monitoring techniques taught in Lesson 6-1, ask the learner to monitor his or her own word-finding skills in areas that were identified as troublesome through retrieval self-analysis. Ask the learner to focus on generating possible modifications that would help to compensate for his or her retrieval difficulties.

WORD-FINDING ACCOMMODATIONS ACTIVITY

Using the self-assessment analysis, have the student collaborate with his or her teachers and family members to identify modifications needed to aid his or her word finding in areas self-identified as challenging.

Word-Finding Accommodations Identification and Lessons

An important aspect of word-finding intervention is reducing the expressive language demands inherent in the learner's academic curriculum, social interactions, and recreation activities. Underlying this component of the program is the value that children with word-finding difficulties deserve equal access to the regular curriculum. Nelson (1998) indicates that providing such access requires the commitment of both the general educator and the specialist (in particular, the speech–language pathologist) to analyze and differentiate the regular curriculum until it matches the language abilities of the learner. She encourages specialists to collaborate with general educators to modify the general education curriculum so that it is accessible to learners with various language skills.

To this end, the word-finding accommodations component of the WFIP–2 is designed to provide differentiated assessment and instruction for learners with word-finding difficulties. The goal is to accommodate these learners' expressive language difficulties so that their achievement is not underestimated due to their word-finding difficulties. Failure to apply accommodations early in a learner's schooling starts a lower achievement effect that compounds over the years. Learners with word-finding difficulties often never recover from this effect.

Assessment for Learners with Word-Finding Difficulties

Individualized assessment and instruction are important parts of an intervention program for learners with word-finding difficulties. As an example, consider Art's present classroom situation.

ART'S STORY

When asked to respond orally, Art, 9 years old, is often unable to express his knowledge in his fourth-grade classroom. In these situations, he is judged as not knowing and being unprepared when in reality he has studied and believes he understands the content. His inability to express himself in class angers and frustrates him. He also finds it difficult to engage in conversations with peers and adults because of his difficulty in accessing words to express his thoughts. He says, "The words are at the edge of my mind." Unfortunately, it is not uncommon for learners like Art to stop trying to express their perspective because they come to believe that they will experience failure. In addition, Art is frequently unable to complete his academic assessments successfully because there is a high retrieval load inherent in the response mode of these assessments (e.g., fill in the blank, write the answer, read out loud). In contrast, when assessment accommodations are implemented and the retrieval load of the assignment is reduced, Art can successfully complete his work, indicating that he has learned the material under study.

Art's experiences demonstrate the need to have differentiated instruction and assessment matched to one's language abilities. For Art and others with word-finding difficulties, this requires strategic application of word-finding accommodations focused on reducing the re-

trieval load embedded in academic instruction and assessment. Following are guidelines to aid in selecting these accommodations for learners with word-finding difficulties.

STRATEGIC APPLICATION OF WORD-FINDING ACCOMMODATIONS

Strategic application of word-finding accommodations requires a review of the linguistic demands inherent in the learner's instruction and a match of the selected accommodations to the language profiles of the learner. Four principles guide the specialist's strategic selection of word-finding accommodations for learners with word-finding difficulties:

1. Create accommodations that reduce the *retrieval load,* not the *work load,* in academic activities.
2. Match word-finding accommodations to the learner's word-finding error patterns.
3. Consider the learner's self-assessment when selecting word-finding accommodations.
4. Implement accommodations across language and literacy domains (e.g., oral, reading, written-language tasks).

Each of these principles is described in detail in this section.

Principle 1. Create accommodations that reduce the retrieval load, not the work load, inherent in academic activities.

Learners challenged with word finding have lexical access difficulties (German, 2000a) and therefore have problems completing tasks that put undue stress on their word-retrieval systems. Therefore, word-finding accommodations for these learners should focus on reducing the retrieval demands inherent in their academic work. Such word-finding-based accommodations (aimed at reducing retrieval load) are preferable to accommodations focused on reducing the instructional level or quantity of academic work. The goal is to create ways for the learner to successfully participate, both quantitatively and qualitatively, in the curriculum.

Word-finding accommodations are designed to maintain the learner at grade level by modifying the task format to match the learner's language abilities. Instructional accommodations include using resource pages, computer files, and other reference materials (e.g., the Internet) to support the learner's word-retrieval processes. Accommodations of assessments include using recognition response modes like multiple-choice frames or "select," "circle," or "highlight the answer" formats.

Because word-finding-based accommodations significantly reduce the focus on the learner's retrieval skills, retrieval difficulties are no longer a barrier to learning. When retrieval demands are reduced, these learners usually can complete grade-level work.

Principle 2. Match word-finding accommodations to the learner's word-finding error patterns.

Learners with word-finding difficulties may produce one or any combination of three word-finding error patterns discussed in Chapter 4. The word-finding accommodations selected should be specific to the word-finding error patterns typically present in a learner's expressive language. Therefore, you should use the knowledge of your learner's word-finding error patterns to guide your selection of word-finding accommodations. To assist you in selection of the most appropriate accommodations for your students, the word-finding accommodations recommended later in this chapter are presented by error pattern.

Principle 3. Consider the learner's self-assessment when selecting word-finding accommodations.

The word-finding accommodations you select should be based on the learner's own assessment of his or her retrieval strengths and weaknesses. Use results from the learner's Word-Finding Self-Assessment Survey (see Chapter 9 and Appendix B) to help determine which of the following language areas creates the greatest challenge to the learner's retrieval skills. It is in these areas that accommodations may need to be implemented.

- Language settings, both school (e.g., classroom, playground) and out-of-school settings (e.g., home, recreation, work)
- Language circumstances, both group (e.g., cooperative learning groups, play groups) and individual (e.g., assignments, reports) language situations
- Retrieval contexts, both single-word and discourse contexts
- Content areas (e.g., reading, language arts, math, science, work areas)

Principle 4. Apply word-finding accommodations across language and literacy domains (e.g., oral, reading, written-language tasks).

Retrieval demands placed on the learner should be modified across language and literacy contexts. To make these accommodations, look across the curriculum to identify where accommodations are most needed for each particular learner. Recognizing the retrieval demands of the various curricula the learner is expected to master is important in establishing the most effective word-finding accommodations. This will require collaboration with the learner's teachers in language arts, science, math, and social studies to identify where support is needed. To aid you in selecting appropriate accommodations, instruction and assessment accommodations recommended later in this chapter focus on reduction of the retrieval load in oral classroom discourse, reading, math, science, and written language.

WORD-FINDING ACCOMMODATIONS FOR THE CLASSROOM

As indicated, the primary goal of the word-finding accommodations component of the WFIP–2 is to establish for learners with word-finding difficulties a language environment that reduces the retrieval load of assessment and instruction activities requiring oral and written responses. The following are specific goals for the word-finding accommodations lessons:

1. To develop collaboration between school personnel (e.g., speech–language pathologists, teachers, specialists), the learner, and family members to plan word-finding accommodations
2. To identify specific word-finding accommodations needed in classroom curriculum, recreational, and home activities
3. To develop resource materials to accommodate learners' word-finding difficulties in the classroom, during recreation, and at home
4. To match technology to the learner's word-finding error patterns to support the learner's oral and written language

This section discusses those four goals and gives examples of word-finding accommodations for the classroom.

Goal 1. Collaborate with school personnel (e.g., speech–language pathologists, teachers), the learner, and family members to plan word-finding accommodations.

Developing collaborative relationships between specialists, parents, and teachers is the first step in designing appropriate word-finding accommodations for students. The collaboration entails discussing the nature of the learner's word-finding difficulties and agreeing on the language areas requiring modification. Although you may be the initiator of this process, its ultimate success is dependent on cooperation among you, the learner, the learner's family members, and the classroom teacher. Without a collaborative effort, the word-finding accommodations component of the WFIP–2 will not be successful.

Goal 2. Identify specific accommodations needed in the classroom, in curriculum, in social interactions during recreation, and at home.

The learner's self-assessment and discussions with his or her teacher should be used to identify activities that need to be modified to reduce the demands on the learner's word retrieval in the classroom. Ask learners who are able to reflect on their word-finding skills to complete the Word-Finding Self-Assessment Survey. The self-analysis provides insights into which language and learning contexts the learner finds most challenging. Concurrently, collaborate with classroom teachers and family members to identify activities that might need to be modified inside and outside of school.

To identify classroom activities that may need to be modified, observe the learner in the classroom, especially during activities that put a high demand on the learner's oral or written retrieval skills. Use the Classroom Observation Form (see Appendix C) to identify activities in the classroom that may put a high demand on the learner's retrieval system. This form focuses on identifying word-finding accommodations for the following classroom activities:

- Oral participation in the classroom
- Vocabulary instruction
- Reading
- Oral classroom work
- Written classroom work
- Homework assignments
- Evaluations

WORD-FINDING ACCOMMODATIONS FOR ORAL PARTICIPATION IN THE CLASSROOM

General education teachers often present material in an interactive format, asking learners questions to check their understanding of the content. Therefore, oral responses to questions are typically required in reading, math, social studies, science, and other classroom subjects. Cazden (1988) described this discourse as a sequence involving topic initiation, learner response, and teacher evaluation. Most often, learners with word-finding problems have been attending and understand the topic initiated by the teacher. However, when called on, they frequently experience a word-finding block, resulting in a negative evaluation on

the part of the teacher. Thus, learners with word-finding difficulties find the oral-response format frustrating because they are unable to retrieve answers to the questions asked during these activities. The extent that these communication breakdowns occur depends on the nature of the vocabulary to be retrieved (German & Newman, 2004) and the pace and nature of the classroom questioning.

In fast-paced oral language activities, learners with word-finding difficulties typically produce one or all of the word-finding error patterns discussed in Chapter 4. During the evaluation phase, the teacher may misperceive these word-finding errors as an indication that the learner is not paying attention or does not know the answer. However, in actuality, the learner may understand the material but is unable to accurately respond to the question due to his or her word-finding difficulties. Such a situation is most evident when the learner blurts out the answer minutes later. Therefore, to minimize these incorrect judgments, the classroom teacher should modify discourse for learners with word-finding difficulties to reduce demands on the learners' retrieval skills.

Individualized test formats and instructional aids for learners with word-finding difficulties also should be employed. Such accommodations aid learning and provide the teacher with a better assessment of the learner's understanding of the material being presented. Classroom oral activity accommodations for learners with word-finding difficulties are indicated in the following list by error pattern, summarized in Table 10.1, and presented in the Recommended Word-Finding Accommodations Form in Appendix C. The goal of each modification is to replace the required oral response with a response format that will allow the learner to demonstrate his or her knowledge. Feel free to add to this list for science, social studies, and other curriculum areas in the learner's school environment. Later sections present accommodations appropriate for reading and math instruction.

- *Accommodations of oral participation to reduce the occurrence of Error Pattern 1: Lemma-Related Semantic Error.* To accommodate learners who may manifest Error Pattern 1 (commonly referred to as a "slip of the tongue" error) when called on in class, recommend that the teacher
  - slow the pace of the oral questioning,
  - signal to the learner to pause and screen out erroneous responses before responding,
  - ask the learner to rehearse the answer before raising his or her hand, and
  - encourage the learner to self-correct if he or she makes a word-finding error when answering.

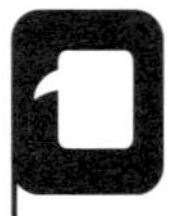

Table 10.1 Recommended Classroom Oral Activity Accommodations by Error Pattern

Word-Finding Error Pattern	Content Area	Activity	Recommended Accommodations	Support Materials
Error Pattern 1	All	Oral questioning	1. Slow pace of questioning. 2. Ask learner to pause before answering, to screen erroneous responses. 3. Ask learner to raise his or her hand only after rehearsing the answer. 4. Ask learner to self-correct errors.	
Error Pattern 2	All	Oral questioning	1. Cue the learner with the initial syllable of the target word. 2. Provide a multiple-choice, true–false, or yes–no response format. 3. Ask the learner to switch to a synonym. 4. Accept volunteer participation only. 5. Inform the learner (minutes before or day before) that you will call on him or her for a particular question.	1. A list of possible questions in advance 2. Resource notebook or electronic file 3. A scaffold of the expected discourse
Error Pattern 3	All	Oral questioning	1. Frame questions in multiple-choice format or recognition response (yes–no or true–false) formats. 2. Ask the learner to switch to a synonym. 3. Accept volunteer participation only.	1. A list of relevant multisyllabic vocabulary in advance 2. Resource notebook or electronic file

- *Accommodations of oral participation to reduce the occurrence of Error Pattern 2: Word-Form Blocked Errors.* To accommodate learners who may manifest Error Pattern 2 (commonly referred to as a "tip of the tongue" error) when called on in class, recommend that the classroom teacher
  - cue the learner with the initial syllable of the target word,
  - provide a multiple-choice way of responding,
  - extend the time allowed for responding,
  - ask the learner to switch to a synonym,
  - only call on the learner when he or she volunteers, or
  - inform the learner (minutes or the day before) that he or she will be called on for a particular question.

- *Accommodations of oral participation to reduce the occurrence of Error Pattern 3: Word-Form Phonologic Errors.* To accommodate for learners who may have difficulty retrieving multisyllabic words when called on in class, recommend that the classroom teacher
  - frame questions in a multiple-choice or recognition format,
  - ask the learner to switch to a synonym, or
  - request volunteer participation only.

WORD-FINDING ACCOMMODATIONS FOR VOCABULARY INSTRUCTION

Typically vocabulary instruction in the classroom focuses on learning word meanings. Activities include defining words, identifying antonyms and synonyms, and creating semantic maps representing the word's taxonomy. These activities help learners develop semantic networks for target vocabulary and result in typical learners' being able to access these learned words in oral and written discourse. However, learners with word-finding difficulties often are not successful in bridging between their vocabulary knowledge and the skills needed for lexical access in oral and written tasks. These students need a dual approach to their vocabulary instruction if they are to efficiently and accurately retrieve their vocabulary in oral and written language activities.

A dual-focus approach to vocabulary instruction includes both acquisition of meanings and corresponding application of mnemonic word-finding strategies. When this approach to vocabulary instruction is used, learners with word-finding difficulties are able to stabilize retrieval of academic vocabulary for oral and written usage.

To guide you in developing the retrieval portion of the dual-focus vocabulary instruction, the example in Figure 10.1 demonstrates retrieval strategy instruction applied to science words in a unit on the heart.

The lesson in Figure 10.1 was designed for a learner who displays Error Pattern 2: Word-Form Blocked Errors (commonly known as "tip of the tongue" errors). Because this learner often stopped midsentence and began to gesture when he or she could not retrieve science vocabulary, a dual-focus approach to vocabulary instruction was beneficial. Following meaning-based instruction on science vocabulary, retrieval-based instruction was provided for the following terms: *heart, pump, atrium, ventricle, blood,* and *circulation.*

Specifically, the familiar-word cue (see Lesson 7-3) was used to stabilize retrieval of the word *heart.* This learner was instructed to think of the familiar-word cue phrase "king of hearts" before saying the word *heart* out loud and rehearsing it in a sentence (e.g., "Thank you from the bottom of my heart."). Similarly, the word *pump* was linked to the familiar-word cue phrase "pumping iron" to cue its retrieval (see Lesson 7-2). The learner then was asked to rehearse the sentence, "My heart pumps blood through my body."

Syllable dividing (Lesson 8-1) and the same-sounds syllable cue (Lesson 8-2) were used to anchor the retrieval of the word *atrium. Atrium* was first divided into three syllables: *a/tri/um.* Next, the same-sounds syllable cue *a* was linked to the first syllable *a* and the same-sounds syllable cue *tree* was linked to the second and third syllables *trium.* These cue words were used because they are similar in sound form to the target word syllables.

Finally, thinking of the retrieval cues, the learner rehearsed saying the target word as a unit and in a sentence: "An atrium is a chamber of the heart." See Figure 10.1 for an illustration of the dual-focused approach to vocabulary instruction applied to other science vocabulary words *ventricle, blood,* and *circulation.* See Appendix A for a master Dual-Focus Vocabulary Instruction Form.

WORD-FINDING ACCOMMODATIONS FOR READING ACTIVITIES

Researchers today believe that difficulties in reading are language-based (Catts & Kamhi, 1999; Snowling & Stackhouse, 1996) and that word-finding difficulties are associated with reading disorders (Bowers & Swanson, 1991; Denckla & Rudel, 1976; McBride-Chang & Franklin, 1996; Wimmer, 1993). For example, Wolf and Goodglass (1986) reported that subtle dysnomia, or naming difficulty, is the most frequent characteristic of children who have dyslexia. Also Murphy, Pollatsek, and

Vocabulary	Comprehension Strategies (Vocabulary Meaning)	Metalinguistic and Mnemonic Retrieval Strategies				
		Syllable Dividing	Same-Sounds Cues	Familiar-Word Cue	Synonym or Category Alternate	Rehearsal
ventricle	One of the two lower chambers of the heart that receives blood from the upper chambers	ven / tri / cle	*vent* to cue *ven*; *trick* to cue *tricle*		chamber	ventricle, ventricle, ventricle
						The ventricles meet at the bottom of the heart.
blood	The red fluid that is pumped from the heart	NA		blood brother		blood, blood, blood,
						Blood flows through your body's veins.
circulation	The movement of blood through the body	Cir / cu / la / tion	*sir* to cue *cir*; *population* to cue *culation*		movement	circulation, circulation, circulation
						Good circulation is important to your health.

Figure 10.1. Completed Dual-Focus Vocabulary Instruction Form for a science unit on the heart.

Well (1988) reported that poor readers displayed word-finding difficulties among other subtle oral-language challenges. Other studies consistently have shown learners with dyslexia and poor reading skills to be slow and inaccurate namers on tests of rapid automatic naming (Katz, 1986; Snowling, Wagtendonk, & Stafford, 1988; Wagner, Torgesen, & Rashotte, 1994; Wolf, 1980, 1986; Wolf & Segal, 1992). In fact, Wolf and Bowers (2000) identified a "double deficit subpattern" among learners with reading disorders, suggesting that naming-speed deficits and phonological deficits co-occur.

In addition, models of lexical access and reading processes indicate that some processes of reading and word finding intersect (Rubin & Liberman, 1983; Wolf, 1980). Clinically this overlap has been observed in analyses of learners' oral reading errors because such analyses often indicate that the reader had tacit knowledge of the target word semantically (e.g., learner reads *king* for *queen*) or phonemically (e.g., learner reads *hospitality* for *hospital*). These observations imply that the reader decoded the target word in the text but may have been unable to read it correctly out loud because of word-finding disruptions.

Difficulties with oral reading can occur in the presence of correct decoding because printed material may be processed before, and possibly independently of, the oral production of the written word. If oral production of words does occur after word decoding, some oral reading errors may actually be based on word-finding errors (German, 2000b; German & Gellar, 2002). In fact, German and Gellar (2003) suggested that word-finding difficulties do interfere with the validity of oral reading assessments. Based on their recommendations, alternate reading assessments need to be considered for learners with word-finding difficulties. Otherwise, accurate assessment of these learners' decoding skills will not occur.

Researchers also have indicated that retrieval or access difficulties may interfere with reading instruction using phonemic awareness (Blachman, 1994; Torgesen, Wagner, & Rashotte, 1994). Smith (2004) indicated that learners with reading and word-finding difficulties have difficulty retrieving letter names, numbers, and the sounds of letters in school. She indicated that these kinds of errors are made even though "these children have full knowledge of the names and sounds they are tying to recall" (Smith, 1991, p. 161). This suggests that individualized reading instruction is needed for these learners.

The next section describes reading assessment accommodations for learners with word-finding difficulties. The accommodations are summarized in the Recommended Word-Finding Accommodations Form in Appendix C (see accommodations listed under Evaluation on the form). You are encouraged to share these accommodation suggestions with the learner's teachers to ensure valid reading assessment as well as meaningful reading instruction.

INDIVIDUALIZED WORD-FINDING ASSESSMENT ACCOMMODATIONS IN READING

The following are recommended reading assessment accommodations for learners with word-finding difficulties:

1. Because oral reading requires oral retrieval of the word being read, oral-reading assessments can be compromised by learner's poor oral retrieval skills. Therefore, it is recommended that neither informal nor formal oral reading assessments be used to determine reading instruction with learners who have word-finding difficulties. Instead, to obtain valid reading evaluations, use silent reading assessments.
2. Because oral reading is laborious for learners with word-finding difficulties, check reading comprehension on silent-reading not oral-reading tasks.
3. Check reading comprehension with questions that use multiple-choice frames or "select, circle, highlight" or "underline the answer" formats. Do not check reading comprehension using questions that require oral or written responses.
4. Assess students' responsiveness to phonemic cueing using the first consonant–vowel combination or syllable.
5. Focus reading fluency activities on silent reading, not oral reading.
6. Conduct word-finding sensitive reading assessments that differentiate phonological awareness from phonological retrieval as indicated in the following section.

Table 10.2 indicates tasks specialized for instruction and assessment in reading for learners with word-finding difficulties.

WORD-FINDING SENSITIVE READING ASSESSMENT

Learners with word-finding difficulties may struggle to access letter sounds and read words orally (i.e., to perform phonological retrieval). Therefore, it is necessary to modify the reading assessment to obtain a valid assessment of their reading skills. Because the Word-Finding Sensitive Reading Assessment (German, 2000b) differentiates phonological retrieval and phonological cued retrieval from phonological awareness, it is recommended to informally assess the reading skills of learners with word-finding difficulties. Figure 10.2 shows the recommended task formats for the Word-Finding Sensitive Reading Assessment. Moving left to right, begin with Phonological Retrieval, continue to Phonological Cued Retrieval, and end with Phonological Awareness.

Table 10.2 Differentiated Instruction and Assessment in Reading for Learners with Word-Finding Difficulties

Word-Finding Error Pattern	Reading Activities	Differentiated Instruction and Assessment for Learners with Word-Finding Difficulties
All error patterns	Oral reading	• Use silent reading. • Use choral reading.
All error patterns	Checking reading comprehension	• Use multiple-choice format or other recognition response formats (true–false, yes–no) for all reading comprehension questions. • Have learner read story silently and highlight portions of text that answer reading comprehension questions. • Have learner read story silently and circle words in text that indicate motivation, feelings, sequence, and so on. • Point to the answer to the question in the text.
All error patterns	Cloze procedure	• Use select-the-answer format for deleted words (learner chooses from the target word and two decoys).
All error patterns	Sound segmentation per word	• Tap, point, color, or draw a line to note different sounds or to note number of syllables.
All error patterns	Sound blending	• Learner points to the picture that represents the blended word heard or read.
All error patterns	Structural analysis	• Circle the root word. • Choose the missing suffix or prefix from a group.

WORD-FINDING ACCOMMODATIONS IN MATH

Math assignments typically include math worksheets or exams that require retrieval of answers. Learners with word-finding difficulties find these assignments and exams difficult because they are unable to consistently retrieve the answers correctly. They may complete one problem correctly yet miss a second problem assessing the same math process or math facts. Designing accommodations for math assessment and instruction for learners with word-finding difficulties involves modifying the oral and written retrieval components of the math tasks. Specifically, a multiple-choice format is used in place of oral drills and writing answers on worksheets, and yes–no, true–false, or "circle the answer" formats are used instead of "fill in the blank" questions on examinations.

Word-Finding Sensitive Reading Assessment of Letter Names

Phonological Retrieval	Phonological Cued Retrieval (Provide first consonant, vowel or syllable.)	Phonological Awareness (Provide two decoys and target letter.)
What is this letter Name? *B*	NA	Point to the letter *B*. *K B T*

Word-Finding Sensitive Reading Assessment of Letter Sounds

Phonological Retrieval	Phonological Cued Retrieval (Provide first consonant, vowel or syllable.)	Phonological Awareness (Provide two decoy letters and the letter of the target sound.)
What sound does this letter make? *B*	NA	Point to the letter that makes the sound *bu.* *J k B*

Word-Finding Sensitive Reading Assessment of Words

Phonological Retrieval	Phonological Cued Retrieval (Provide first consonant, vowel or syllable.)	Phonological Awareness (Provide two decoys and the target word.)
Read this word out loud: *apple*	I will give you a cue *ap* to help you read this word: ____________	Point to this word: *apple.* *apple orange tackle*
Sound this word out: *carnival*	NA	Point to the syllable that makes the sound *car.* (Follow suit with each syllable.) *car ni val*

Word-Finding Sensitive Reading Assessment of Auditory Synthesis

Phonological Retrieval	Phonological Cued Retrieval (Provide first consonant, vowel or syllable.)	Phonological Awareness (Provide two decoy pictures and a picture of the target word.)
What word is this? *com put ter*	NA	Point to the picture that goes with this word: *com put ter.*

(*continues*)

Figure 10.2. Word-finding sensitive reading assessment of letter names, words, auditory synthesis, and auditory analysis.

 Figure 10.2 *Continued.*

Word-Finding Sensitive Reading Assessment of Auditory Analysis

Phonological Retrieval	Phonological Cued Retrieval (Provide first consonant, vowel or syllable.)	Phonological Awareness (Learner indicates with finger.)
Divide this word into syllables: *gardener*	NA	How many syllables do your hear in *gardener*? 1, 2, or 3

Resource notebooks and cue cards are used to cue procedures and steps inherent in math operations. Table 10.3 summarizes the word-finding accommodations for math. These accommodations also are presented in the Recommended Word-Finding Accommodations Form in Appendix C. You are encouraged to share these suggestions for math accommodations with the learner's math teachers to ensure valid assessment and meaningful math instruction.

WORD-FINDING ACCOMMODATIONS FOR TYPICAL CLASSROOM ASSIGNMENTS

Classroom assignments often include oral reports or oral presentations of individual or group work. Learners with word-finding difficulties find these assignments troublesome because they have difficulty finding the words to express their thoughts. Oral assignments of this nature usually result in one of two unsuccessful experiences for these learners. Either they attempt the assignment, do poorly, and then are judged unprepared, or they avoid the assignment and are judged irresponsible. However, when appropriate accommodations are in place, learners with word-finding difficulties can complete their classroom work. For example, instead of traditional oral reports, the learner can use electronic slide presentations, digital movies, or electronic portfolios.

Other assignments that typically place high demands on a learner's word-finding system include worksheets requiring retrieval of answers for fill-in-the-blank items or written brief paragraphs. Providing multiple-choice questions instead of fill-in-the-blank items or having learners highlight the answer in the text accommodates learners' word-finding difficulties. Table 10.4 summarizes recommended accommodations for modifying oral and written classroom work. These accommodations also

Table 10.3 Differentiated Instruction and Assessment in Math for Learners with Word-Finding Difficulties

Word-Finding Error Pattern	Math Activity	Differentiated Instruction and Assessment for Learners with Word-Finding Difficulties
All Error Patterns	Story problems or learning math processes	1. Learners develop and use a resource notebook or an electronic file of formulas, key math words, and so on. 2. Learners develop a hardcopy or electronic file containing cue lists for steps needed to complete math operations.
All Error Patterns	Oral math drills	Learner circles the correct answer using multiple-choice frames.
All Error Patterns	Math calculations	1. Learner uses a calculator or software program. 2. Teacher provides worksheets with multiple-choice frames.
	Fractions	Learner colors in, points to, or cuts out the section representing the fraction.
All Error Patterns	Place value	1. Learner puts given numerals in the correct place value column. 2. Learner points to the correct place value. 3. Learner uses a chart with place value indicated across the top.
All Error Patterns	Telling time	Teacher uses recognition response (point-to or yes–no) format.

are presented in the Recommended Word-Finding Accommodations Form in Appendix C.

WORD-FINDING ACCOMMODATIONS FOR HOMEWORK

Homework assignments often include memorization tasks or written language tasks that put high demands on a learner's word-finding skills. Consequently, students with word-finding difficulties often do not complete their homework. As a result, these learners are misjudged as (a) lacking the skill to understand or carry out the assignment or (b) being unmotivated or irresponsible because the work is not completed. However, when appropriate modifications are made to homework assignments, learners with word-finding difficulties are able to complete their

Table 10.4 Recommended Word-Finding Accommodations for Oral and Written Classroom Work

Word-Finding Error Pattern	Content Area	Activity	Recommended Accommodations
All	All	Oral reports or presentations	1. Substitute with media or digital presentations using presentation software. 2. Supplement with cards, transparencies, or other visuals. 3. Supplement or substitute with demonstrations. 4. Assign collaborative work with other learners.
All	All	Worksheets	1. Create electronic work sheets. 2. Provide multiple-choice question frames. 3. Recommend highlighting of answers in text. 4. Recommend use of resource material to support answering fill-in-the-blank or essay questions.

work and experience success on assignments that previously they would not have attempted.

Table 10.5 presents recommended accommodations in homework assignments based on the learner's word-finding profile. The focus of each accommodation is a reduction of the *retrieval load,* not the *work load* of the activity.

WORD-FINDING ACCOMMODATIONS FOR EXAMINATIONS

Typically, testing situations put high demands on a learner's word-finding skills. Whether exams are in oral or written form, they usually require single-word responses or written essays. Many tests encompass short answer or fill-in-the-blank formats that measure a learner's recall of facts and definitions. Although learners with word-finding difficulties may have studied for the exams and have an understanding of the material being tested, the nature of the exam format makes it difficult for them to demonstrate their knowledge.

Modification of traditional examination formats yields a truer evaluation of a learners' achievement. The goal of each modification is to replace the oral or written response typically required with a recognition–

Table 10.5 Recommended Accommodations for Homework Assignments

Error Pattern	Content Area	Activity	Recommended Accommodations
All error patterns	All	Memorization tasks	Have the learner develop a resource electronic file or notebook to which he or she can refer.
All error patterns	All	Answering questions	1. Have the learner indicate the page number of the answer to the question. 2. Copy text material and have the learner underline or highlight the answers.
Difficulty retrieving specific words	All	Writing short essays	1. Copy text material and have the learner highlight the answer. 2. Have the learner find Web sites that address the material under study. 3. Have the learner cut and paste from electronic reference sites.

response format. This format removes the focus on written or oral retrieval of specific words. For example, using methods of performance assessment as an alternative to traditional assessment can benefit the learner with word-finding difficulties. A performance assessment can be specific to the processes involved in the subject matter, such as conducting an experiment.

To aid in the development of accommodated exams for learners with word-finding difficulties, Table 10.6 presents recommended accommodations in assessment formats for learners with word-finding difficulties. These accommodations are also presented in the Recommended Word-Finding Accommodations Form in Appendix C.

RESOURCE MATERIALS AND TECHNOLOGY

Goal 3. Develop resource materials to accommodate for the learners' word-finding difficulties in the classroom, in social or recreational settings, and at home.

Table 10.6 Recommended Accommodations for Assessments

Word-Finding Profile	Content Area	Activity	Accommodations
All error patterns	All	Exams	1. Allow use of student-developed resources, electronic files, or notebooks for each content area. 2. Use electronic exams. 3. Change the exam format: a. Use multiple-choice frames. b. Use recognition-response (yes–no or true–false) format. c. Highlight the correct response in text. d. Indicate the page number and line of the answer. 4. Use open-book exams in class. 5. Give a take-home exam. 6. Allow the learner extra time to complete the exam. 7. Substitute exams with projects using technology, such as digital movies, electronic flow charts, or presentation software.

Two types of support materials that are helpful for learners with word-finding difficulties are cue lists and electronic resource files or notebooks. Both these materials support a learner's word-finding skills, but they differ in when and how they are used. Electronic formats are recommended for these support materials, but hardcopy is also appropriate.

ELECTRONIC OR HARDCOPY CUE LISTS

Cue lists consist of a series of brief statements that cue the learner for various math processes and science procedures. The lists support learners during math and science assignments and exams where retrieval of multistep math processes or formulas or science procedures are required. They also can serve as cues for retrieval during class discussion. Because these cue lists are useful in numerous situations across the curriculum, their application is easiest when they are electronic and organized by content area or activity. Encourage your learners to use their cue lists to support retrieval of process and procedural steps when doing homework or taking exams in these content areas. Figure 10.3 presents an example of a cue list for a math assignment involving rounding numbers. You can use it as a model for developing other cue lists in math.

ROUNDING NUMBERS

Problem: Round 690

Cue List	Sample Answer
1. Find the place to round	6 is hundreds
2. Go to the number on the right	9 is on the right
3. Decide if number stays the same or goes up (5 or greater goes up)	9 is greater
4. Write the new number in zeroes at the end.	700 is answer

Figure 10.3. Sample cue list to aid retrieval of procedural steps for rounding numbers.

ELECTRONIC RESOURCE FILES OR NOTEBOOKS

The resource file or notebook is a support material you and the learner create. It contains the major vocabulary, concepts, and facts associated with each topic of study. It serves as a resource for the learner when completing class assignments and homework, and when preparing for and taking exams. Material that needs to be rehearsed prior to classroom discussions can also be embedded in the resource file or notebook.

Because the learner can refer to the resource file or notebook when needed, this resource reduces the demand on the learner's oral and written retrieval in that content area. It changes the focus of class activities from retrieval of information to organization and manipulation of that information. Like the cue list, this resource is most easily used in electronic form. Learners can create electronic folders for each content area and store important curriculum concepts, for example, in files in corresponding folders. This resource can be developed jointly with all professionals.

SELECTING TECHNOLOGY ACCOMMODATIONS

Goal 4. Match technology to the learner's word-finding error patterns to accommodate for his or her word-finding difficulties in oral and written language.

Technology accommodations allow learners greater access to the curriculum than do traditional accommodations (Masterson, Apel, & Wood, 2002), primarily because traditional accommodations typically reduce the workload rather than facilitating students while they do their work.

In contrast, the use of technology offers the advantage of both supporting direct instruction as well as providing the retrieval cues and prompts necessary for students with word-finding difficulties.

For technology accommodations to be successful, their selection as a curriculum accommodation must also be strategic. MacArthur (2000) recommended that technology interface with specially designed instruction. For learners with word-finding difficulties, specially designed instruction involves all of the following:

- managing issues of computer access
- matching instruction to the learner's word-finding error patterns
- integrating technology with the learner's curriculum

A variety of input options are available to address the issue of computer access (Wood & Masterson, 1999). Learners with word-finding difficulties should be matched to appropriate methods early in their education so they become automatic in their computer access. Matching technology to the learner's word-finding error patterns and academic tasks ensures that the accommodations are appropriate and effective. Thus, the rest of this section presents recommended technology applications for both oral language and written language tasks based on their appropriateness for learners with specific word-finding error patterns.

WORD-PROCESSING PROGRAMS

Once learners have mastered computer access, they should be matched to a word-processing program to support their retrieval in oral and written language activities. Various notebook computers provide word-processing tools at a low cost. For learners with word-finding difficulties, developing proficiency with word processing will facilitate use of presentation software for oral language assignments as well as promote the use of cue lists, discourse menus, and resource files for classroom work and exams.

Word processing also supports written language development. Increased ease of revising (Graham & Harris, 2002), higher productivity (Nichols, 1996), improved use of expository texts (Snyder, 1993), and higher writing scores (Owston & Wideman, 1997) have all been reported for users of word-processing software. Therefore, we can expect that word-processing proficiency will also aid students with word-finding difficulties in their essay writing, note taking, information gathering, and e-mailing.

PRESENTATION SOFTWARE

Software developed for presentations and speech can greatly benefit learners with word-finding difficulties. Used to provide the learner with visuals, presentation software cues the learner's word retrieval as he or she presents. For example, learners who frequently manifest the word-finding Error Pattern 1: Lemma-Related Semantic Errors (commonly known as "slip of the tongue" errors) typically produce fast inaccurate responses. These learners need to slow their discourse when talking in order to inhibit interfering words. Presentation software acts a visual to support this slowing process. Learners who manifest this word-finding error pattern are directed to segment their sentences into phrases to slow the speaking rate and establish appropriate pausing. They can easily accomplish this by keying each phrase on a different slide. Then as they present their report, they can advance their slides at a pace that ensures accurate retrieval.

Similarly, learners who manifest word-finding Error Pattern 2: Word-Form Blocked Errors (commonly known as "tip of the tongue" errors) can also benefit from using presentation software during oral presentations. Because learners with this error pattern typically produce no responses or slow inaccurate target word substitutions, they benefit from visual aids that cue retrieval of evasive target words. For example, they can list important vocabulary on their slides. Same-sounds (see Lesson 7-1) or familiar-word (see Lesson 7-3) cues applied earlier to anchor retrieval of target vocabulary can also be included on these slides as reminders. Because the slides are visible only to the speaker, the audience is unaware that the speaker is cueing his or her retrieval during the presentation. See Figure 10.4 for an example of a PowerPoint slide created to aid a speaker who typically manifests word-finding Error Pattern 2.

Using presentation software during oral presentations also can help learners reduce word-form phonologic errors such as those in word-finding Error Pattern 3 (commonly known as "twist of the tongue" errors). These learners typically have difficulty retrieving multisyllabic words and, therefore, benefit from visual aids that cue retrieval of evasive syllables. These learners can list important vocabulary on their slides, make troublesome syllables of multisyllabic words appear in boldface type, or list words segmented by syllable to aid fluent access. Same-sounds syllable cues (see Lesson 8-2) linked to troublesome syllables also can be included on the slides. Again, because the slides are visible only to the speaker, the audience is unaware that the speaker is cueing his or her retrieval during the presentation. See Figure 10.5 for an example

My Presentation on Clouds
Retrieval Strategies
• cu mu lus (cumulate junk)
• cir rus (circus)
• stra tus (strap)
There are three different types of clouds I studied:
• cumulus,
• cirrus, and
• stratus

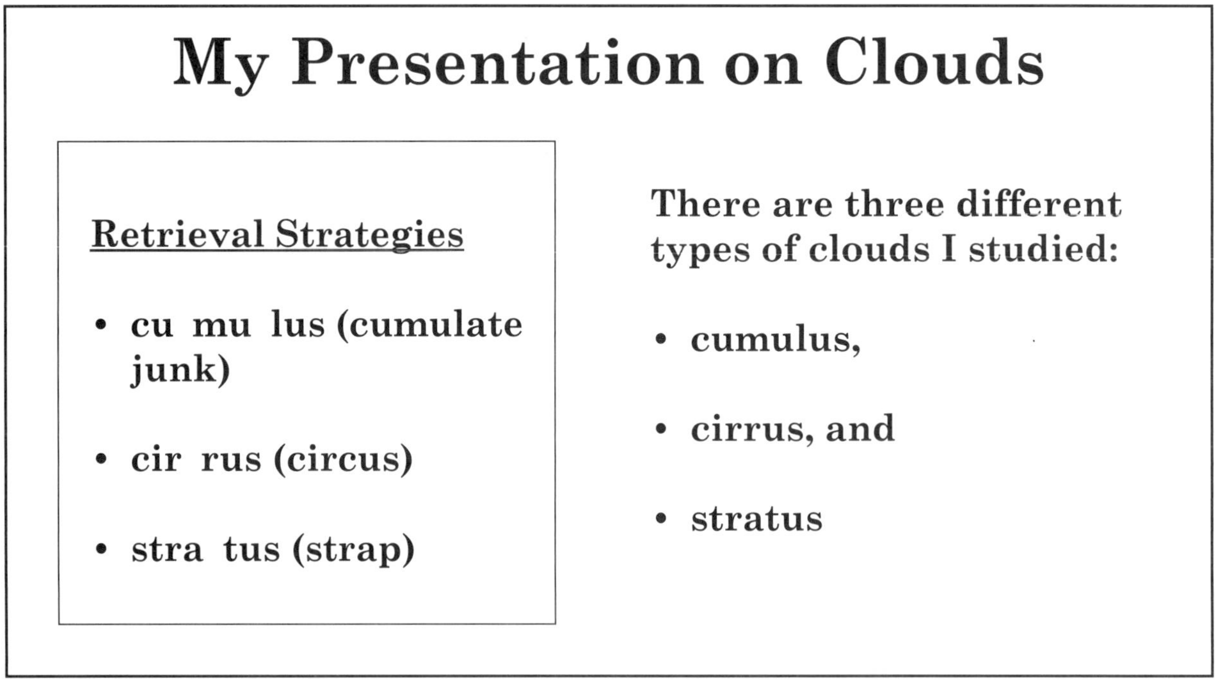

Figure 10.4. PowerPoint slide adapted to include familiar-word and same-sounds cues retrieval strategies to support retrieval of science vocabulary.

of a PowerPoint slide created to aid a speaker who typically manifests word-finding Error Pattern 3.

TECHNOLOGY FOR RETRIEVAL STRATEGY INSTRUCTION

Retrieval strategy instruction, described in Chapter 4, also can be supported by technology. For example, Web sites are available that provide synonyms and category words, similar-sounding words, and co-occurring words for learners who need synonyms and category names for the synonym and category substituting strategy (see Lesson 7-4), similar-sounding words for the same-sounds cue strategy (see Lesson 7-1), or co-occurring words and phrases for the familiar-word cue strategy (see Lesson 7-3). For learners who manifest word-finding Error Pattern 3, talking dictionaries can be used to facilitate the syllable-dividing strategy (see Lesson 8-1) and to provide models for rehearsal of multisyllabic vocabulary. To visit these Web sites, see specific URLs and descriptors in the corresponding lesson plans in Chapters 6, 7, and 8. Finally, electronic note programs that place multicolor small-sized windows on the desktop can be created to display important retrieval cues to remind learners of their academic or social vocabulary.

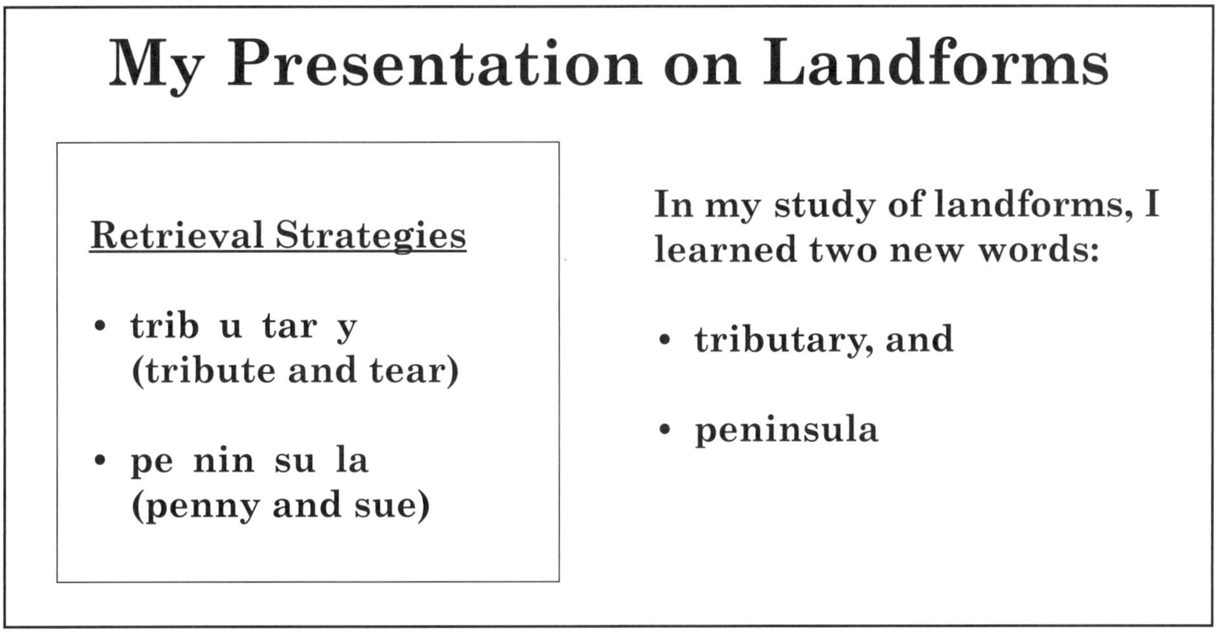

My Presentation on Landforms
Retrieval Strategies
• trib u tar y (tribute and tear)
• pe nin su la (penny and sue)
In my study of landforms, I learned two new words:
• tributary, and
• peninsula

Figure 10.5. PowerPoint slide adapted to include syllable-dividing and syllable same-sounds cue retrieval strategies to support retrieval of social studies vocabulary.

SOFTWARE TO REDUCE WORD-FINDING ERROR PATTERN 1 IN WRITTEN LANGUAGE

GRAMMAR CHECKERS

Grammar checkers can support the writing skills of learners who manifest word-finding Error Pattern 1: Lemma-Related Semantic Errors. Typically learners who manifest this word-finding error pattern in written language produce semantic substitutions or omissions resulting in grammatical errors in their written work (Scott &Windsor, 2000). The semantic substitutions are similar to those observed in their oral language (e.g., learners write *car* for *truck* or *stop* for *start,* or make omissions in the noun or verb phrase of the sentence). Grammatical errors in their written language may include omission of plural *-s* markers, present participles, past tense *-ed* markers, and substitution of regular for irregular verb forms (Scott, 2002).

Identification of these written language errors is facilitated by the grammar checker during the editing phase of a learner's work. However, successful use of this software typically requires collaboration among the specialist, the learner, and the teacher. After basic instruction on how to use the correct grammar software, learners with word-finding difficulties can use this software to edit their written work in the following ways:

- reviewing their written drafts with a grammar checker
- correcting the grammar errors, target word substitutions, and omissions identified
- underlining identified errors they are unsure how to correct

TEXT-TO-SPEECH SOFTWARE

Text-to-speech software is standard on many computers today. It orally reads highlighted text in the word-processing document. Tutors and parents often read learners' written work out loud to them because learners with word-finding difficulties can typically recognize their word or grammatical errors when they hear their written draft read. With the use of text-to-speech technology, learners can carry out this same technique independently, letting the computer read their written work out loud. Learners with word-finding difficulties should be instructed to carry out the following steps during the editing process when using the text-to-speech software:

1. Print a hardcopy of the written draft.
2. Activate the text-to-speech software to read the electronic file out loud.
3. Follow along, reading the hardcopy silently while the text-to-speech software reads the electronic file out loud.
4. Circle heard errors on the hardcopy of the written text.
5. Correct circled errors in the electronic file before printing out the final draft.

Use of both the grammar checker and the text-to-speech software can increase the learner's awareness of his or her word-finding errors in written language, as well as teach the learner how to identify and correct word-finding errors in written language. The end result will be an improved document.

SOFTWARE TO REDUCE WORD-FINDING ERROR PATTERN 2 IN WRITTEN LANGUAGE

TEXT-TO-SPEECH SOFTWARE

Text-to-speech software also can support the writing skills of learners who manifest word-finding Error Pattern 2: Word-Form Blocked Errors. Typically these learners may produce target word substitutions, circumlocutions, indefinite pronouns, omissions, and overuse of personal pronouns in their written discourse. These written-language errors occur when the learner has a word-finding block while engaged in the writing task. These blocks are similar to those observed in the learner's oral language (e.g., learners may write semantic substitutions like *calculator* for *computer,* produce functional circumlocutions like "You can go on the Internet with it," use indefinite pronouns such as "You put the thingy on the thing," display omissions such as "She was happy to get the um, er ... for her birthday," and overuse pronouns such as "They went with them and he bought her a ticket after they saw them"). Identification of these word-finding-based written-language errors is facilitated by use of the text-to-speech software during the editing phase of the learners' work. To identify their word-finding-based written-language errors, learners should follow the steps in the previous section when editing their written work. As learners listen to the computer read their text out loud, you can help them understand the inappropriateness of their word-finding errors.

PREDICTION SOFTWARE

Prediction software enables learners to key in the first letter or syllable of a target word to generate a list of words beginning with those same letters. The learner then selects from the ensuing word list the vocabulary he or she wants to insert. Because this application provides users with word choices, it supports their lexical selection and spelling processes (Masterson, Apel, & Wood, 2002) and is therefore an appropriate accommodation for learners who have difficulty accessing vocabulary while writing. Further, because teachers can insert vocabulary specific to the unit under study, content vocabulary difficult to retrieve and spell can be made accessible to learners with word-finding difficulties. These learners should be taught to include prediction software as one of their written language tools.

SOFTWARE TO REDUCE WORD-FINDING ERROR PATTERN 3 IN WRITTEN LANGUAGE

PREDICTION SOFTWARE

Because prediction software is a technology that enables users to access word lists with only the first letter and or syllable of a word, learners can accommodate for their difficulty in retrieving multisyllabic words by using this software when writing. For those challenging multisyllabic words, learners can key in the first syllable of the word and then select the target word from the choices. When this application is individualized to include the multisyllabic vocabulary specific to the content under study, the learner's retrieval skills are supported in content specific written language assignments.

TEXT-TO-SPEECH SOFTWARE

Text-to-speech software can also support the writing skills of learners when they manifest difficulty retrieving multisyllabic words. Because these learners produce phonemic substitutions for multisyllabic words orally (e.g., *copuer* for *computer*), they typically have difficulty accessing the spellings of these words when writing. To avoid writing these target words incorrectly, learners may write circumlocutions (e.g., "You go on the Internet with it" for *computer*) and indefinite pronouns or leave blanks for these difficult-to-retrieve multisyllabic words. Identification of these written language errors is facilitated by text-to-speech software. Learners with this word-finding error pattern should follow the steps in the previous section when editing their written work.

SPELLING CHECKERS

Learners who have difficulty retrieving multisyllabic words in oral language typically have difficulty writing the correct spellings of these words. Even though they may be able to identify correct spellings on recognition response tasks (i.e., they can select the correct spelling between two decoys), they are not consistently able to retrieve the complete form of the word in order to spell it correctly. Spelling checker software can be used in the editing phase of a learner's written work to identify misspellings of multisyllabic words and provide correct spelling options.

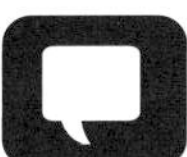

LESSON 10-1

IDENTIFYING NEEDED WORD-FINDING ACCOMMODATIONS

Use this lesson to identify needed accommodations. Lessons 10-1 and 10-2 may be combined.

RETRIEVAL CONTEXT: Retrieval of specific words in sentences and discourse

ERROR PATTERN: All word-finding error patterns

ACCOMMODATION BENCHMARK (OBJECTIVE): To identify accommodations needed in classroom discussions, classroom work, and classroom activities

PARTICIPANTS: Learner and specialist or teacher

TIME: 15 to 20 minutes

SETTING: Small language group in language room or in general education or special education class

MATERIALS:

- Classroom Observation Form (Appendix C)
- Recommended Word-Finding Accommodations Form (Appendix C)
- Word-Finding Self-Assessment Survey (Appendix B)
- Learner's class schedule
- List of learner's teachers and subjects
- Copies of homework assignments and examinations

ACTIVITIES

1. Explain to the learner that some aspects of the learning environment may put high demands on his or her word-finding skills.

2. Provide examples of different classroom activities that put high demands on the learner's word-finding skills (e.g., oral questioning, oral reports, participating in group discussions).

3. Explain to the learner that, together, you are going to request modification in these school activities that put high demands on his or her word-finding skills.

4. Review the Classroom Observation Form for examples of classroom activities that may need to be modified.

5. Review with the learner the portion of the Word-Finding Self-Assessment Survey that focuses on the learning environment to identify accommodations needed in classroom discussions, work, and activities.

GENERALIZATION ACTIVITY

For the next lesson, ask the learner to observe his or her classrooms, noting the activities discussed in Step 4 of the activities. The goal is to teach learners to evaluate their own learning environment in order to become aware of the high retrieval demands inherent in their academic work.

WORD-FINDING SELF-ADVOCACY GOALS

1. The learner will become sensitive to those aspects of his or her learning environment that may need to be modified to reduce demands on his or her retrieval skills.

2. The learner will self-monitor his or her learning environment for activities that put high demands on his or her retrieval skills.

LESSON 10-2

IDENTIFYING WORD-FINDING ACCOMMODATIONS FOR HOMEWORK AND EXAMINATIONS

Use this lesson to identify needed accommodations. Lessons 10-1 and 10-2 may be combined.

RETRIEVAL CONTEXT: Retrieval of specific words in sentences and discourse

ERROR PATTERN: All word-finding error patterns

ACCOMMODATION BENCHMARK (OBJECTIVE): To identify, with the learner, accommodations needed in homework assignments and in course examinations

PARTICIPANTS: Learner and specialist or teacher

TIME: 15 to 20 minutes

SETTING: Small language group in language room or in general education or special education class

MATERIALS:
- Classroom Observation Form (Appendix C)
- Recommended Word-Finding Accommodations Form (Appendix C)
- Word-Finding Self-Assessment Survey (Appendix B)
- Learner's class schedule
- List of learner's teachers and subjects
- Copies of homework assignments and examinations

RECOMMENDED TECHNOLOGY: Select from the technology supports presented earlier in this chapter.

ACTIVITIES

1. Discuss the learner's observations of his or her learning environment and review the results of his or her Word-Finding Self-Assessment Survey.

2. Review the Classroom Observation Form and the Recommended Word-Finding Accommodations Form for examples of homework assignments and examinations that may need to be modified to reduce the inherent retrieval load of those activities.

GENERALIZATION ACTIVITY

For the next lesson, ask the learner to note the format of homework assignments and examinations relative to demands on his or her retrieval skills. Ask the learner to observe where he or she could be supported with instructional technology.

WORD-FINDING SELF-ADVOCACY GOALS

1. The learner will become sensitive to those aspects of homework and examinations that may need to be modified to reduce demands on his or her retrieval skills.

2. The learner will monitor his or her homework and examinations for demands that these activities put on his or her retrieval skills.

LESSONS 10-3 THROUGH 10-6

SPECIALIST–TEACHER DIALOGUE

Use these lessons to identify needed accommodations.

RETRIEVAL CONTEXT: Retrieval of specific words in sentences and discourse

ERROR PATTERN: All word-finding error patterns

ACCOMMODATION BENCHMARK (OBJECTIVE): To identify, with the teacher, accommodations needed in classroom discussions, activities, homework assignments, and course examinations to support learning

PARTICIPANTS: Specialist and teachers

TIME: 15-minute conference with each of the learner's teachers

SETTING: General education or special education classroom

MATERIALS:

- Classroom Observation Form (Appendix C)
- Recommended Word-Finding Accommodations Form (Appendix C)
- Word-Finding Self-Assessment Survey (Appendix B)
- Learner's class schedule
- List of learner's teachers and subjects
- Copies of homework assignments and examinations

RECOMMENDED TECHNOLOGY: Select from the technology supports presented earlier in this chapter.

ACTIVITIES

1. During the learner's scheduled language lessons, arrange to visit the classrooms you think may need to be modified for

the learner with word-finding difficulties. While observing in these classrooms, complete the Classroom Observation Form.

2. Following the observations, arrange to meet with the teacher whose classroom you observed. During your conferences with the teacher, share the Classroom Observation Form for that teacher's classroom and findings from the learner's Word-Finding Self-Assessment Survey.

3. Collaborate with the teachers to identify accommodations that would facilitate the student's learning in their classrooms. Together, complete the Recommended Word-Finding Accommodations Form for each teacher's corresponding classroom.

GENERALIZATION ACTIVITY

The learner is asked to note those aspects of the learning environment that he or she believes put a high demand on his or her retrieval skills.

WORD-FINDING SELF-ADVOCACY GOAL

The learner will become aware of the word-finding accommodations everyone agreed to implement to reduce the demands on his or her retrieval.

LESSON 10-7

IMPLEMENTING CLASSROOM ACCOMMODATIONS

Use this lesson to implement classroom accommodations.

RETRIEVAL CONTEXT: Retrieval of specific words in sentences and discourse

ERROR PATTERN: All word-finding error patterns

ACCOMMODATION BENCHMARK (OBJECTIVE): To decide on the accommodations that will be implemented for the learner during classroom discussions, activities, homework assignments, and course examinations

PARTICIPANTS: Learner, specialist, and teacher or teachers

TIME: 15 to 20 minutes

SETTING: Small language group in language room or in general education or special education class

MATERIALS:

- Classroom Observation Form (Appendix C)
- Recommended Word-Finding Accommodations Form (Appendix C)
- Word-Finding Self-Assessment Survey (Appendix B)
- Learner's class schedule
- List of learner's teachers and subjects

RECOMMENDED TECHNOLOGY: Select from the technology supports presented earlier in this chapter.

ACTIVITIES

1. Review accommodations selected during conferences with the classroom teachers and the learner.

2. Review the Classroom Observation Form and the Recommended Word-Finding Accommodations Form for examples of accommodations that are recommended based on your conferences.

3. Discuss with the learner the specific accommodations you and the teachers would like to implement in each of the areas under consideration. Depending on the age of the learner, you may want to ask his or her opinion of the suggested accommodations. In particular, older learners should be a part of this decision process.

GENERALIZATION ACTIVITY

The learner (if he or she is old enough) meets with you and his or her classroom teachers to jointly discuss and determine what classroom accommodations will be implemented.

WORD-FINDING SELF-ADVOCACY GOALS

1. The learner will become aware of those aspects of the learning environment that will be modified to reduce demands on his or her retrieval skills.

2. The learner will become aware of the methods that will be used to modify classroom activities and will participate in conferences focused on implementing classroom accommodations.

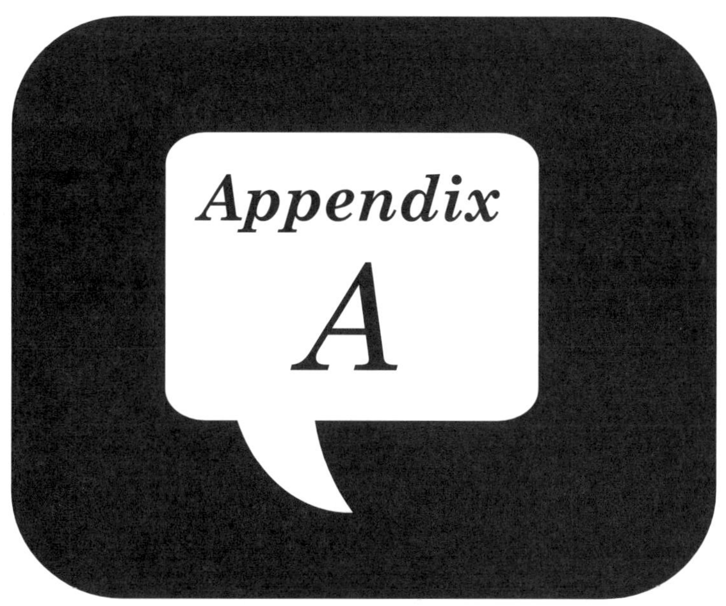

Word-Finding Retrieval Strategy Instruction Forms

Specialists and teachers may copy these forms for use with the WFIP–2.

RETRIEVAL STRATEGY LESSON PLAN

Specialist ______________________ Date __________ Plan for __________ to __________
month/day/year month/day/year

Part 1: Assigning Lessons

Instructions: Check the retrieval strategies to be taught to each learner.

Retrieval Strategy	WFIP–2 Lesson	Learner's Name				
Error Pattern 1						
Preferred Strategies						
Self-monitoring	6-1					
Self-correcting	6-2					
Pausing	6-3					
Same-sounds meaning cue + rehearsal	7-2					
Supplementary Strategies						
Imagery cueing + rehearsal	6-4					
Gesture cueing + rehearsal	6-5					
Error Pattern 2						
Preferred Strategies						
Same-sounds cue + rehearsal	7-1					
Same-sounds meaning cue + rehearsal	7-2					
Familiar-word cue + rehearsal	7-3					

Retrieval Strategy	WFIP–2 Lesson	Learner's Name				
Synonym or category substituting + rehearsal	7-4, 7-5					
Supplementary Strategies						
Graphemic cueing	7-6					
Error Pattern 3						
Preferred Strategies						
Syllable dividing + rehearsal	8-1					
Same-sounds syllable cue + rehearsal	8-2					
Synonym or category substituting + rehearsal	7-4, 7-5					

Part 2: Selecting Content

Instructions: Indicate the academic subject and vocabulary for each learner.

Lesson Content	Learner's Name					
Academic subject						
Specific words treated						

VOCABULARY AND RETRIEVAL STRATEGY PRACTICE FORM INSTRUCTIONS

The Vocabulary and Retrieval Strategy Practice Form is designed to aid learners in reviewing and rehearsing the vocabulary and retrieval strategies they have been taught in their WFIP–2 lessons.

Instructions: The specialists and learner complete this Vocabulary and Retrieval Strategies Practice Form for those target words needing additional practice. Complete Columns 1 through 3 at the end of the language lesson. Complete Columns 4 and 5 at home or at the beginning of the language lesson.

1. Write the target words that have been identified as needing additional practice in Column 1.
2. Segment the target words in Column 2.
3. Write the same-sounds cue, the same-sounds meaning cue, the familiar-word cue, or alternate word (i.e., synonym or category substitute) in Column 3 or Column 4.
4. In Column 5 use a checkmark to indicate that the learner has applied the retrieval strategy in Column 3 or Column 4 to say the target word from Column 1.
5. In Column 6 use a checkmark to indicate that the learner has applied the retrieval strategy in Column 3 or Column 4 to say the target word from Column 1 in a sentence.

VOCABULARY AND RETRIEVAL STRATEGY PRACTICE FORM

Column 1	Column 2	Column 3	Column 4	Column 5	Column 6
	Metalinguistic and Mnemonic Retrieval Strategies				
Target Vocabulary Word	Syllable Dividing	Same-Sounds and Familiar-Word Cues	Synonym and Category Alternates	Say the Target Word as a Unit	Say the Target Word in a Sentence
1.					
2.					
3.					
4.					
5.					
6.					
7.					
8.					
9.					
10.					

NAME | CONTENT AREA | DATE

1 Target Word
2 Syllable-Dividing
3 Think Same-Sounds Syllable or Familiar-Word Cues
4 Rehearse Target Word as a Unit
5 Rehearse Target Word in a Sentence

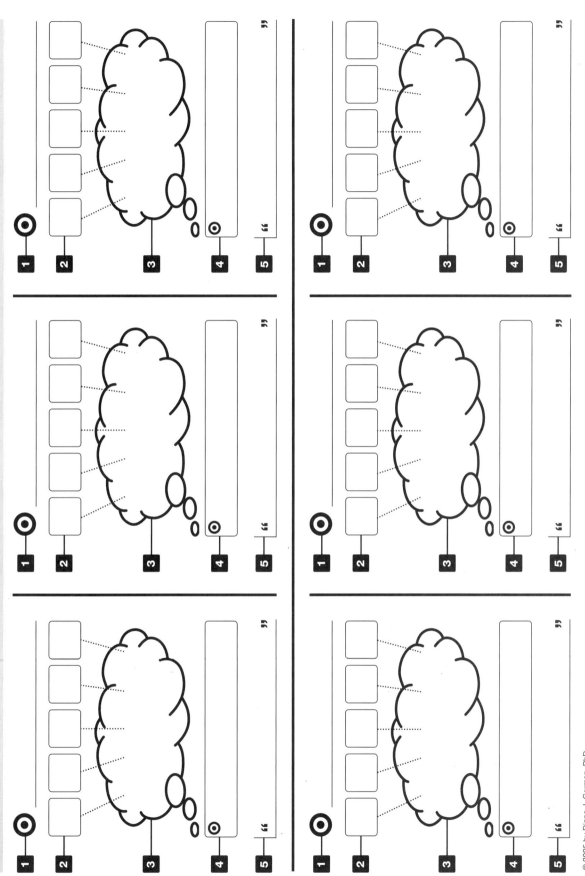

VOCABULARY SUBJECT: TENNIS

Objective: To teach learners to apply the syllable-dividing and same-sounds cues to tennis vocabulary

Instructions: The tennis vocabulary is presented in the list on this page and embedded in the completed Syllable-Dividing and Same-Sounds Syllable Cue Study Forms that follow. Have the learner practice the selected tennis vocabulary using the syllable-dividing and same-sounds cue retrieval strategies.

net	set
racquet	match
court	singles
tennis ball	doubles
serve	deuce
volley	love
lob	advantage
ace	baseline

WFIP-2 SYLLABLE-DIVIDING AND SAME-SOUNDS SYLLABLE CUE STUDY FORM

NAME CONTENT AREA Sports Vocabulary, Tennis DATE

1 Target Word
2 Syllable-Dividing
3 Think Same-Sounds Syllable or Familiar-Word Cues
4 Rehearse Target Word as a Unit
5 Rehearse Target Word in a Sentence

1. net
2. net | | | |
3. nest
4. net, net, net
5. "I hit the ball into the net."

1. racquet
2. rac | quet | | |
3. racquetball or rack
4. racquet, racquet, racquet
5. "I hit the ball with the racquet."

1. court
2. court | | | |
3. corn
4. court, court, court
5. "I like to play tennis on a clay court."

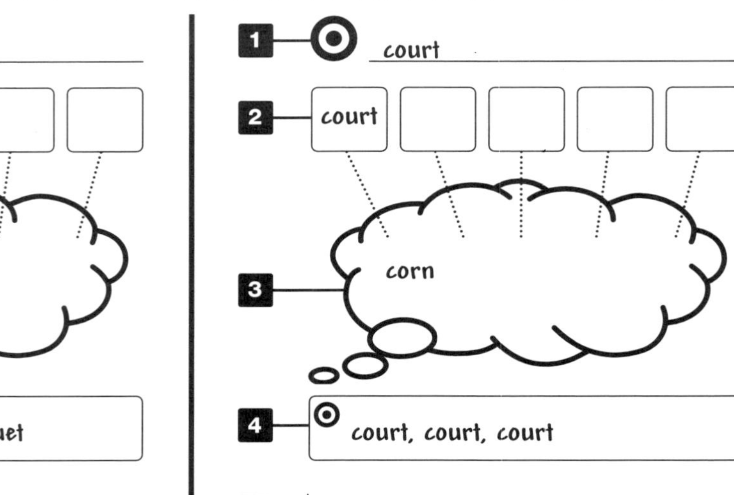

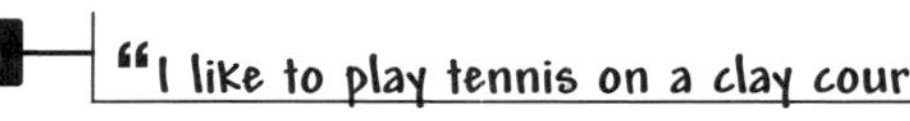

1. tennis ball
2. ten | nis | ball | |
3. ten
4. tennis ball, tennis ball, tennis ball
5. "There are three tennis balls in a can."

1. serve
2. serve | | | |
3. Serve dinner
4. serve, serve, serve
5. "I served the ball."

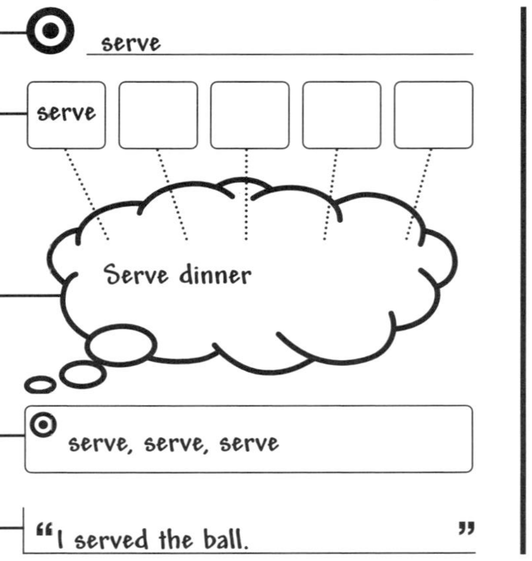

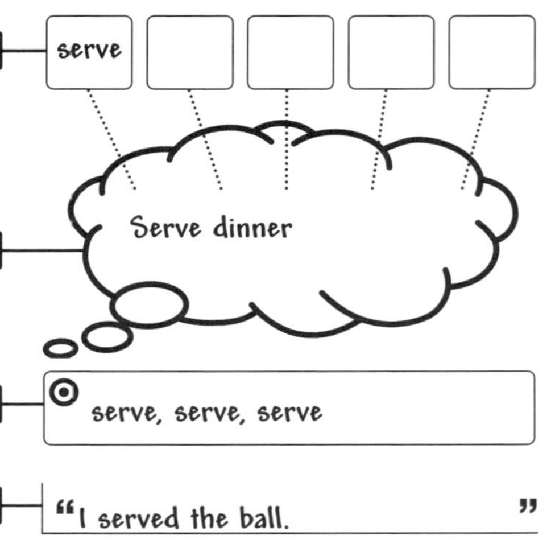

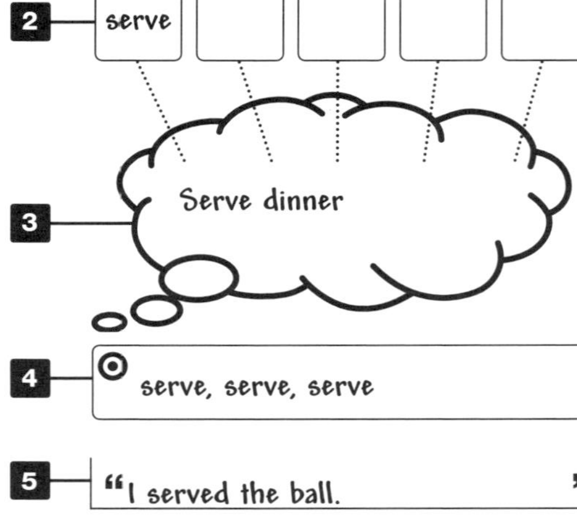

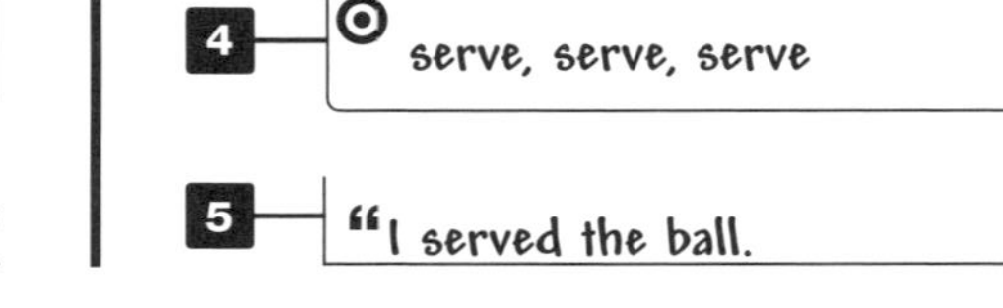

1. volley
2. vol | ley | | |
3. volleyball
4. volley, volley, volley
5. "They volleyed the ball back and forth."

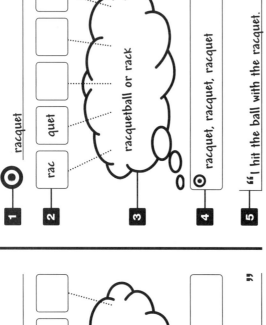

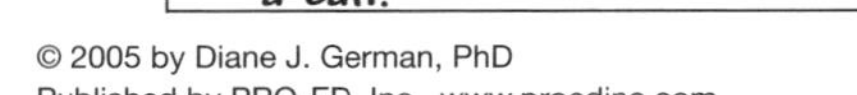

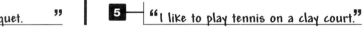

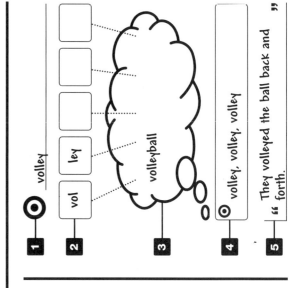

NAME CONTENT AREA Sports Vocabulary, Tennis DATE

1 Target Word
2 Syllable-Dividing
3 Think Same-Sounds Syllable or Familiar-Word Cues
4 Rehearse Target Word as a Unit
5 Rehearse Target Word in a Sentence

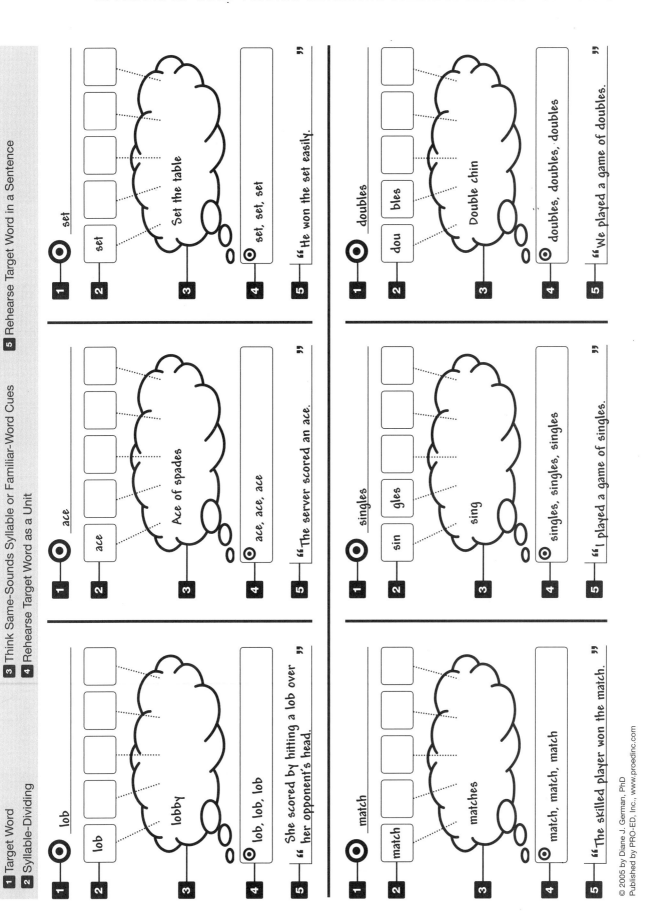

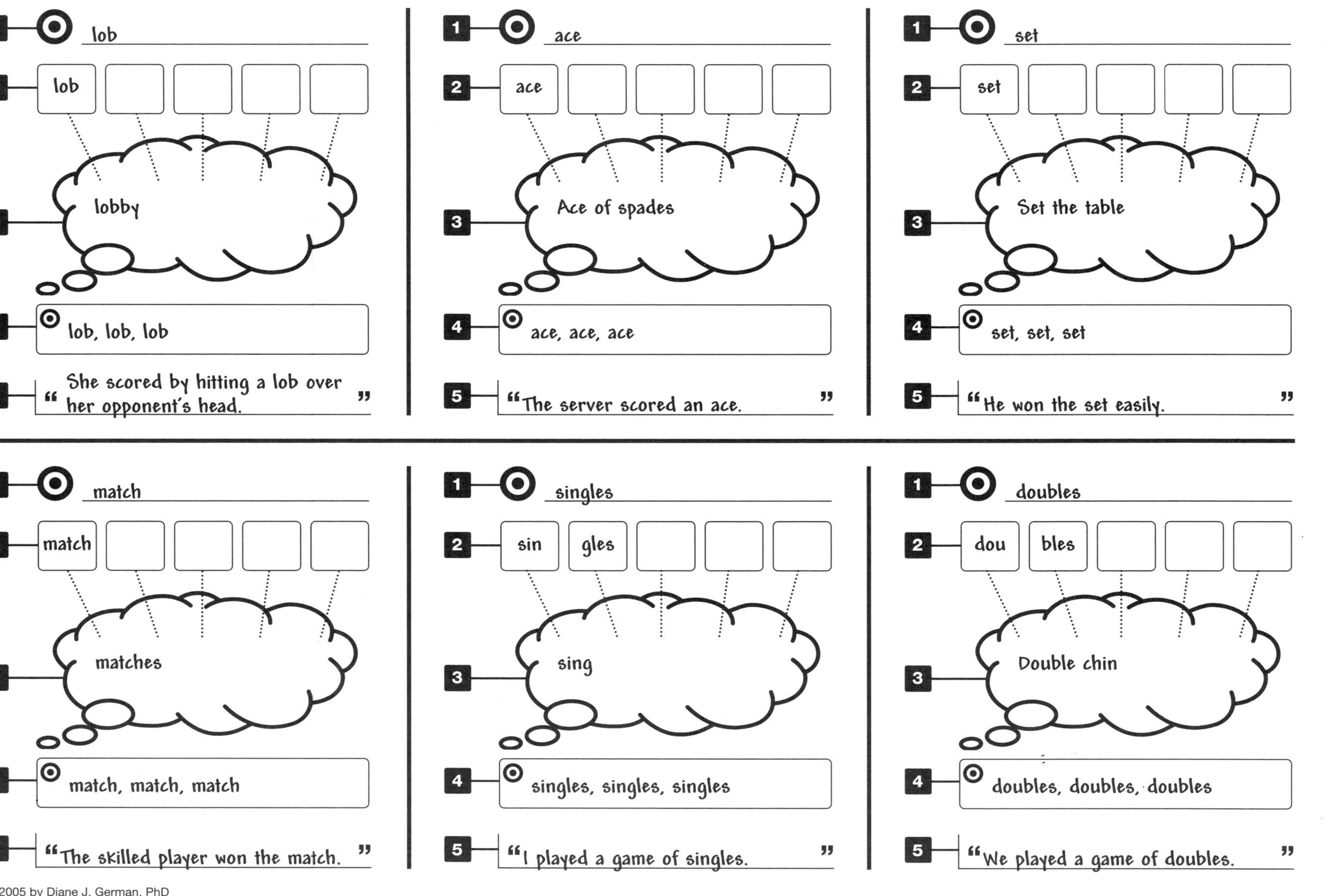

1 lob
2 lob
3 lobby
4 lob, lob, lob
5 "She scored by hitting a lob over her opponent's head."

1 ace
2 ace
3 Ace of spades
4 ace, ace, ace
5 "The server scored an ace."

1 set
2 set
3 Set the table
4 set, set, set
5 "He won the set easily."

1 match
2 match
3 matches
4 match, match, match
5 "The skilled player won the match."

1 singles
2 sin | gles
3 sing
4 singles, singles, singles
5 "I played a game of singles."

1 doubles
2 dou | bles
3 Double chin
4 doubles, doubles, doubles
5 "We played a game of doubles."

WFIP–2 SYLLABLE-DIVIDING AND SAME-SOUNDS SYLLABLE CUE STUDY FORM

NAME ______ CONTENT AREA Sports Vocabulary, Tennis DATE ______

1 Target Word
2 Syllable-Dividing
3 Think Same-Sounds Syllable or Familiar-Word Cues
4 Rehearse Target Word as a Unit
5 Rehearse Target Word in a Sentence

1 deuce
2 deuce
3 do
4 deuce, deuce, deuce
5 "Score two successive points to get a deuce."

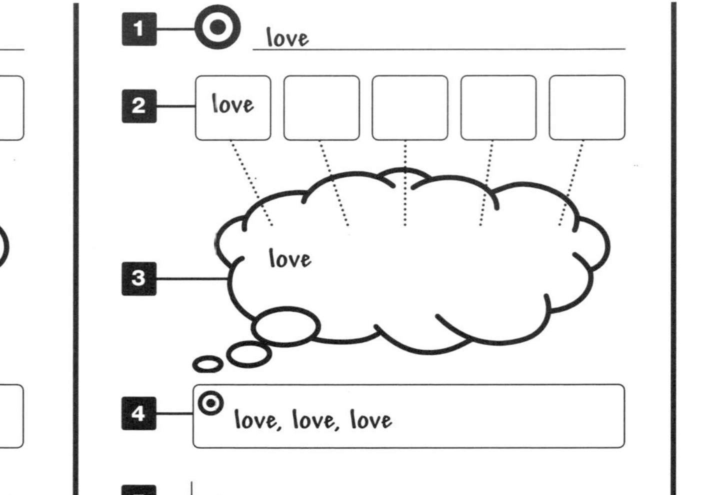

1 love
2 love
3 love
4 love, love, love
5 "The score was 40–love."

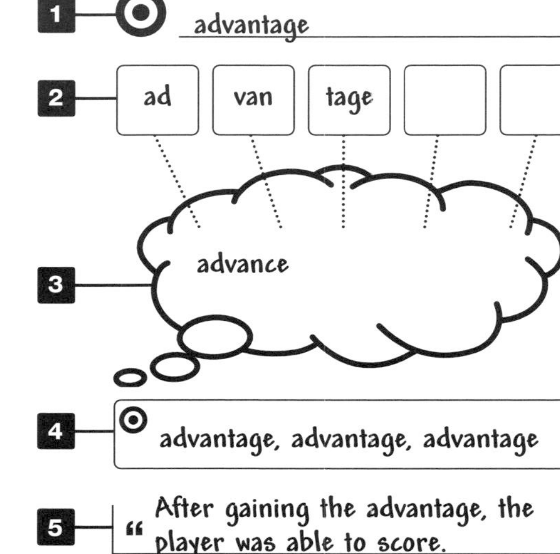

1 advantage
2 ad | van | tage
3 advance
4 advantage, advantage, advantage
5 "After gaining the advantage, the player was able to score."

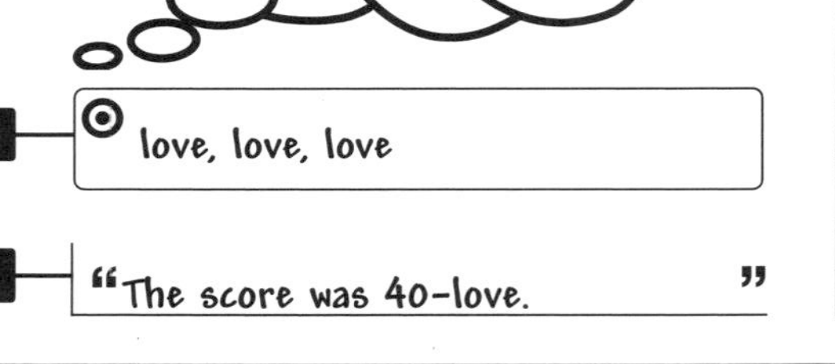

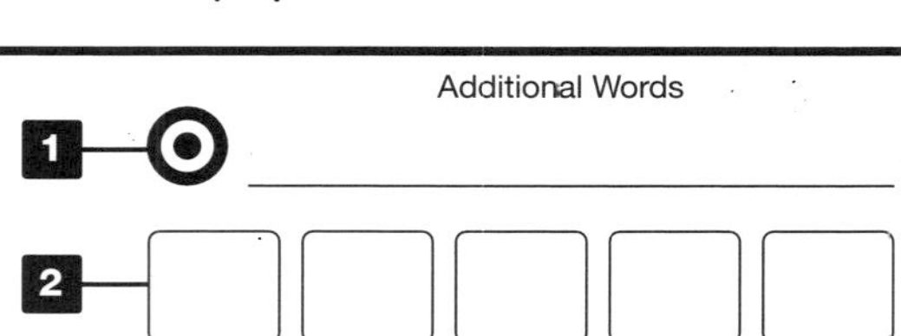

1 baseline
2 base | line
3 base
4 baseline, baseline, baseline
5 "His return landed just beyond the baseline."

Additional Words

1
2
3
4
5 " "

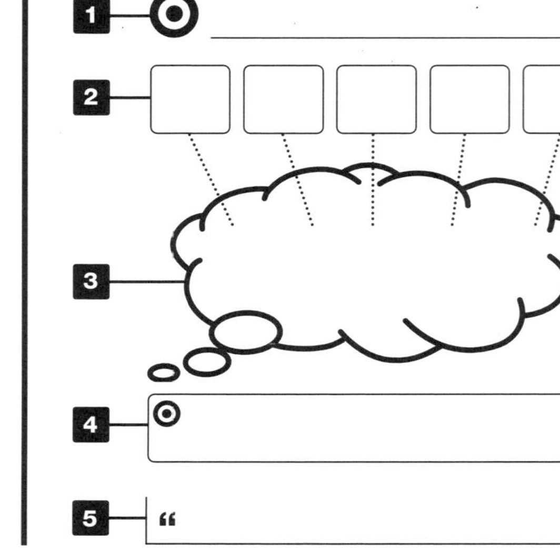

Additional Words

1
2
3
4
5 " "

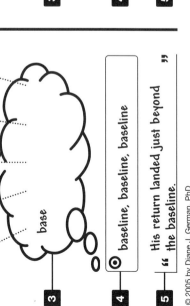

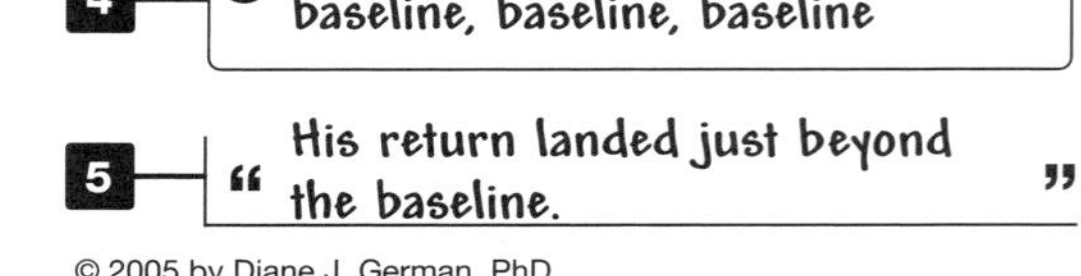

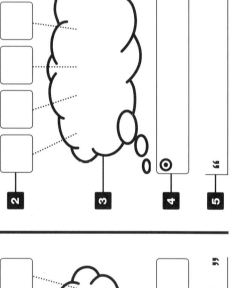

VOCABULARY SUBJECT: SOCCER

Objective: To teach learners to apply the syllable-dividing and same-sounds cues to soccer vocabulary

Instructions: The soccer vocabulary is presented in the list on this page and embedded in the completed Syllable-Dividing and Same-Sounds Syllable Cue Study Forms that follow. Have the learner practice the selected soccer vocabulary using the syllable-dividing and same-sounds cue retrieval strategies.

soccer ball	shin guards	corner kick
header	cleats	punt
throw-in	goalie	juggle
goal	midfield	dribble

WFIP–2 SYLLABLE-DIVIDING AND SAME-SOUNDS SYLLABLE CUE STUDY FORM

NAME CONTENT AREA Sports Vocabulary, Soccer DATE

1 Target Word
2 Syllable-Dividing
3 Think Same-Sounds Syllable or Familiar-Word Cues
4 Rehearse Target Word as a Unit
5 Rehearse Target Word in a Sentence

1 soccer ball

2 soc | cer | ball | |

3 Socket or sock

4 soccer ball, soccer ball, soccer ball

5 "Soccer balls are black and white."

1 header

2 head | er | | |

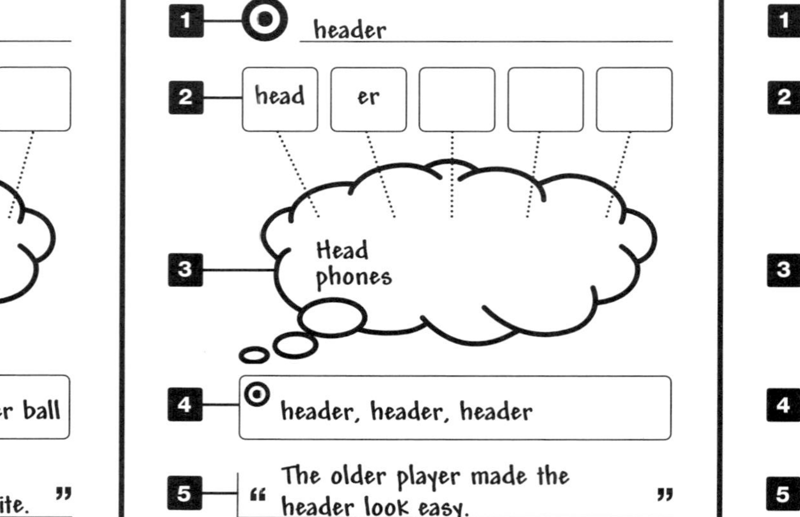

4 header, header, header

5 "The older player made the header look easy."

1 throw-in

2 throw | in | | |

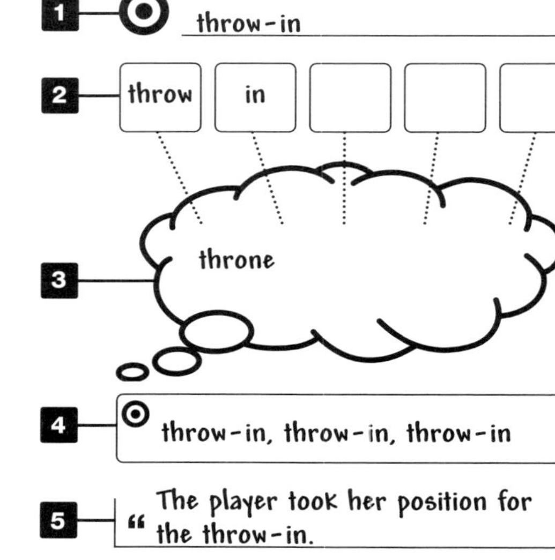

4 throw-in, throw-in, throw-in

5 "The player took her position for the throw-in."

1 goal

2 goal | | | |

3 gold

4 goal, goal, goal

5 "We won by one goal."

1 shin guards

2 shin | guards | | |

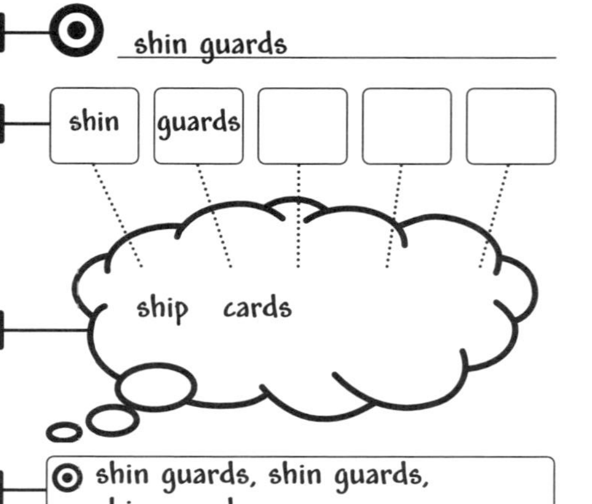

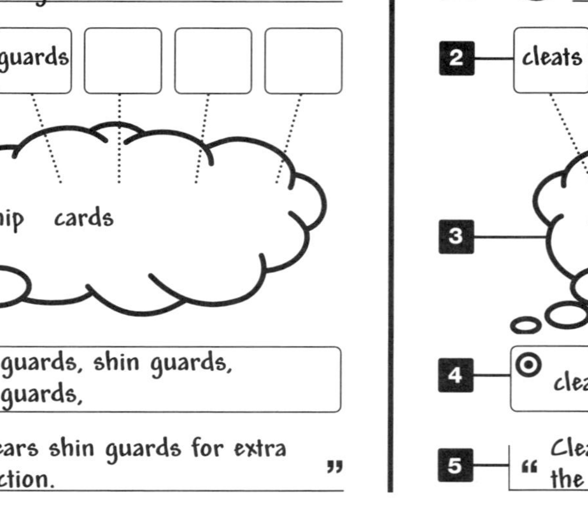

4 shin guards, shin guards, shin guards,

5 "He wears shin guards for extra protection."

1 cleats

2 cleats | | | |

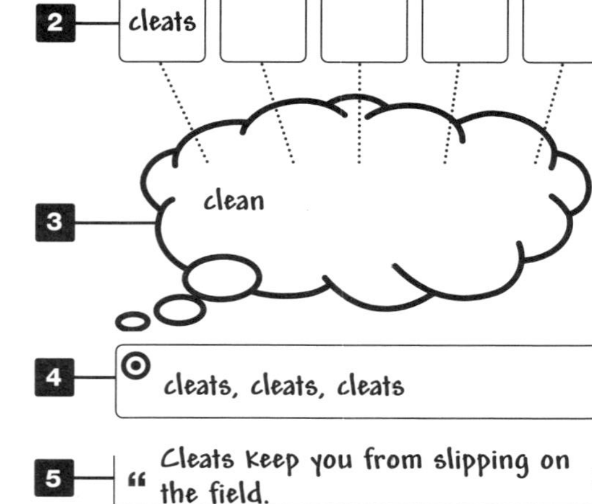

4 cleats, cleats, cleats

5 "Cleats keep you from slipping on the field."

NAME CONTENT AREA Sports Vocabulary, Soccer DATE

1 Target Word
2 Syllable-Dividing
3 Think Same-Sounds Syllable or Familiar-Word Cues
4 Rehearse Target Word as a Unit
5 Rehearse Target Word in a Sentence

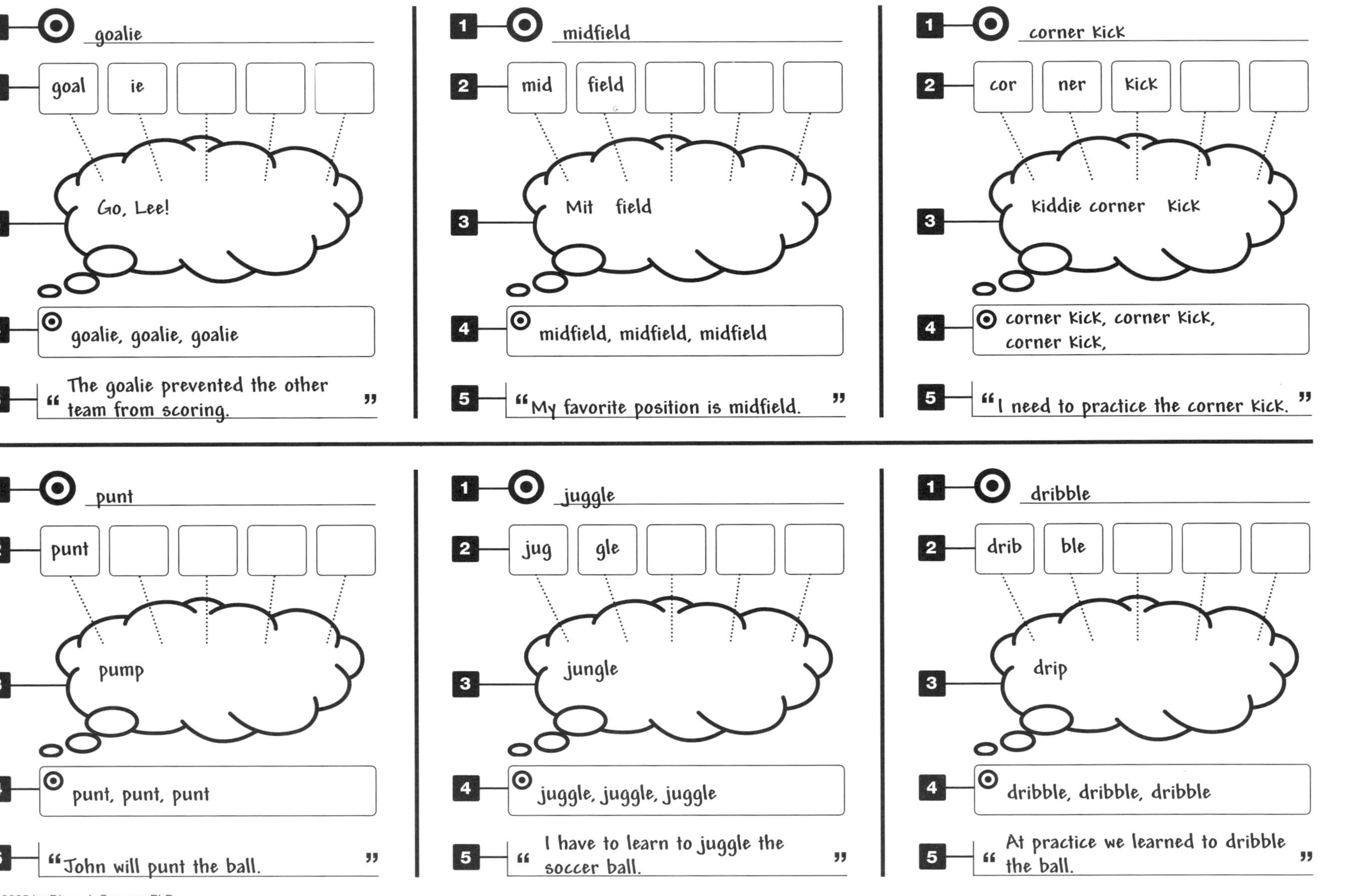
1 goalie
2 goal | ie
3 Go, Lee!
4 goalie, goalie, goalie
5 "The goalie prevented the other team from scoring."
1 midfield
2 mid | field
3 Mit field
4 midfield, midfield, midfield
5 "My favorite position is midfield."
1 corner kick
2 cor | ner | kick
3 kiddie corner kick
4 corner kick, corner kick, corner kick,
5 "I need to practice the corner kick."
1 punt
2 punt
3 pump
4 punt, punt, punt
5 "John will punt the ball."
1 juggle
2 jug | gle
3 jungle
4 juggle, juggle, juggle
5 "I have to learn to juggle the soccer ball."
1 dribble
2 drib | ble
3 drip
4 dribble, dribble, dribble
5 "At practice we learned to dribble the ball."

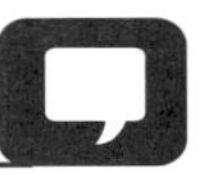

VOCABULARY SUBJECT: HOCKEY

Objective: To teach learners to apply the syllable-dividing and same-sounds cues to hockey vocabulary

Instructions: The hockey vocabulary is presented in the list on this page and embedded in the completed Syllable-Dividing and Same-Sounds Syllable Cue Study Forms that follow. Have the learner practice the selected hockey vocabulary using the syllable-dividing and same-sounds cue retrieval strategies.

stick	Zamboni	defense
puck	goalie	ice rink
skate	penalty	referee
helmet	power play	period
offside	face-off	
offense	slap shot	

1 Target Word
2 Syllable-Dividing
3 Think Same-Sounds Syllable or Familiar-Word Cues
4 Rehearse Target Word as a Unit
5 Rehearse Target Word in a Sentence

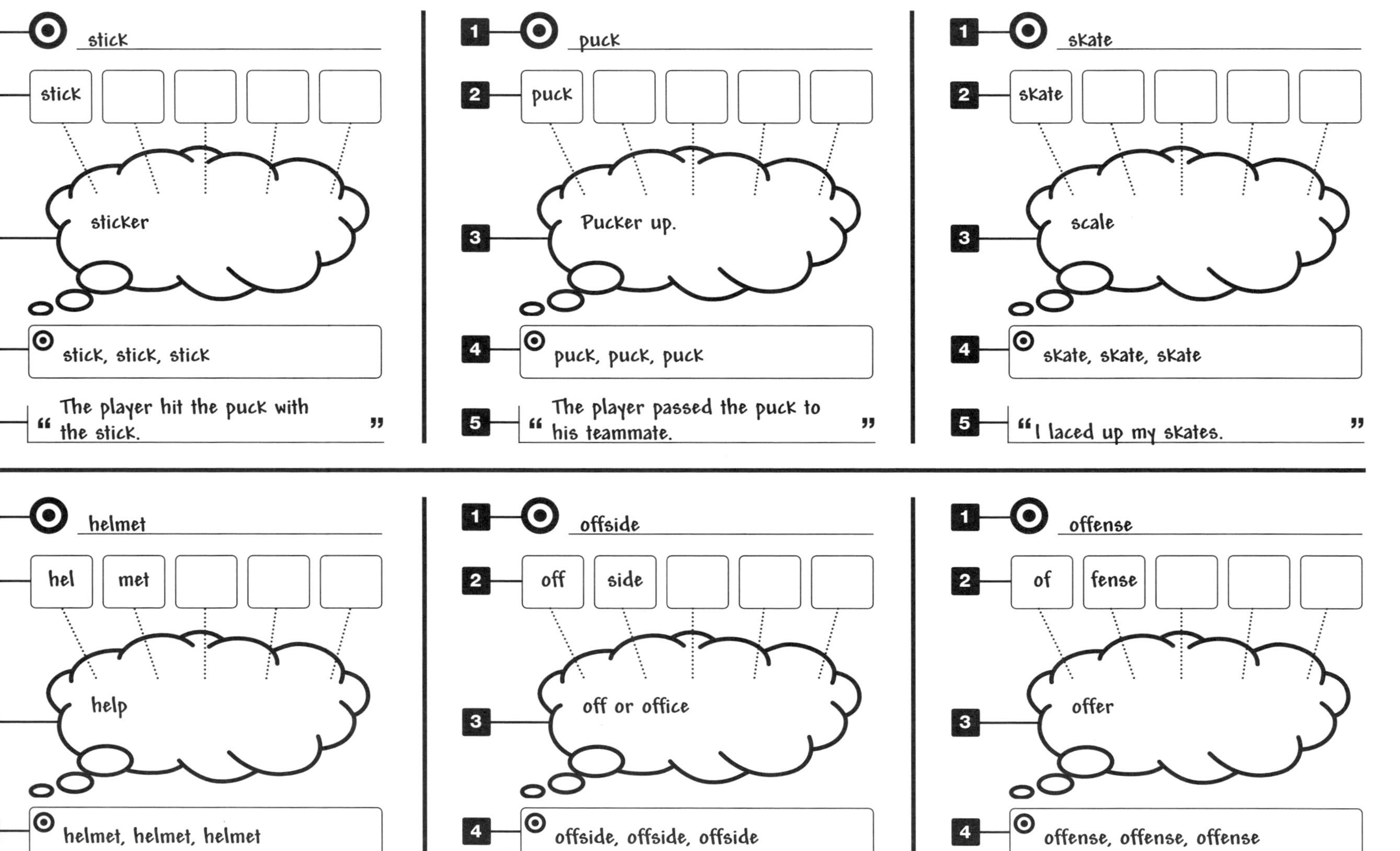
1 stick
2 stick
3 sticker
4 stick, stick, stick
5 "The player hit the puck with the stick."
1 puck
2 puck
3 Pucker up.
4 puck, puck, puck
5 "The player passed the puck to his teammate."
1 skate
2 skate
3 scale
4 skate, skate, skate
5 "I laced up my skates."
1 helmet
2 hel met
3 help
4 helmet, helmet, helmet
5 "A smart player always wears a helmet."
1 offside
2 off side
3 off or office
4 offside, offside, offside
5 "The play was called offside."
1 offense
2 of fense
3 offer
4 offense, offense, offense
5 "The offense tried to score a goal."

Published by PRO-ED, Inc., www.proedinc.com

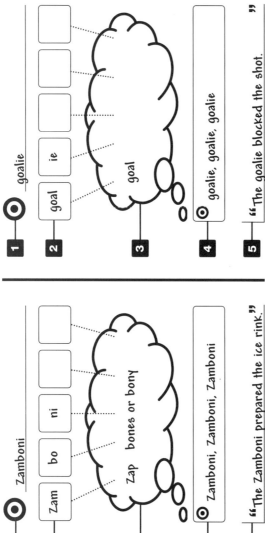

WFIP–2 SYLLABLE-DIVIDING AND SAME-SOUNDS SYLLABLE CUE STUDY FORM

NAME ____ CONTENT AREA Sports Vocabulary, Hockey DATE ____

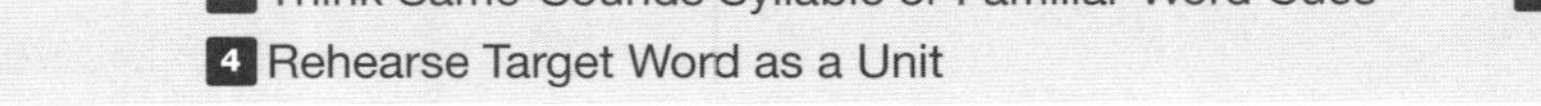

1 Target Word
2 Syllable-Dividing
3 Think Same-Sounds Syllable or Familiar-Word Cues
4 Rehearse Target Word as a Unit
5 Rehearse Target Word in a Sentence

1 Zamboni
2 Zam | bo | ni | |
3 Zap bones or bony
4 Zamboni, Zamboni, Zamboni
5 "The Zamboni prepared the ice rink."

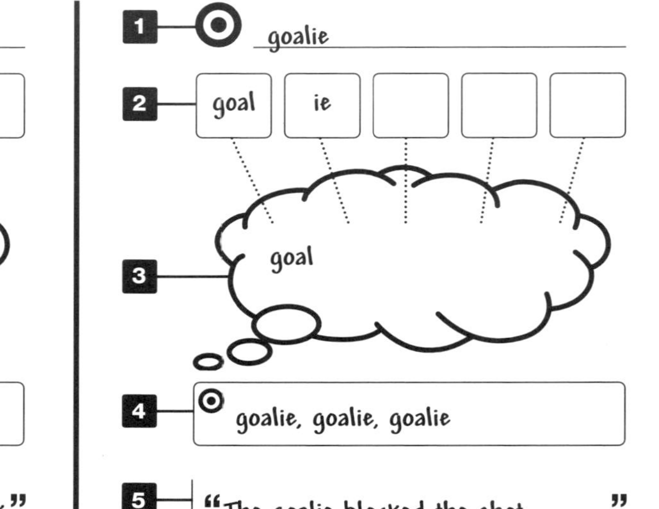

1 goalie
2 goal | ie | | |
3 goal
4 goalie, goalie, goalie
5 "The goalie blocked the shot. "

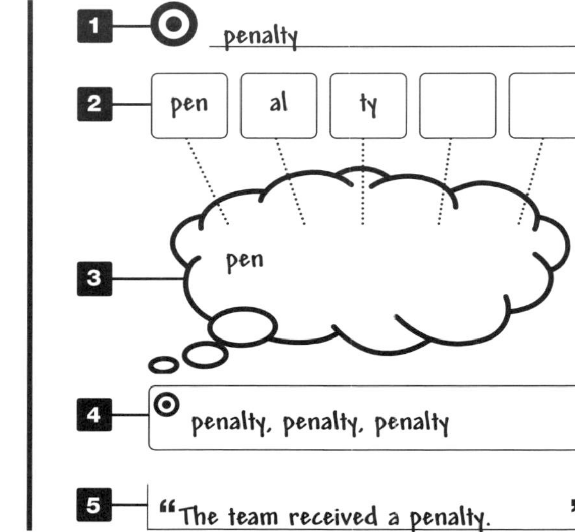

1 penalty
2 pen | al | ty | |
3 pen
4 penalty, penalty, penalty
5 "The team received a penalty. "

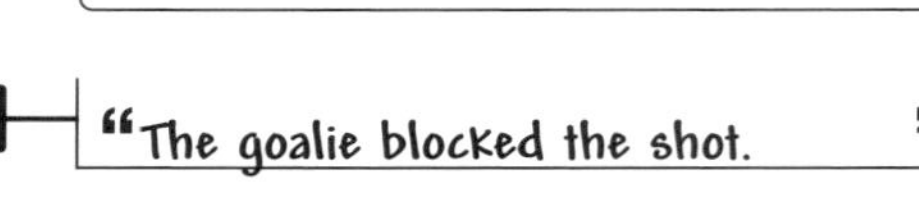

1 power play
2 pow | er | play | |
3 powder
4 power play, power play, power play
5 " The visiting team scored during a power play. "

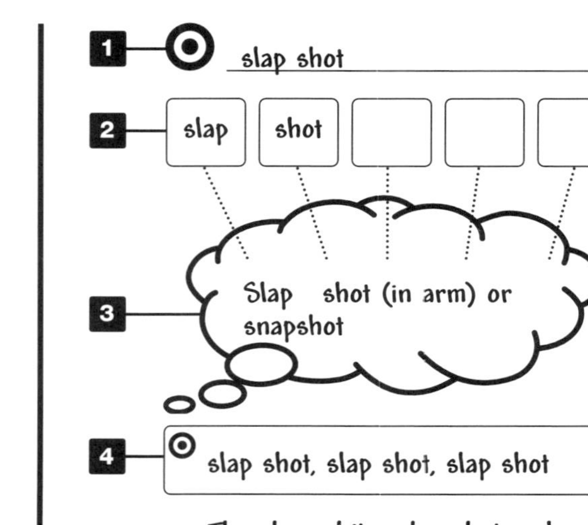

1 face-off
2 face | off | | |
3 face or fake
4 face-off, face-off, face-off
5 " The referee dropped the puck in the opening face-off. "

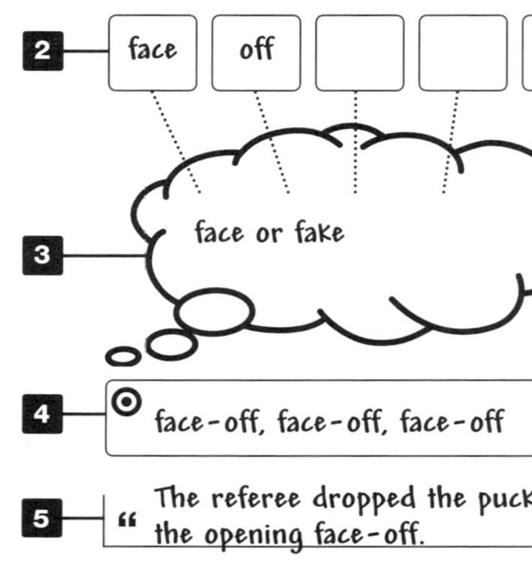

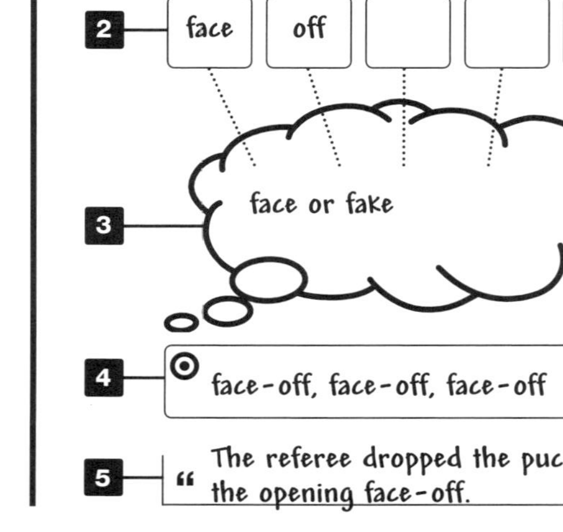

1 slap shot
2 slap | shot | | |
3 Slap shot (in arm) or snapshot
4 slap shot, slap shot, slap shot
5 " The player hit a slap shot and scored a goal. "

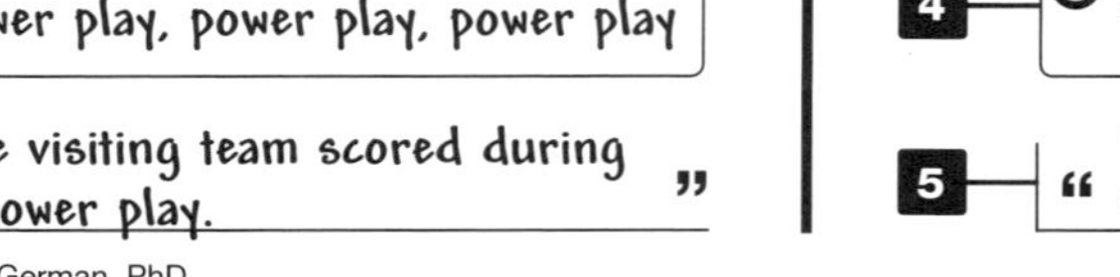

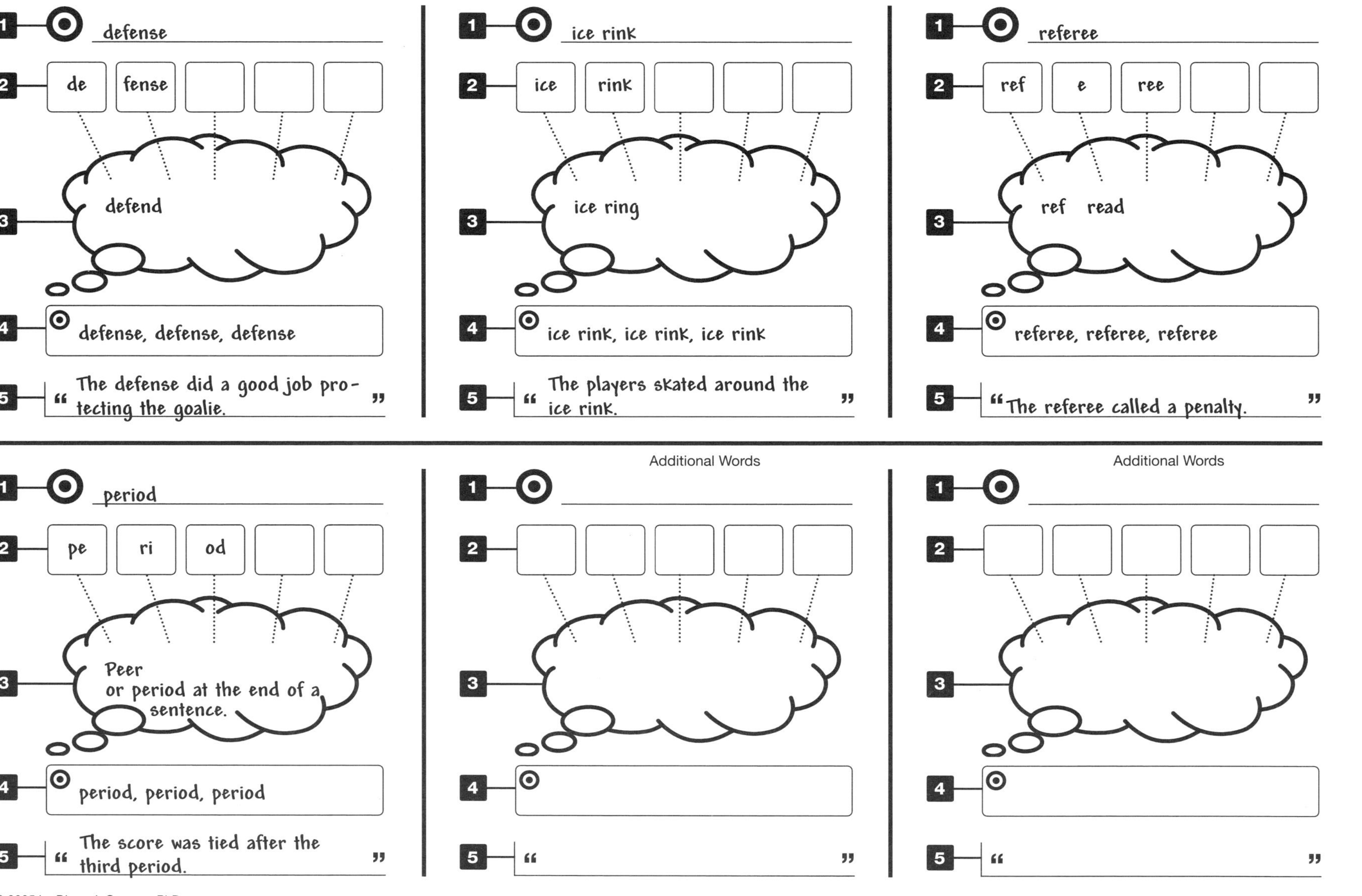

NAME CONTENT AREA Sports Vocabulary, Hockey DATE

1 Target Word
2 Syllable-Dividing
3 Think Same-Sounds Syllable or Familiar-Word Cues
4 Rehearse Target Word as a Unit
5 Rehearse Target Word in a Sentence

1 defense
2 de | fense
3 defend
4 defense, defense, defense
5 "The defense did a good job protecting the goalie."

1 ice rink
2 ice | rink
3 ice ring
4 ice rink, ice rink, ice rink
5 "The players skated around the ice rink."

1 referee
2 ref | e | ree
3 ref read
4 referee, referee, referee
5 "The referee called a penalty."

1 period
2 pe | ri | od
3 Peer or period at the end of a sentence.
4 period, period, period
5 "The score was tied after the third period."

Additional Words

1
2
3
4
5 " "

Additional Words

1
2
3
4
5 " "

VOCABULARY SUBJECT: BASEBALL

Objective: To teach learners to apply the syllable-dividing and same-sounds cues to baseball vocabulary.

Instructions: The baseball vocabulary is presented in the list on this page and embedded in the completed Syllable-Dividing and Same-Sounds Syllable Cue Study Forms that follow. Have the learner practice the selected baseball vocabulary using the syllable-dividing and same-sounds cue retrieval strategies.

bat	foul ball	umpire
glove	fly ball	runner
stands	short stop	fielder
dugout	baseman	rookie
strike	catcher	
home run	pitcher	

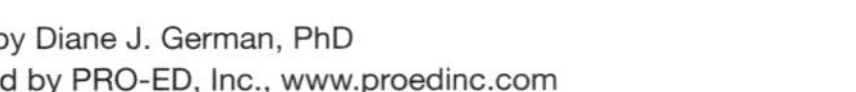

NAME CONTENT AREA Sports Vocabulary, Baseball DATE

1 Target Word
2 Syllable-Dividing
3 Think Same-Sounds Syllable or Familiar-Word Cues
4 Rehearse Target Word as a Unit
5 Rehearse Target Word in a Sentence

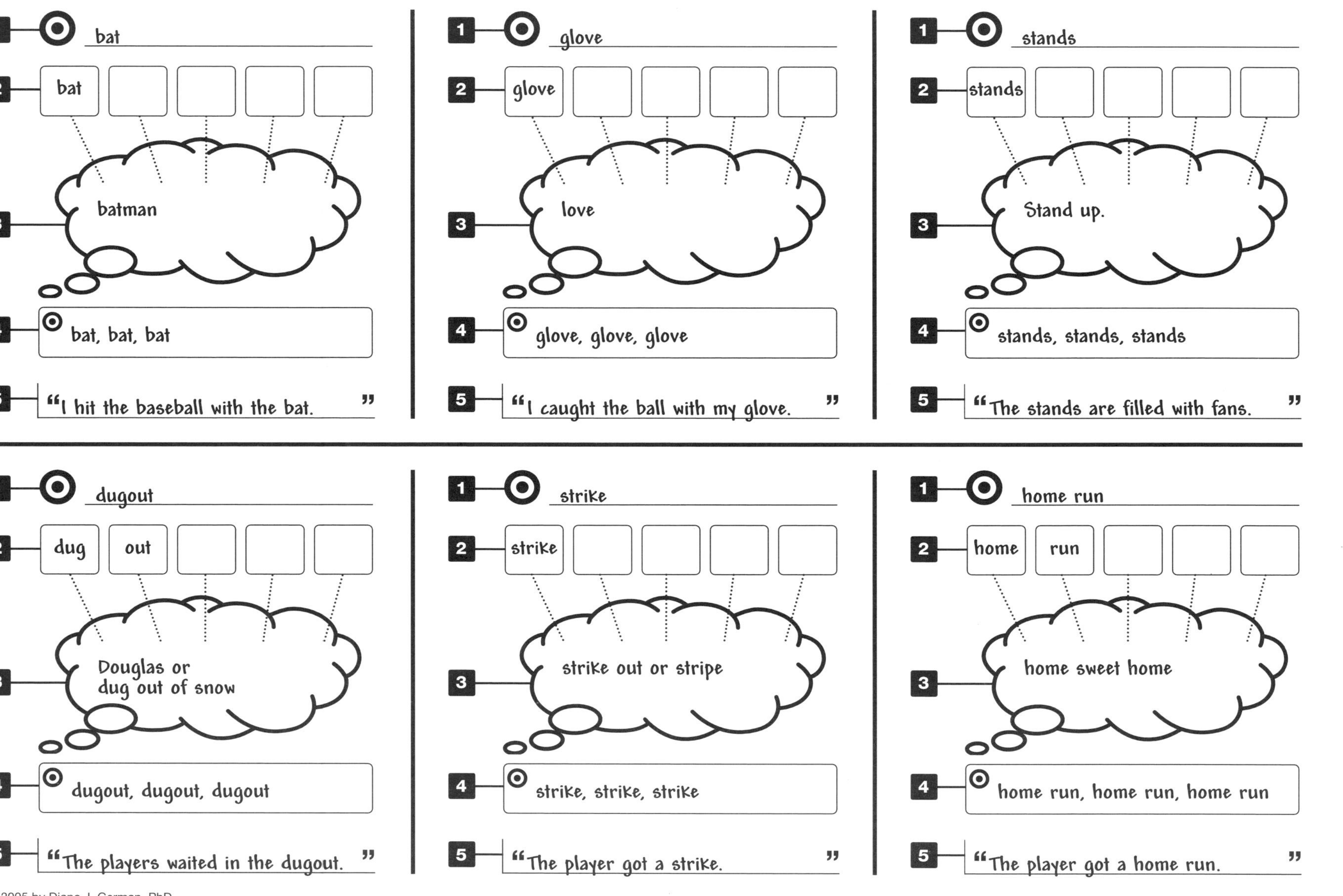

WFIP–2 SYLLABLE-DIVIDING AND SAME-SOUNDS SYLLABLE CUE STUDY FORM

NAME CONTENT AREA Sports Vocabulary, Baseball DATE

1 Target Word
2 Syllable-Dividing
3 Think Same-Sounds Syllable or Familiar-Word Cues
4 Rehearse Target Word as a Unit
5 Rehearse Target Word in a Sentence

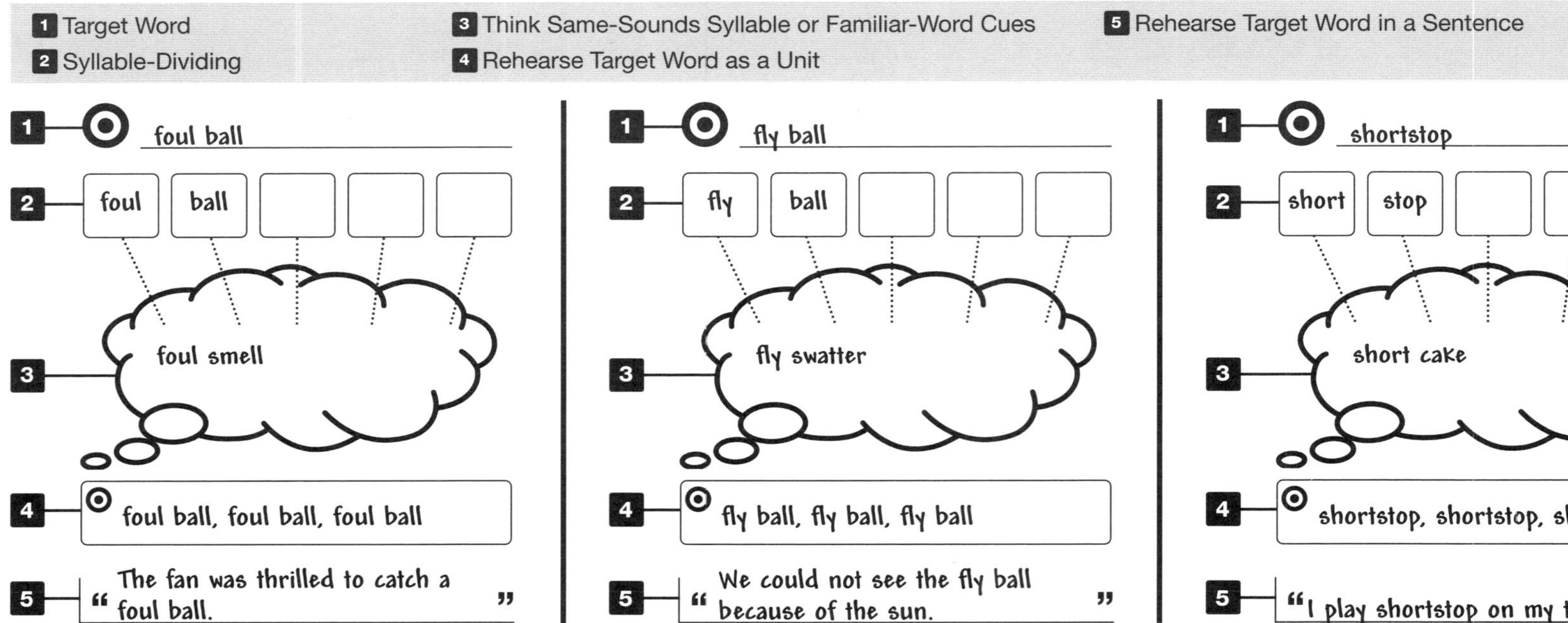

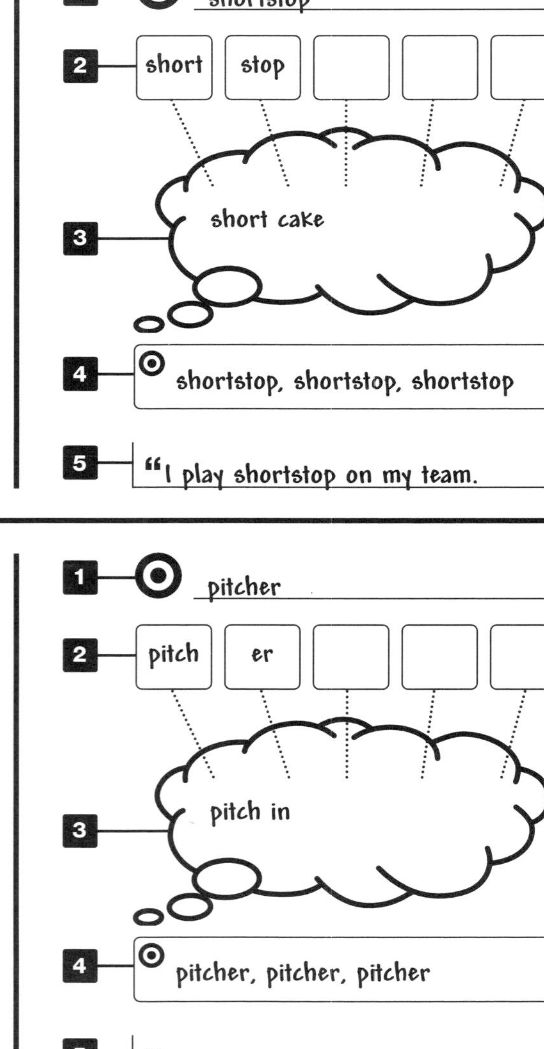

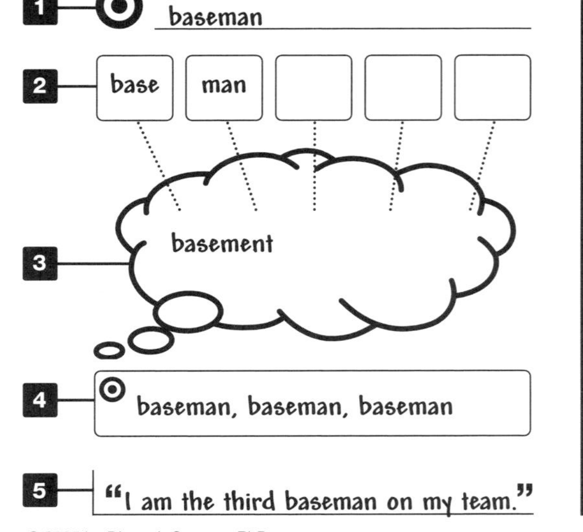

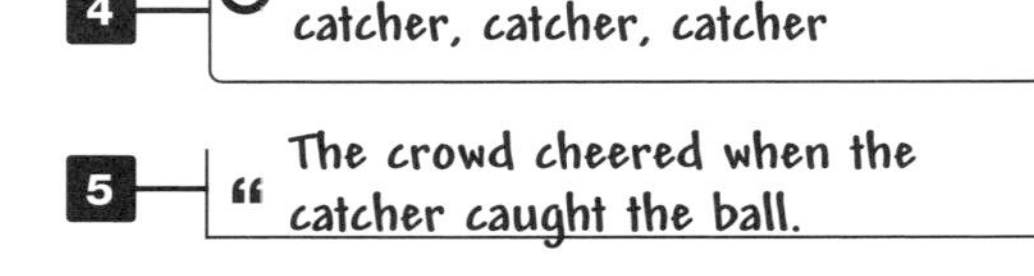

1. foul ball
2. foul | ball
3. foul smell
4. foul ball, foul ball, foul ball
5. "The fan was thrilled to catch a foul ball."

1. fly ball
2. fly | ball
3. fly swatter
4. fly ball, fly ball, fly ball
5. "We could not see the fly ball because of the sun."

1. shortstop
2. short | stop
3. short cake
4. shortstop, shortstop, shortstop
5. "I play shortstop on my team."

1. baseman
2. base | man
3. basement
4. baseman, baseman, baseman
5. "I am the third baseman on my team."

1. catcher
2. catch | er
3. ketchup
4. catcher, catcher, catcher
5. "The crowd cheered when the catcher caught the ball."

1. pitcher
2. pitch | er
3. pitch in
4. pitcher, pitcher, pitcher
5. "The pitcher threw a curve ball."

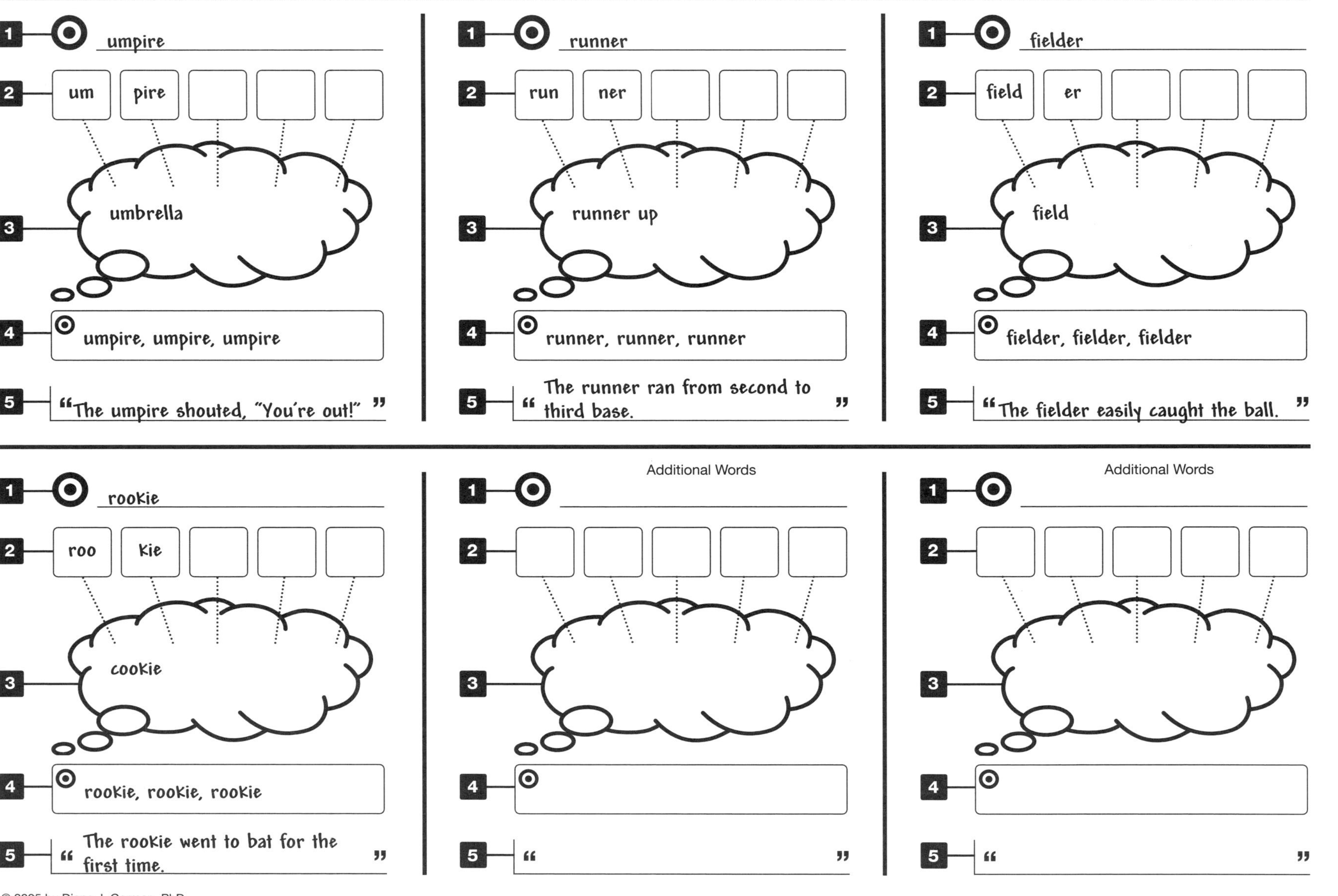

1 Target Word
2 Syllable-Dividing
3 Think Same-Sounds Syllable or Familiar-Word Cues
4 Rehearse Target Word as a Unit
5 Rehearse Target Word in a Sentence

1 umpire
2 um | pire
3 umbrella
4 umpire, umpire, umpire
5 "The umpire shouted, "You're out!""

1 runner
2 run | ner
3 runner up
4 runner, runner, runner
5 "The runner ran from second to third base."

1 fielder
2 field | er
3 field
4 fielder, fielder, fielder
5 "The fielder easily caught the ball."

1 rookie
2 roo | kie
3 cookie
4 rookie, rookie, rookie
5 "The rookie went to bat for the first time."

Additional Words
1
2
3
4
5 " "

Additional Words
1
2
3
4
5 " "

Published by PRO-ED, Inc., www.proedinc.com

VOCABULARY SUBJECT: FOOTBALL

Objective: To teach learners to apply the syllable-dividing and same-sounds cues to football vocabulary

Instructions: The football vocabulary is presented in the list on this page and embedded in the completed Syllable-Dividing and Same-Sounds Syllable Cue Study Forms that follow. Have the learner practice the selected football vocabulary using the syllable-dividing and same-sounds cue retrieval strategies.

stadium	quarter	sideline
goalpost	yard line	end zone
scoreboard	touchdown	fumble
halfback	kickoff	interception
tackle	coach	
huddle	overtime	

NAME CONTENT AREA Sports Vocabulary, Football DATE

1 Target Word **2** Syllable-Dividing **3** Think Same-Sounds Syllable or Familiar-Word Cues **4** Rehearse Target Word as a Unit **5** Rehearse Target Word in a Sentence

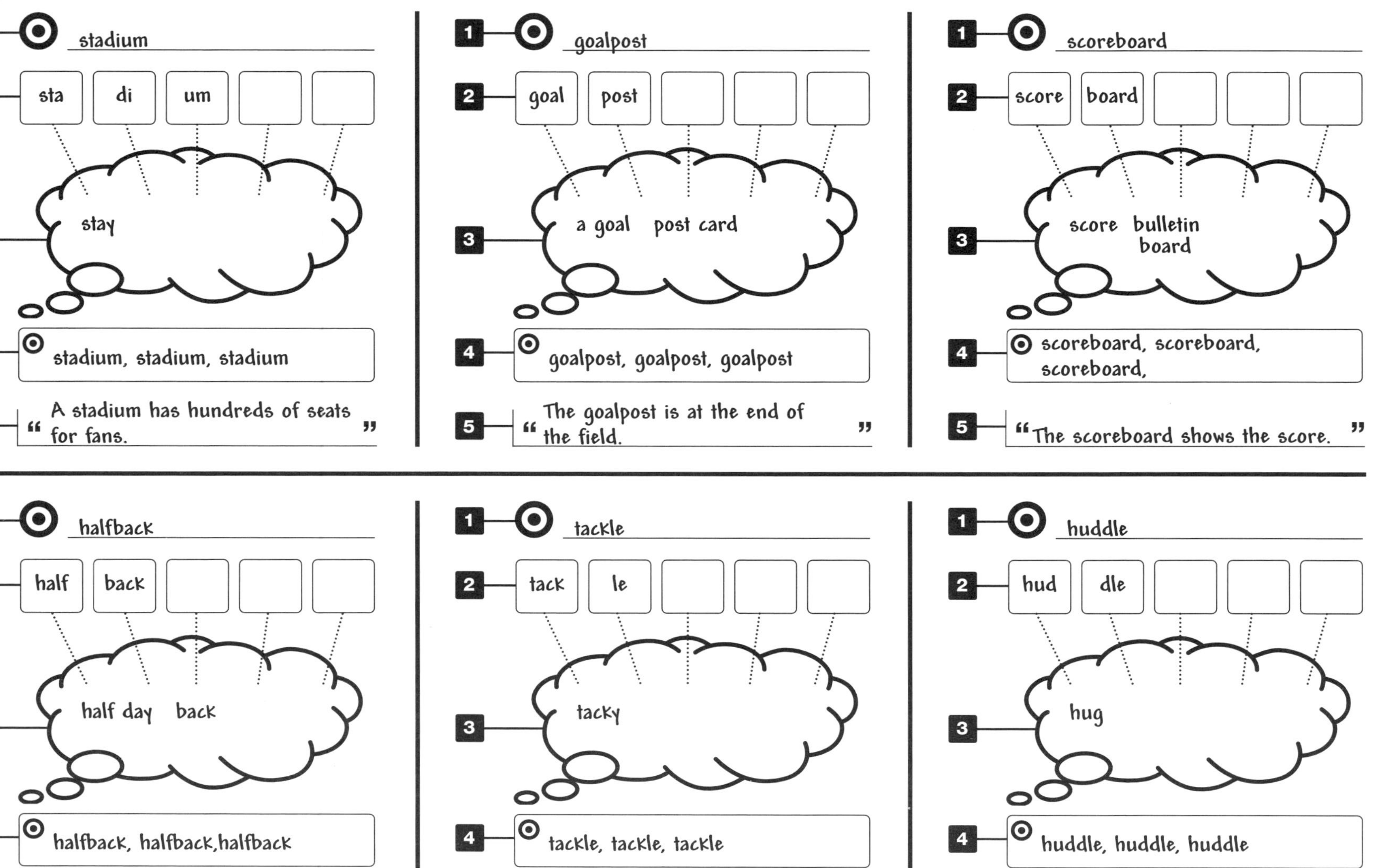

1 stadium
2 sta | di | um
3 stay
4 stadium, stadium, stadium
5 "A stadium has hundreds of seats for fans."

1 goalpost
2 goal | post
3 a goal post card
4 goalpost, goalpost, goalpost
5 "The goalpost is at the end of the field."

1 scoreboard
2 score | board
3 score bulletin board
4 scoreboard, scoreboard, scoreboard,
5 "The scoreboard shows the score."

1 halfback
2 half | back
3 half day back
4 halfback, halfback,halfback
5 "A halfback stands behind a player."

1 tackle
2 tack | le
3 tacky
4 tackle, tackle, tackle
5 "A tackle may cause players to get hurt."

1 huddle
2 hud | dle
3 hug
4 huddle, huddle, huddle
5 "The players were in the huddle."

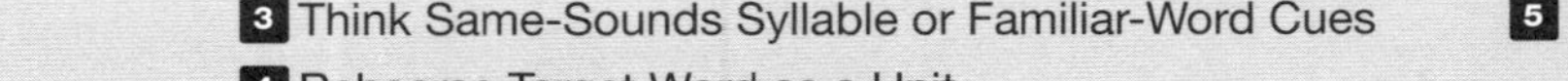

WFIP–2 SYLLABLE-DIVIDING AND SAME-SOUNDS SYLLABLE CUE STUDY FORM

NAME ______ **CONTENT AREA** Sports Vocabulary, Football **DATE** ______

1 Target Word
2 Syllable-Dividing
3 Think Same-Sounds Syllable or Familiar-Word Cues
4 Rehearse Target Word as a Unit
5 Rehearse Target Word in a Sentence

1 quarter
2 quar | ter
3 quarter (money)
4 quarter, quarter, quarter
5 "One period of play is called a quarter."

1 yard line
2 yard | line

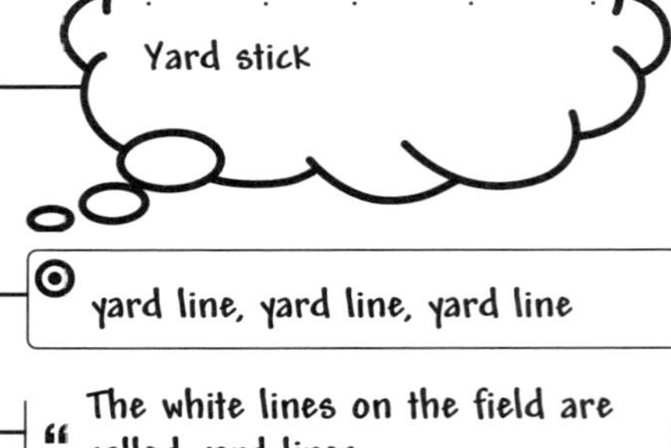

3 Yard stick
4 yard line, yard line, yard line
5 "The white lines on the field are called yard lines."

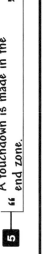

1 touchdown
2 touch | down

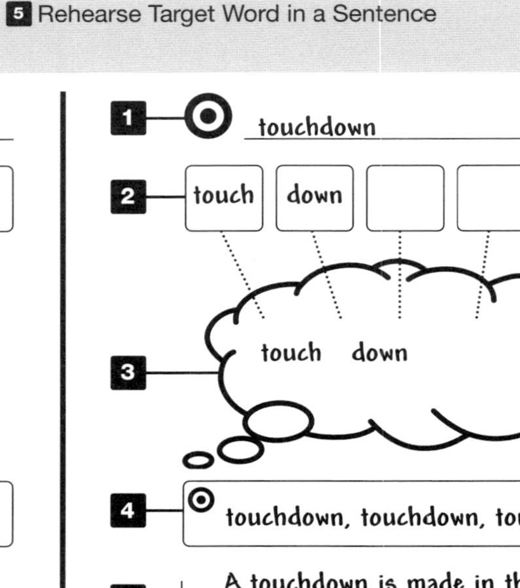

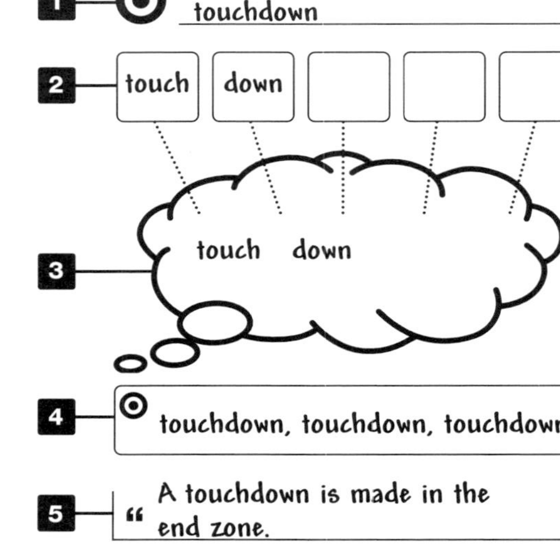

3 touch down
4 touchdown, touchdown, touchdown
5 "A touchdown is made in the end zone."

1 kickoff
2 kick | off

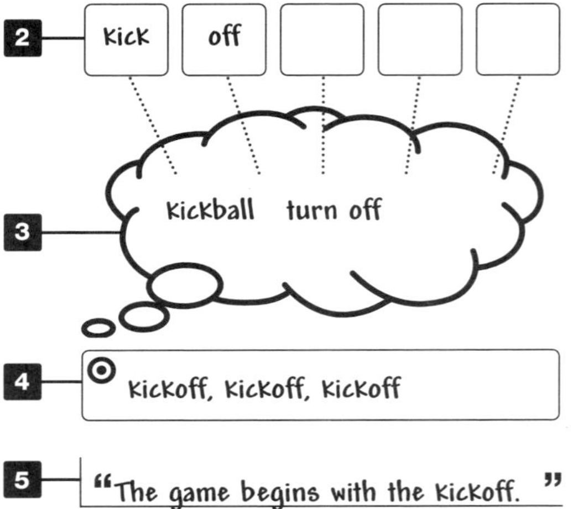

3 kickball turn off
4 kickoff, kickoff, kickoff
5 "The game begins with the kickoff."

1 coach
2 coach

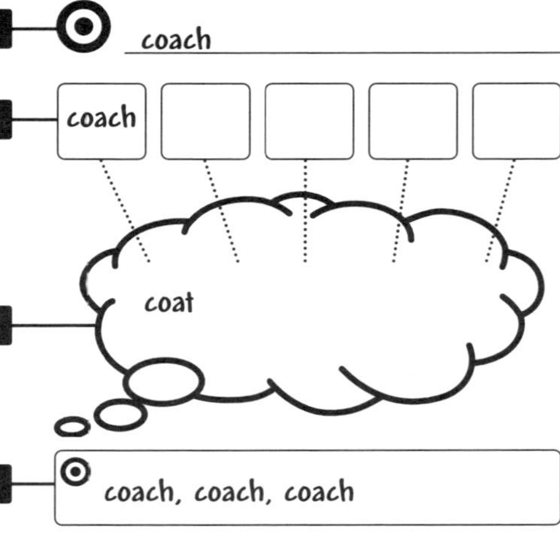

3 coat
4 coach, coach, coach
5 "The coach is the boss."

1 overtime
2 o | ver | time

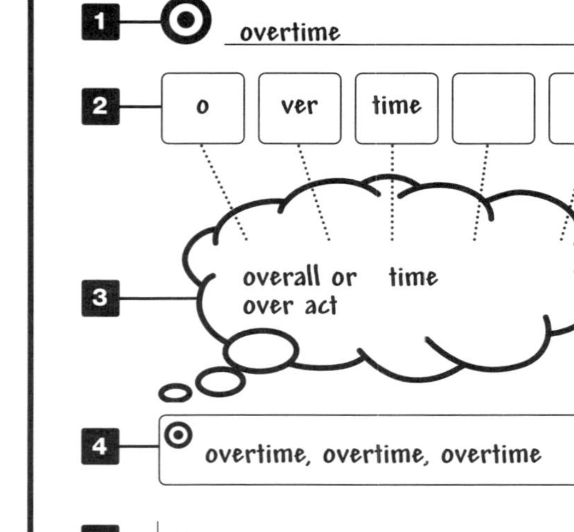

3 overall or over act time
4 overtime, overtime, overtime
5 "The game went into overtime."

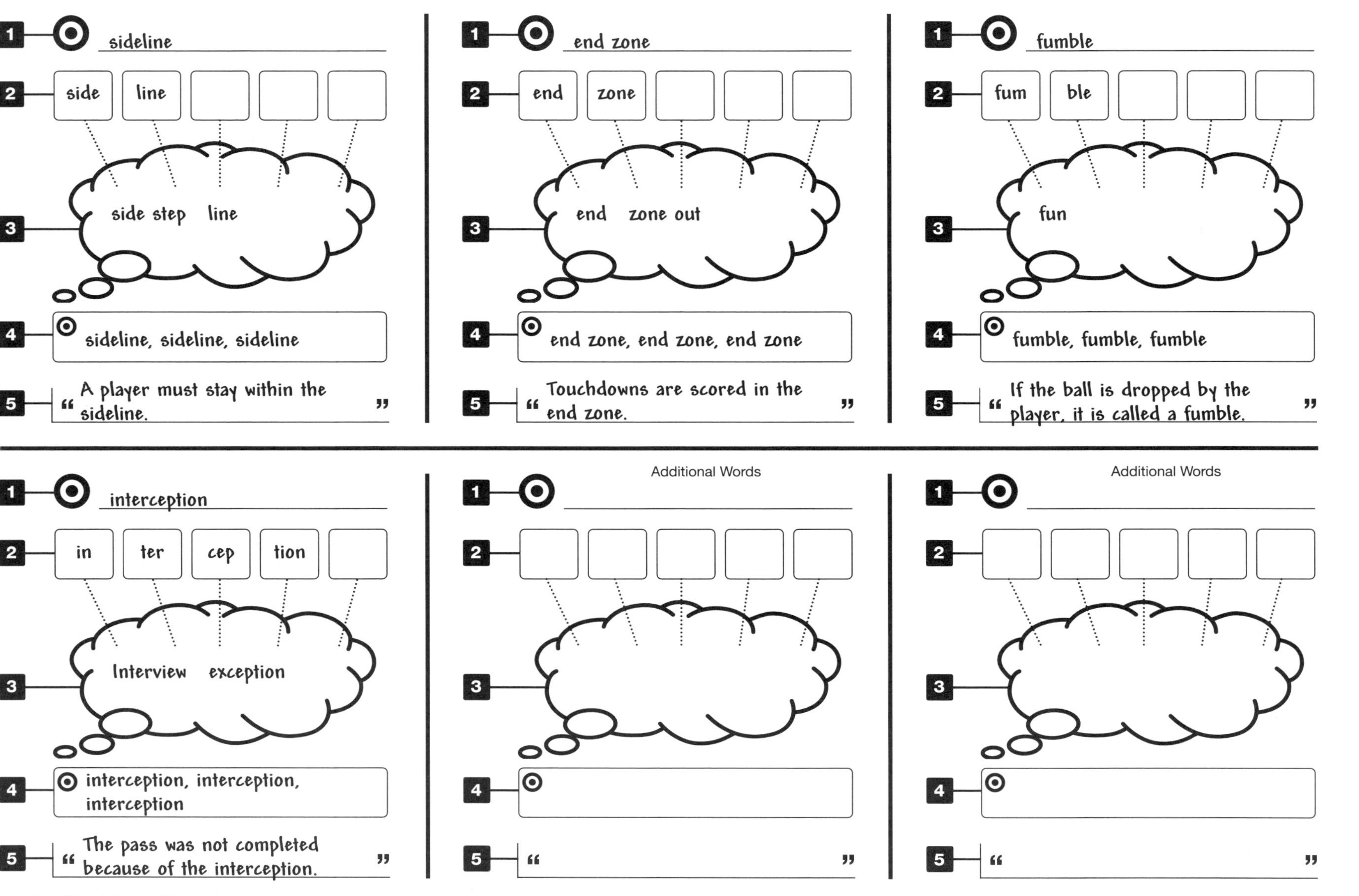
1 Target Word
2 Syllable-Dividing
3 Think Same-Sounds Syllable or Familiar-Word Cues
4 Rehearse Target Word as a Unit
5 Rehearse Target Word in a Sentence
1 sideline
2 side line
3 side step line
4 sideline, sideline, sideline
5 "A player must stay within the sideline."
1 end zone
2 end zone
3 end zone out
4 end zone, end zone, end zone
5 "Touchdowns are scored in the end zone."
1 fumble
2 fum ble
3 fun
4 fumble, fumble, fumble
5 "If the ball is dropped by the player, it is called a fumble."
1 interception
2 in ter cep tion
3 Interview exception
4 interception, interception, interception
5 "The pass was not completed because of the interception."
Additional Words
1
2
3
4
5 " "
Additional Words
1
2
3
4
5 " "

VOCABULARY SUBJECT: GOLF

Objective: To teach learners to apply the syllable-dividing and same-sounds cues to golf vocabulary

Instructions: The golf vocabulary is presented in the list on this page and embedded in the completed Syllable-Dividing and Same-Sounds Syllable Cue Study Forms that follow. Have the learner practice the selected golf vocabulary using the syllable-dividing and same-sounds cue retrieval strategies.

iron	bogey	sand trap
wood	par	drive
putter	birdie	chip
caddie	eagle	fairway

NAME CONTENT AREA Sports Vocabulary, Golf DATE

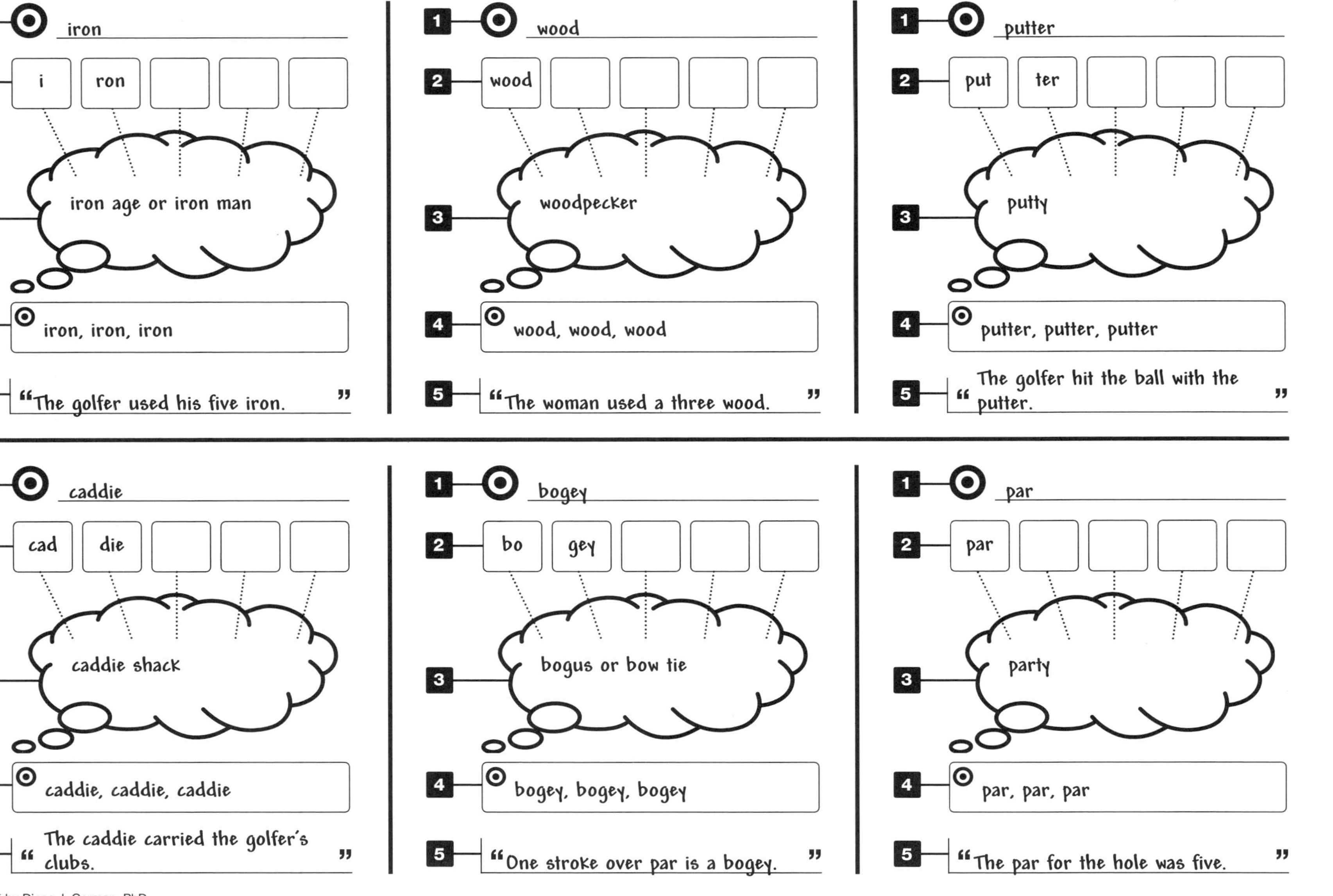

1 Target Word
2 Syllable-Dividing
3 Think Same-Sounds Syllable or Familiar-Word Cues
4 Rehearse Target Word as a Unit
5 Rehearse Target Word in a Sentence

1 iron
2 i | ron
3 iron age or iron man
4 iron, iron, iron
5 "The golfer used his five iron."

1 wood
2 wood
3 woodpecker
4 wood, wood, wood
5 "The woman used a three wood."

1 putter
2 put | ter
3 putty
4 putter, putter, putter
5 "The golfer hit the ball with the putter."

1 caddie
2 cad | die
3 caddie shack
4 caddie, caddie, caddie
5 "The caddie carried the golfer's clubs."

1 bogey
2 bo | gey
3 bogus or bow tie
4 bogey, bogey, bogey
5 "One stroke over par is a bogey."

1 par
2 par
3 party
4 par, par, par
5 "The par for the hole was five."

Published by PRO-ED, Inc., www.proedinc.com

WFIP–2 SYLLABLE-DIVIDING AND SAME-SOUNDS SYLLABLE CUE STUDY FORM

NAME ____ CONTENT AREA Sports Vocabulary, Golf DATE ____

1 Target Word
2 Syllable-Dividing
3 Think Same-Sounds Syllable or Familiar-Word Cues
4 Rehearse Target Word as a Unit
5 Rehearse Target Word in a Sentence

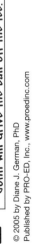

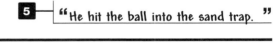

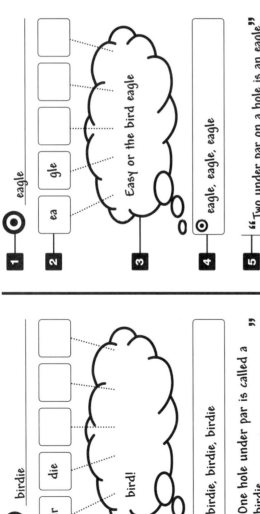

1 birdie
2 bir | die | | |
3 bird!
4 birdie, birdie, birdie
5 "One hole under par is called a birdie."

1 eagle
2 ea | gle | | |
3 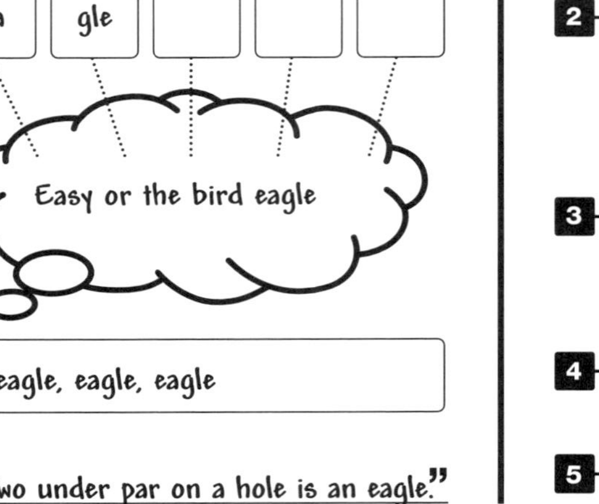

4 eagle, eagle, eagle
5 "Two under par on a hole is an eagle."

1 sand trap
2 sand | trap | | |
3 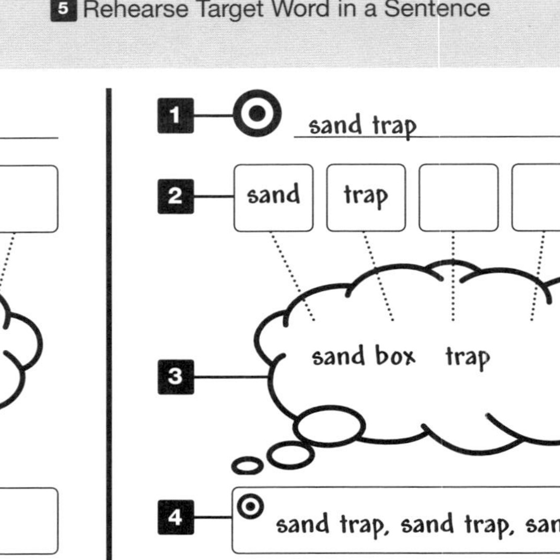

4 sand trap, sand trap, sand trap
5 "He hit the ball into the sand trap."

1 drive
2 drive | | | |
3 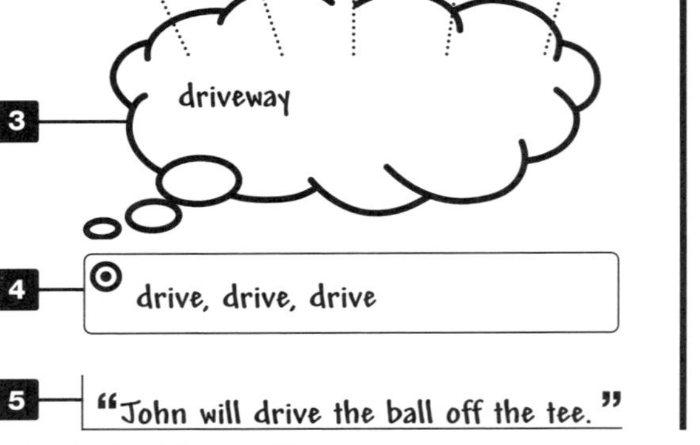

4 drive, drive, drive
5 "John will drive the ball off the tee."

1 chip
2 chip | | | |
3 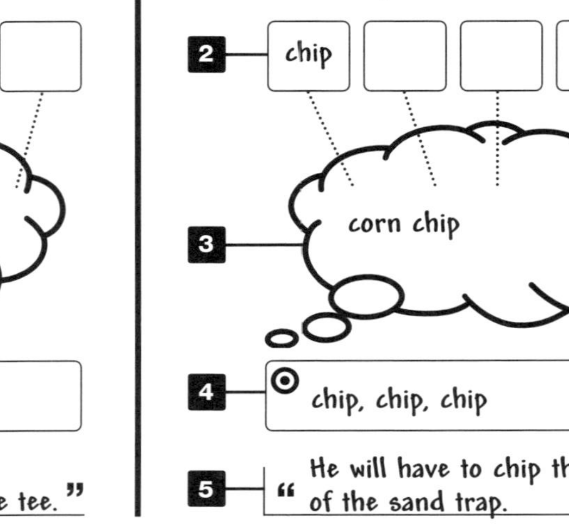
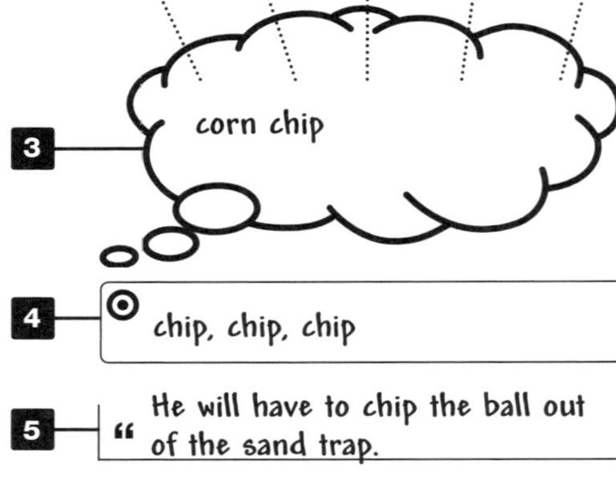

4 chip, chip, chip
5 "He will have to chip the ball out of the sand trap."

1 fairway
2 fair | way | | |
3 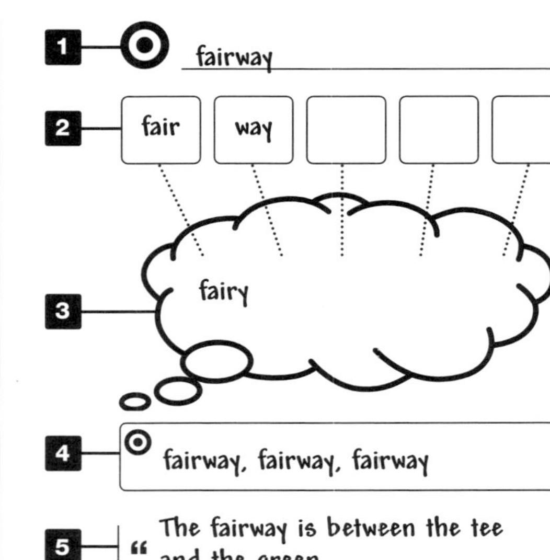

4 fairway, fairway, fairway
5 "The fairway is between the tee and the green."

VOCABULARY SUBJECT: SWIMMING

Objective: To teach learners to apply the syllable-dividing and same-sounds cues to swimming vocabulary

Instructions: The swimming vocabulary is presented in the list on this page and embedded in the completed Syllable-Dividing and Same-Sounds Syllable Cue Study Forms that follow. Have the learner practice the selected swimming vocabulary using the syllable-dividing and same-sounds cue retrieval strategies.

pool	freestyle	sidestroke
lane	backstroke	flipturn
goggles	butterfly	heat
flippers	breaststroke	meet

WFIP-2 SYLLABLE-DIVIDING AND SAME-SOUNDS SYLLABLE CUE STUDY FORM

NAME CONTENT AREA Sports Vocabulary, Swimming DATE

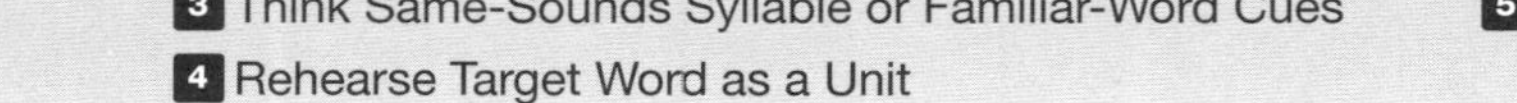

1 Target Word
2 Syllable-Dividing
3 Think Same-Sounds Syllable or Familiar-Word Cues
4 Rehearse Target Word as a Unit
5 Rehearse Target Word in a Sentence

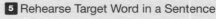

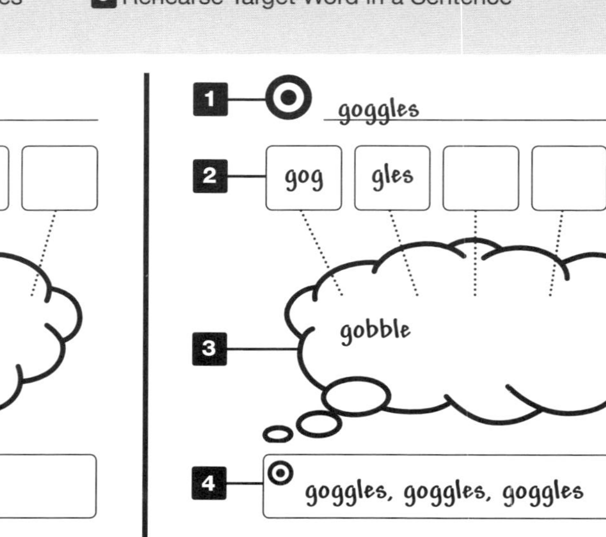
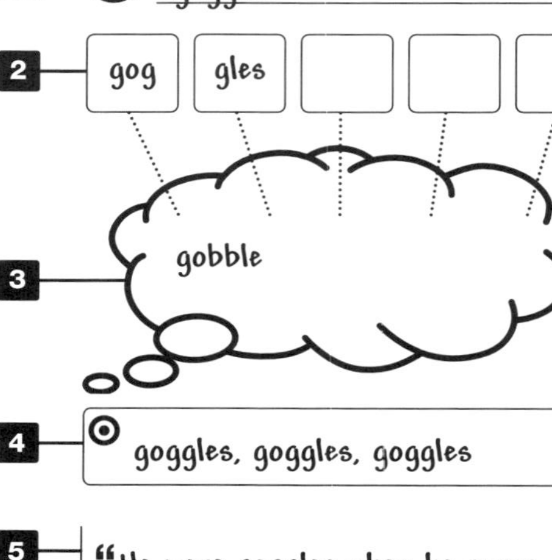

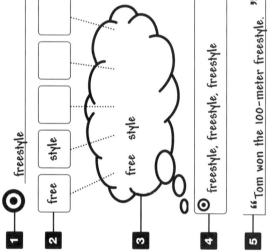

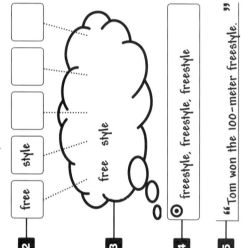

1 pool
2 pool
3 swimming pool or pool table
4 pool, pool, pool
5 "We all jumped in the pool to swim."

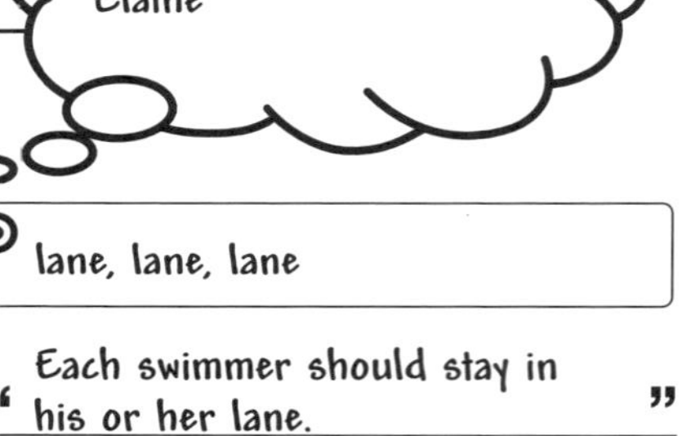

1 lane
2 lane
3 Elaine
4 lane, lane, lane
5 "Each swimmer should stay in his or her lane."

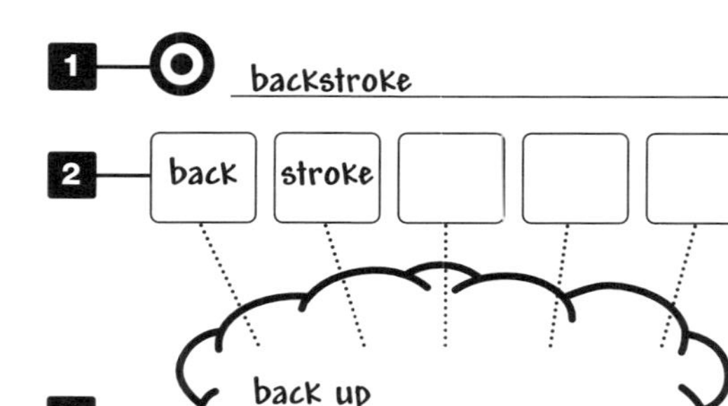
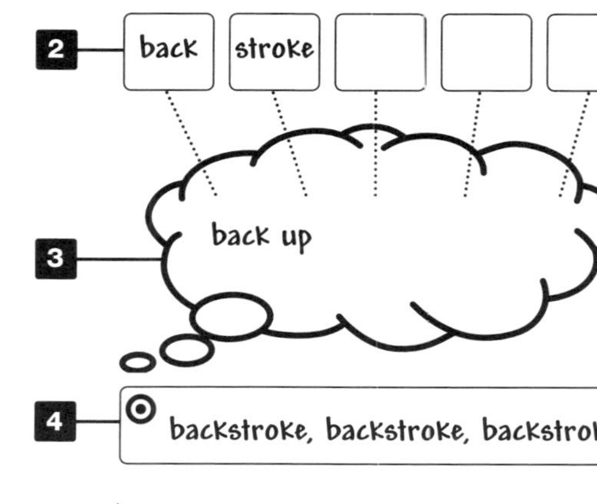

1 goggles
2 gog | gles
3 gobble
4 goggles, goggles, goggles
5 "He wore goggles when he swam."

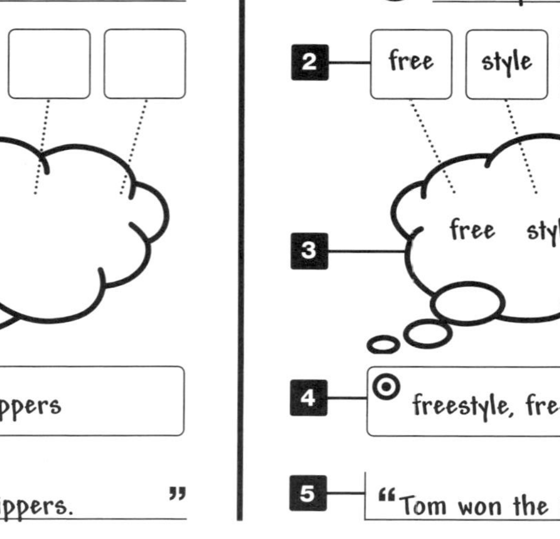

1 flippers
2 flip | pers
3 flip
4 flippers, flippers, flippers
5 "The swimmer wore flippers."

1 freestyle
2 free | style
3 free style
4 freestyle, freestyle, freestyle
5 "Tom won the 100-meter freestyle."

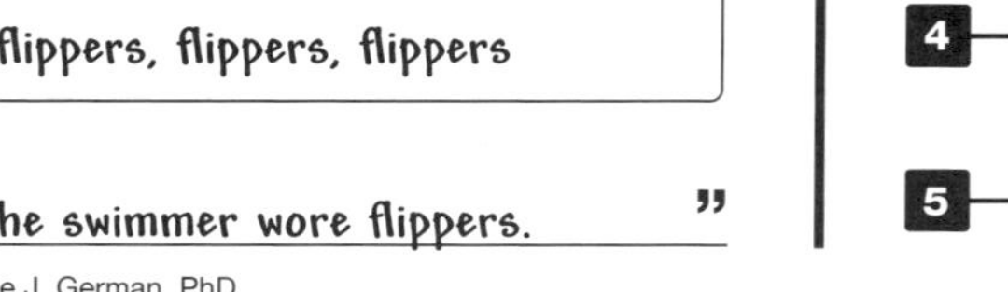
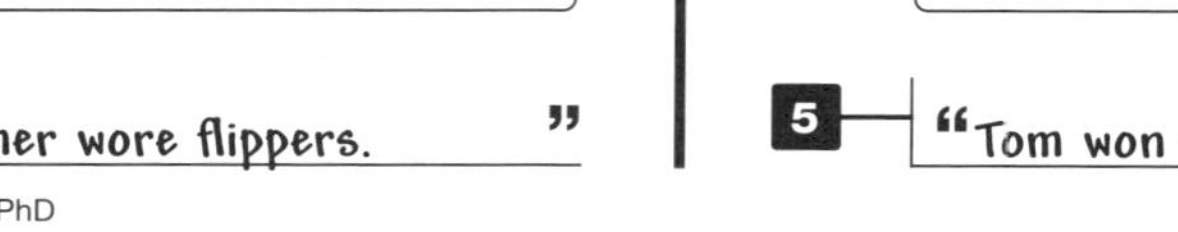

1 backstroke
2 back | stroke
3 back up
4 backstroke, backstroke, backstroke
5 "He had a fast backstroke."

NAME CONTENT AREA Sports Vocabulary, Swimming DATE

1 Target Word
2 Syllable-Dividing
3 Think Same-Sounds Syllable or Familiar-Word Cues
4 Rehearse Target Word as a Unit
5 Rehearse Target Word in a Sentence

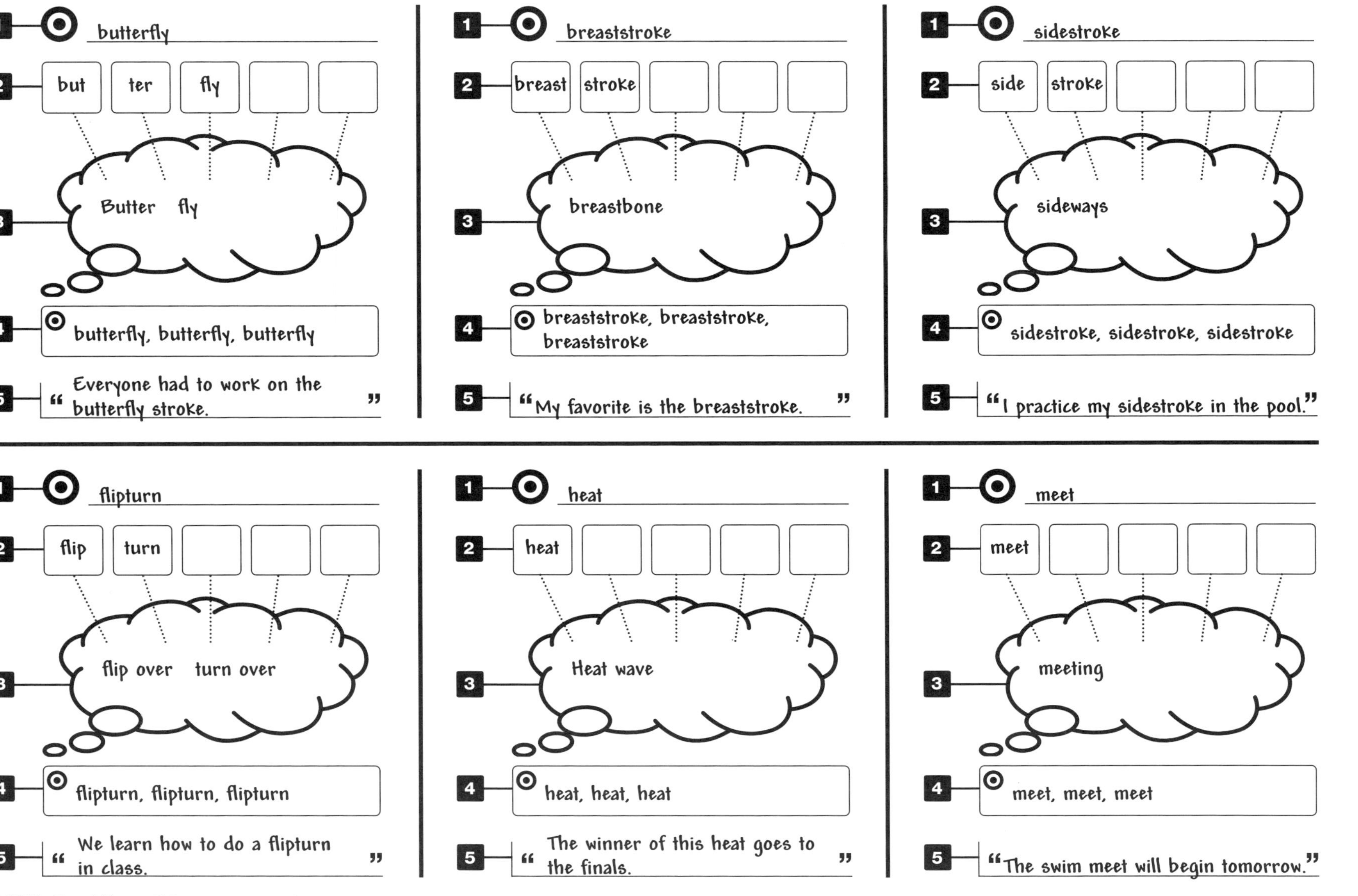
1 butterfly
2 but | ter | fly
3 Butter fly
4 butterfly, butterfly, butterfly
5 "Everyone had to work on the butterfly stroke."
1 breaststroke
2 breast | stroke
3 breastbone
4 breaststroke, breaststroke, breaststroke
5 "My favorite is the breaststroke."
1 sidestroke
2 side | stroke
3 sideways
4 sidestroke, sidestroke, sidestroke
5 "I practice my sidestroke in the pool."
1 flipturn
2 flip | turn
3 flip over turn over
4 flipturn, flipturn, flipturn
5 "We learn how to do a flipturn in class."
1 heat
2 heat
3 Heat wave
4 heat, heat, heat
5 "The winner of this heat goes to the finals."
1 meet
2 meet
3 meeting
4 meet, meet, meet
5 "The swim meet will begin tomorrow."

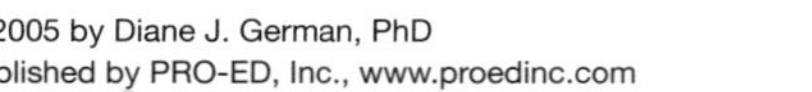

VOCABULARY SUBJECT: WEATHER

Objective: To teach learners to apply the syllable-dividing and same-sounds cues to weather vocabulary

Instructions: The weather vocabulary is presented in the list on this page and embedded in the completed Syllable-Dividing and Same-Sounds Syllable Cue Study Forms that follow. Have the learner practice the selected weather vocabulary using the syllable-dividing and same-sounds cue retrieval strategies.

weather	meteorologist	air
cumulus	sphere	pressure
cirrus	air resistance	gas
stratus	wind vane	thermometer

NAME CONTENT AREA Science DATE

1 Target Word
2 Syllable-Dividing
3 Think Same-Sounds Syllable or Familiar-Word Cues
4 Rehearse Target Word as a Unit
5 Rehearse Target Word in a Sentence

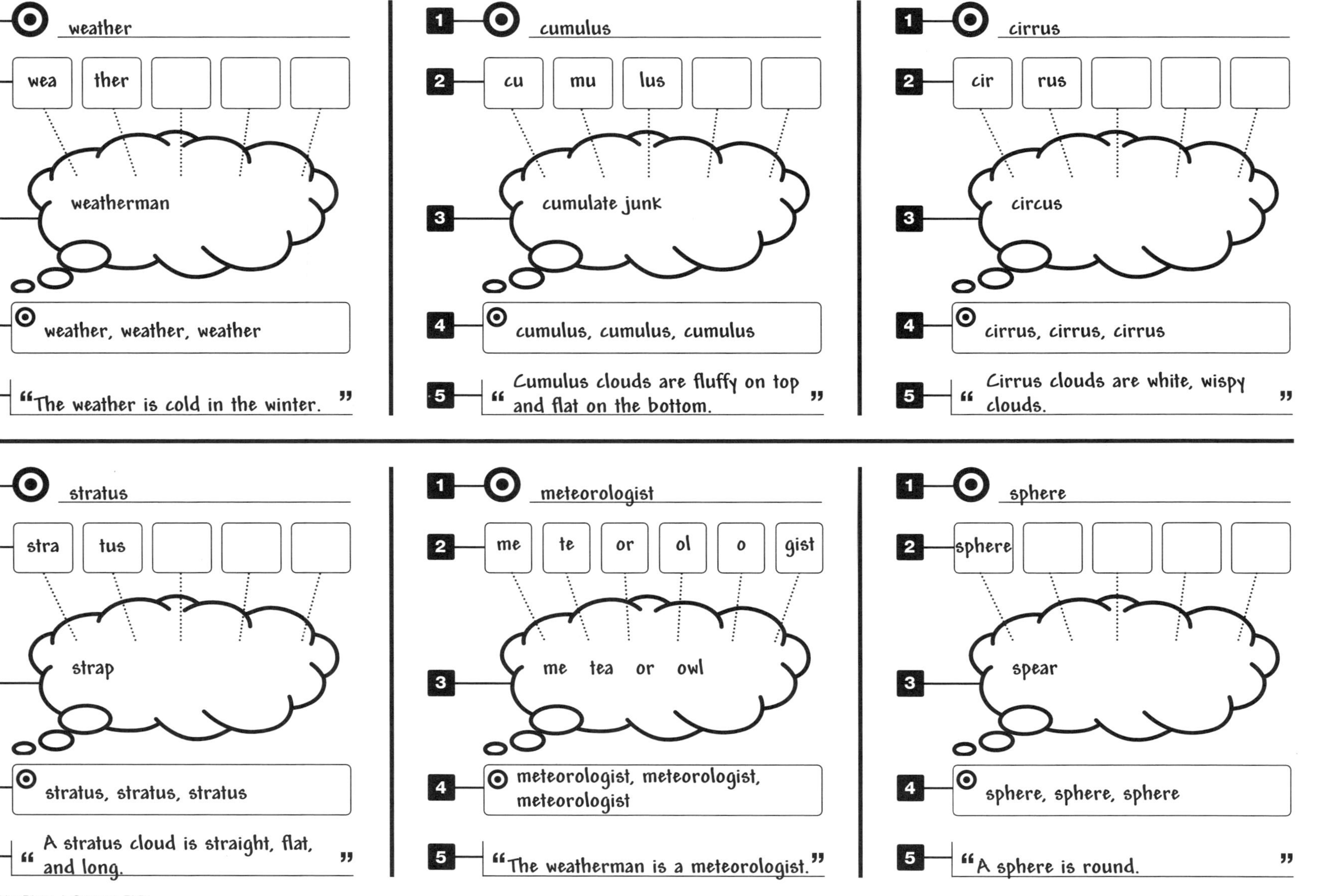

1 weather
2 wea | ther
3 weatherman
4 weather, weather, weather
5 "The weather is cold in the winter."
1 cumulus
2 cu | mu | lus
3 cumulate junk
4 cumulus, cumulus, cumulus
5 "Cumulus clouds are fluffy on top and flat on the bottom."
1 cirrus
2 cir | rus
3 circus
4 cirrus, cirrus, cirrus
5 "Cirrus clouds are white, wispy clouds."
1 stratus
2 stra | tus
3 strap
4 stratus, stratus, stratus
5 "A stratus cloud is straight, flat, and long."
1 meteorologist
2 me | te | or | ol | o | gist
3 me tea or owl
4 meteorologist, meteorologist, meteorologist
5 "The weatherman is a meteorologist."
1 sphere
2 sphere
3 spear
4 sphere, sphere, sphere
5 "A sphere is round."

WFIP–2 SYLLABLE-DIVIDING AND SAME-SOUNDS SYLLABLE CUE STUDY FORM

NAME CONTENT AREA *Science* DATE

1 Target Word
2 Syllable-Dividing
3 Think Same-Sounds Syllable or Familiar-Word Cues
4 Rehearse Target Word as a Unit
5 Rehearse Target Word in a Sentence

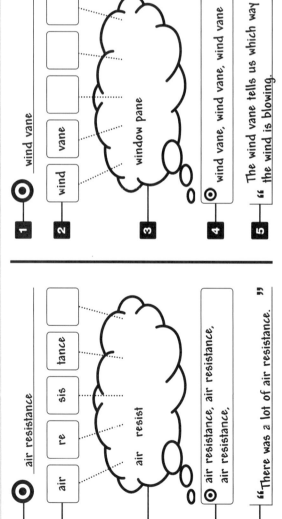

1 air resistance

2 air | re | sis | tance

3 air resist

4 air resistance, air resistance, air resistance,

5 "There was a lot of air resistance."

1 wind vane

2 wind | vane

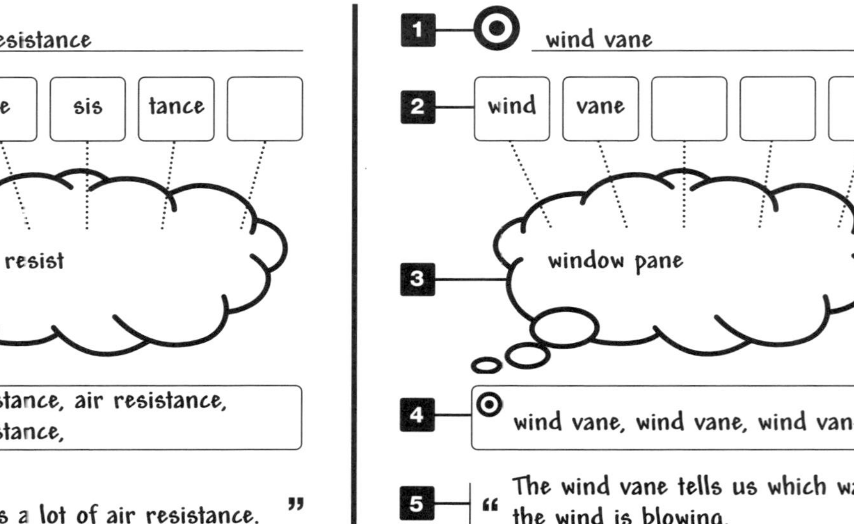

4 wind vane, wind vane, wind vane

5 "The wind vane tells us which way the wind is blowing."

1 air

2 air

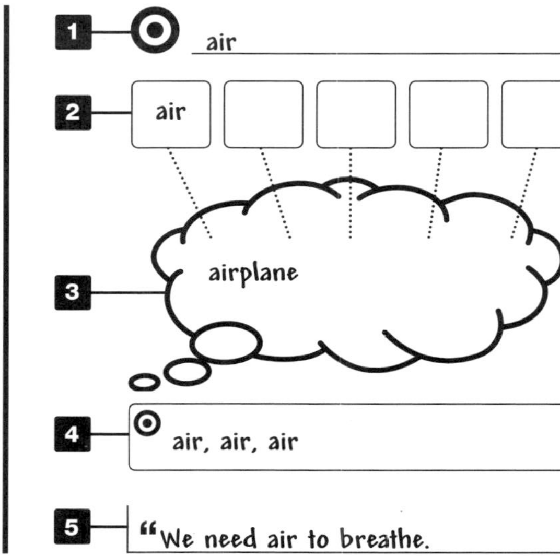

4 air, air, air

5 "We need air to breathe."

1 pressure

2 pres | sure

3 press or present

4 pressure, pressure, pressure

5 "The weatherman reported the barometric pressure."

1 gas

2 gas

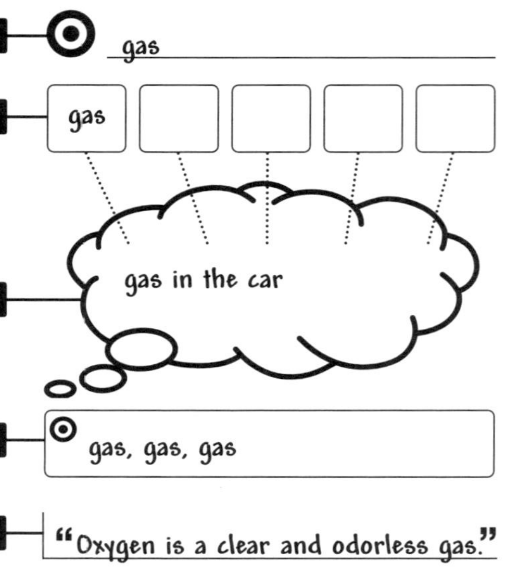

4 gas, gas, gas

5 "Oxygen is a clear and odorless gas."

1 thermometer

2 ther | mom | e | ter

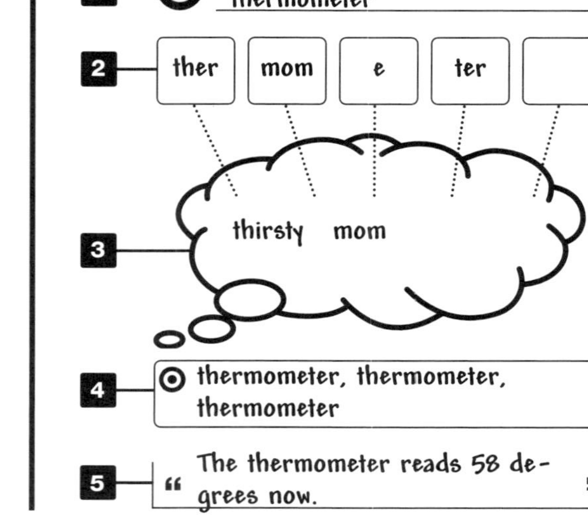

4 thermometer, thermometer, thermometer

5 "The thermometer reads 58 degrees now."

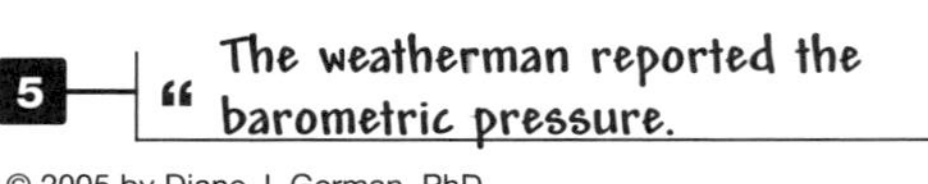

VOCABULARY SUBJECT: LANDFORMS

Objective: To teach learners to apply the syllable-dividing and same-sounds cues to landforms vocabulary

Instructions: The landforms vocabulary is presented in the list on this page and embedded in the completed Syllable-Dividing and Same-Sounds Syllable Cue Study Forms that follow. Have the learner practice the selected landforms vocabulary using the syllable-dividing and same-sounds cue retrieval strategies.

mountain	volcano	glacier
valley	strait	gulf
desert	swamp	peninsula
island	tributary	canyon
river	plain	cave
lake	plateau	channel
ocean	pond	cliff
sea	prairie	tundra

WFIP–2 SYLLABLE-DIVIDING AND SAME-SOUNDS SYLLABLE CUE STUDY FORM

NAME

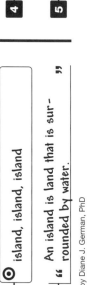

CONTENT AREA Social Studies: Landforms

DATE

1 Target Word
2 Syllable-Dividing
3 Think Same-Sounds Syllable or Familiar-Word Cues
4 Rehearse Target Word as a Unit
5 Rehearse Target Word in a Sentence

1 mountain
2 moun | tain
3 Mountain dew
4 mountain, mountain, mountain
5 "A mountain is taller than a hill."

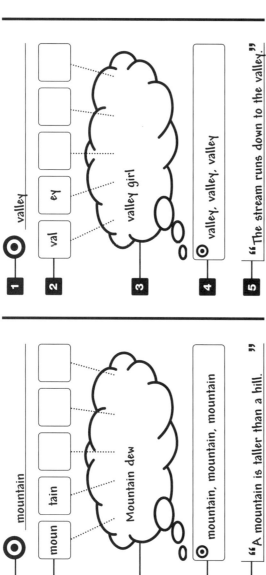

1 valley
2 val | ey
3
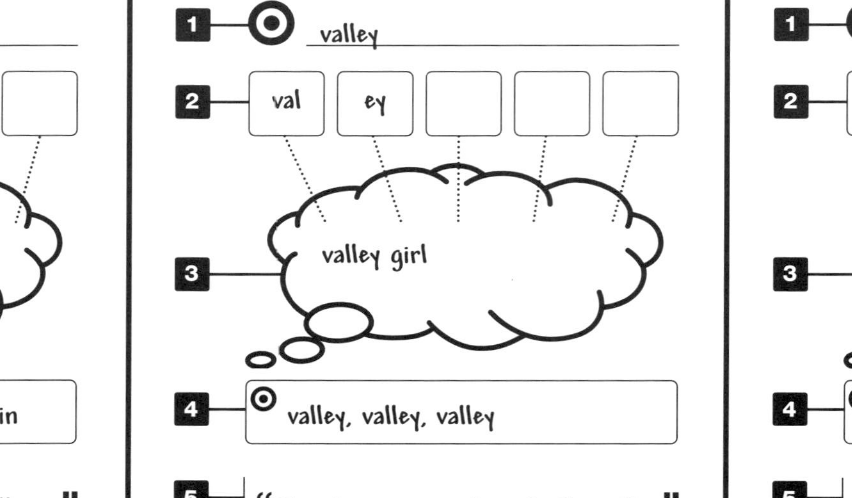

4 valley, valley, valley
5 "The stream runs down to the valley."

1 desert
2 des | ert
3
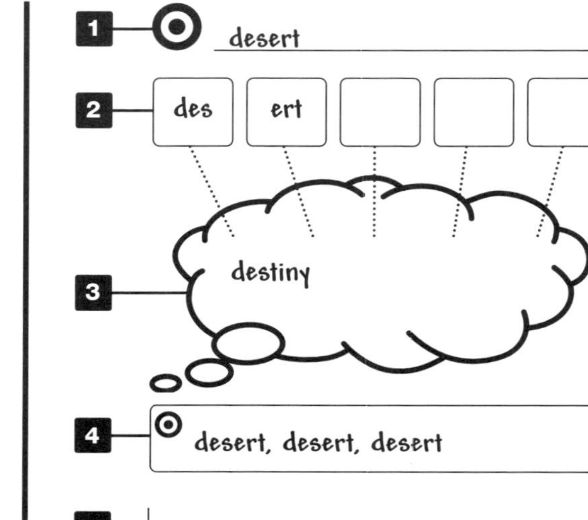

4 desert, desert, desert
5 "The desert is very hot and dry."

1 island
2 is | land
3
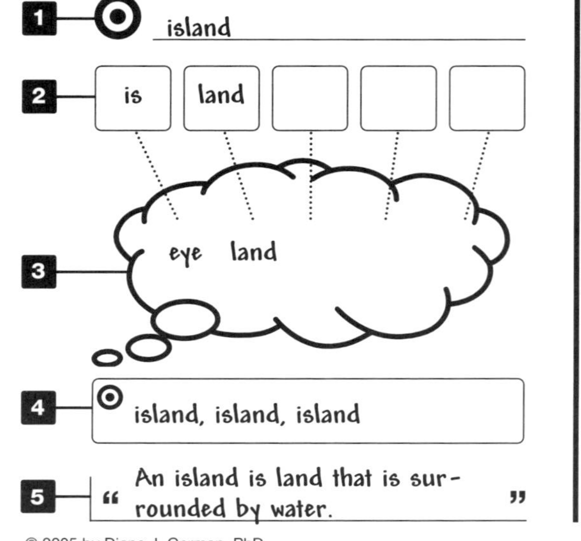

4 island, island, island
5 "An island is land that is surrounded by water."

1 river
2 riv | er
3 river bed or green river
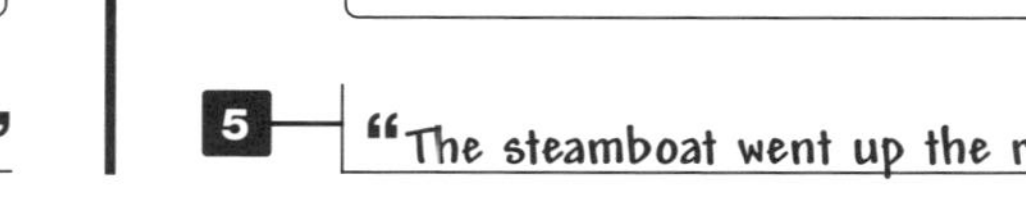
4 river, river, river
5 "The steamboat went up the river."

1 lake
2 lake
3
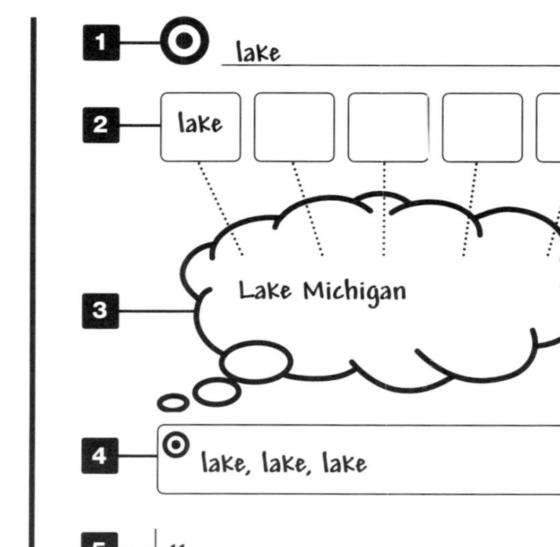

4 lake, lake, lake
5 "A lake is not as large as an ocean."

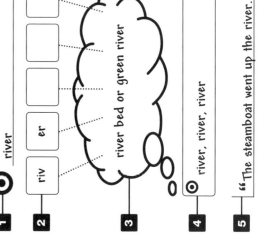

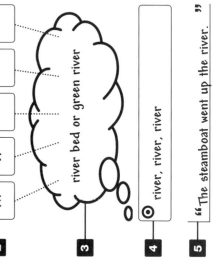

NAME CONTENT AREA Social Studies: Landforms DATE

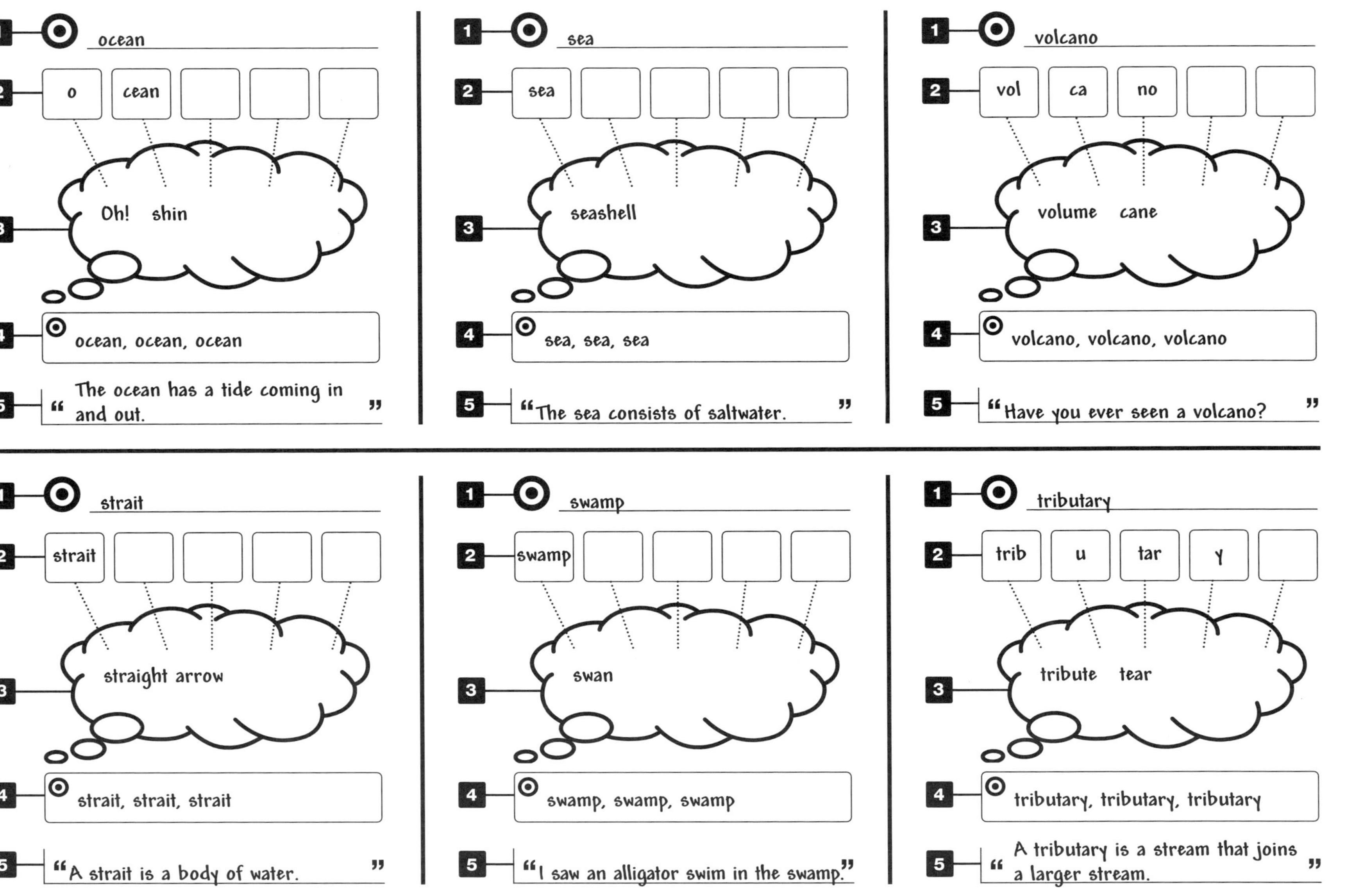

1 Target Word
2 Syllable-Dividing
3 Think Same-Sounds Syllable or Familiar-Word Cues
4 Rehearse Target Word as a Unit
5 Rehearse Target Word in a Sentence
1 ocean
2 o cean
3 Oh! shin
4 ocean, ocean, ocean
5 "The ocean has a tide coming in and out."
1 sea
2 sea
3 seashell
4 sea, sea, sea
5 "The sea consists of saltwater."
1 volcano
2 vol ca no
3 volume cane
4 volcano, volcano, volcano
5 "Have you ever seen a volcano?"
1 strait
2 strait
3 straight arrow
4 strait, strait, strait
5 "A strait is a body of water."
1 swamp
2 swamp
3 swan
4 swamp, swamp, swamp
5 "I saw an alligator swim in the swamp."
1 tributary
2 trib u tar y
3 tribute tear
4 tributary, tributary, tributary
5 "A tributary is a stream that joins a larger stream."

WFIP–2 SYLLABLE-DIVIDING AND SAME-SOUNDS SYLLABLE CUE STUDY FORM

NAME ____ CONTENT AREA Social Studies: Landforms DATE ____

1 Target Word
2 Syllable-Dividing
3 Think Same-Sounds Syllable or Familiar-Word Cues
4 Rehearse Target Word as a Unit
5 Rehearse Target Word in a Sentence

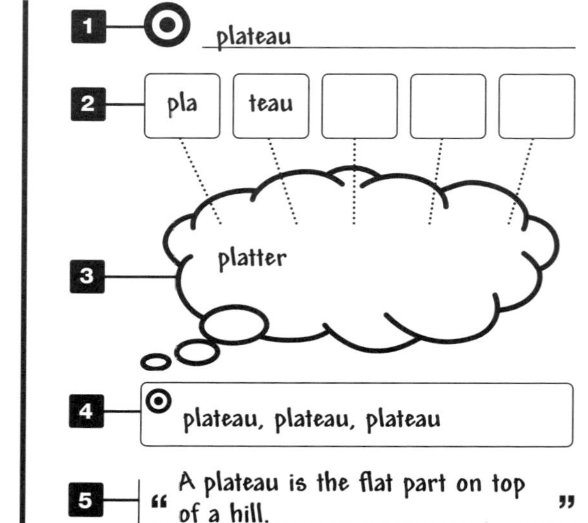
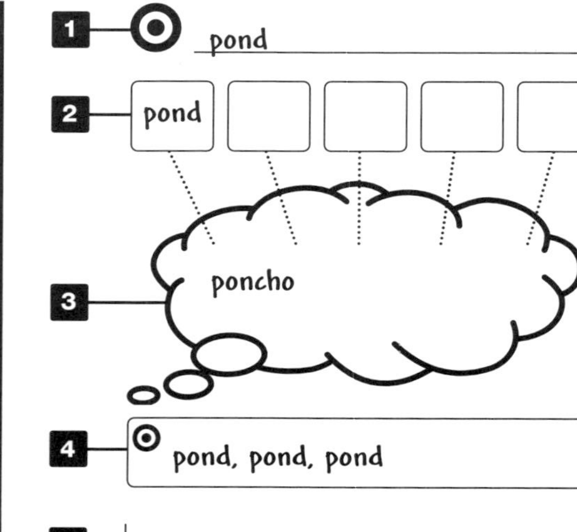
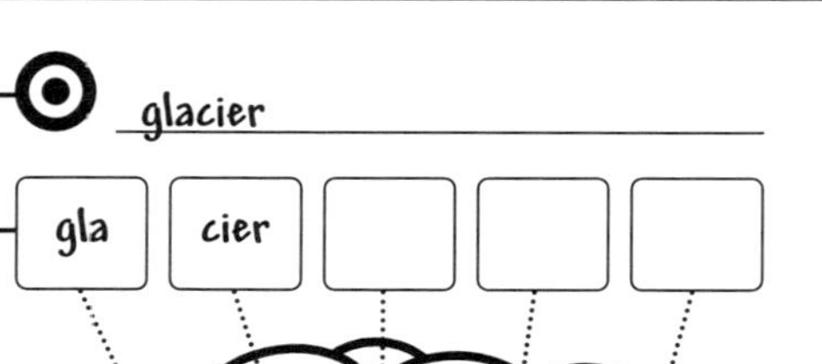

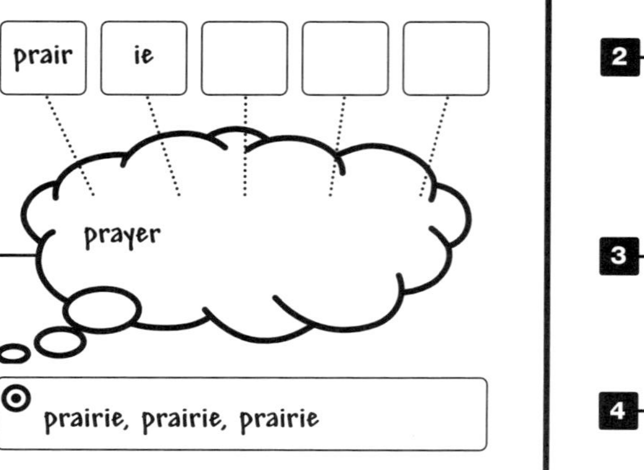
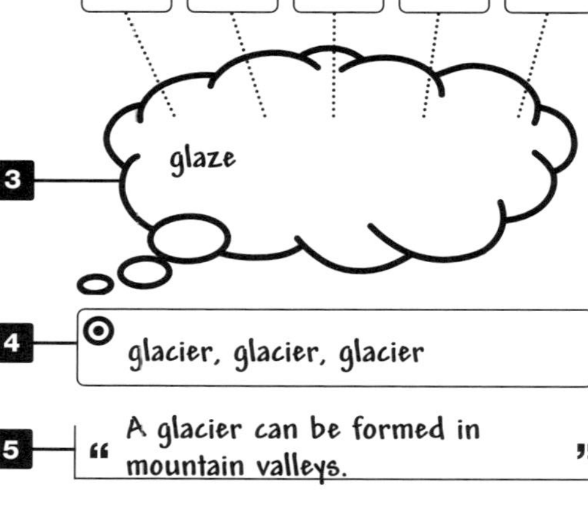
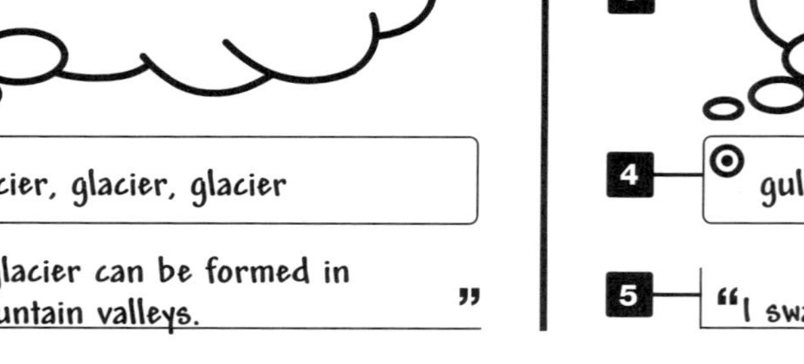

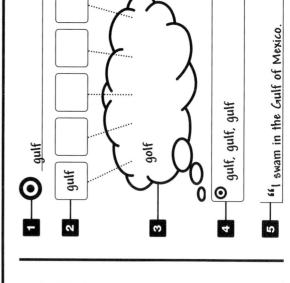

1 plain
2 plain | | | |
3 plane
4 plain, plain, plain
5 "In the midwest the land is made mostly of plains."

1 plateau
2 pla | teau | | |
3 platter
4 plateau, plateau, plateau
5 "A plateau is the flat part on top of a hill."

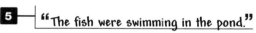

1 pond
2 pond | | | |
3 poncho
4 pond, pond, pond
5 "The fish were swimming in the pond."

1 prairie
2 prair | ie | | |
3 prayer
4 prairie, prairie, prairie
5 "Some animals live on the prairie."

1 glacier
2 gla | cier | | |
3 glaze
4 glacier, glacier, glacier
5 "A glacier can be formed in mountain valleys."

1 gulf
2 gulf | | | |
3 golf
4 gulf, gulf, gulf
5 "I swam in the Gulf of Mexico."

NAME **CONTENT AREA** Social Studies: Landforms **DATE**

1 Target Word
2 Syllable-Dividing
3 Think Same-Sounds Syllable or Familiar-Word Cues
4 Rehearse Target Word as a Unit
5 Rehearse Target Word in a Sentence

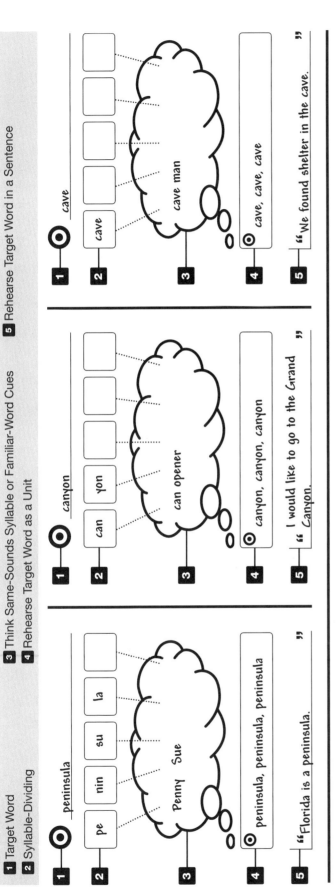

1 peninsula
2 pe | nin | su | la |
3 Penny Sue
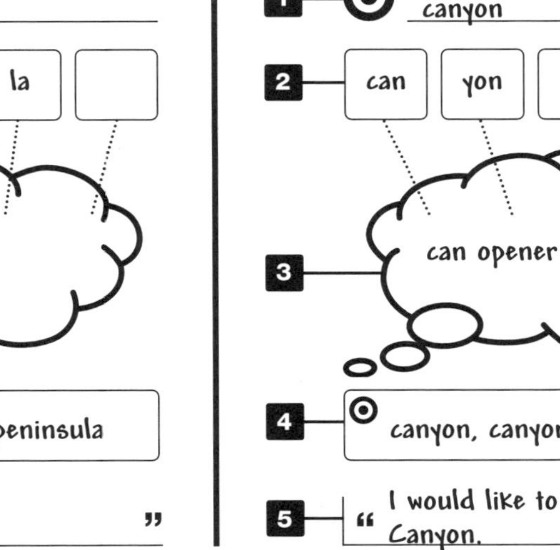
4 peninsula, peninsula, peninsula
5 "Florida is a peninsula."

1 canyon
2 can | yon | | |
3 can opener
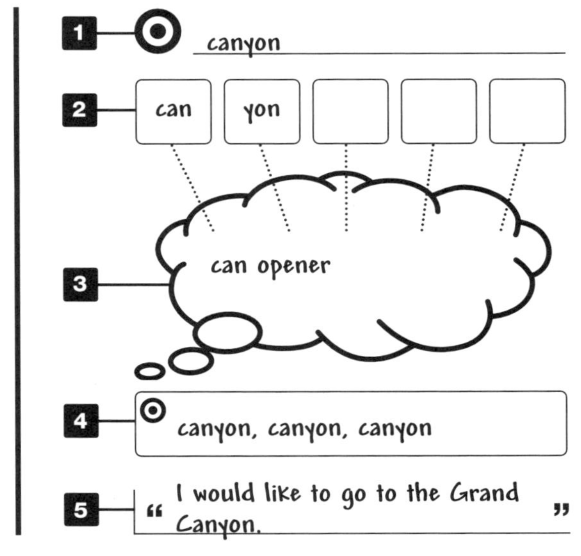
4 canyon, canyon, canyon
5 "I would like to go to the Grand Canyon."

1 cave
2 cave | | | |
3 cave man
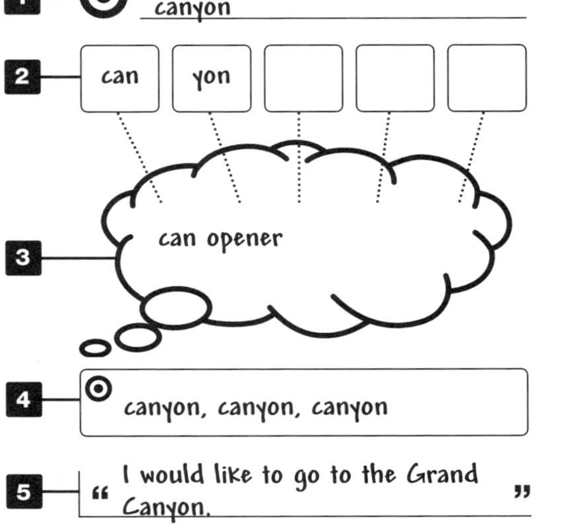
4 cave, cave, cave
5 "We found shelter in the cave."

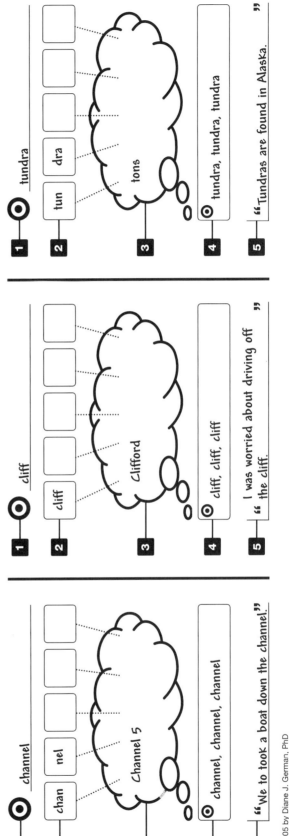

1 channel
2 chan | nel | | |
3 Channel 5
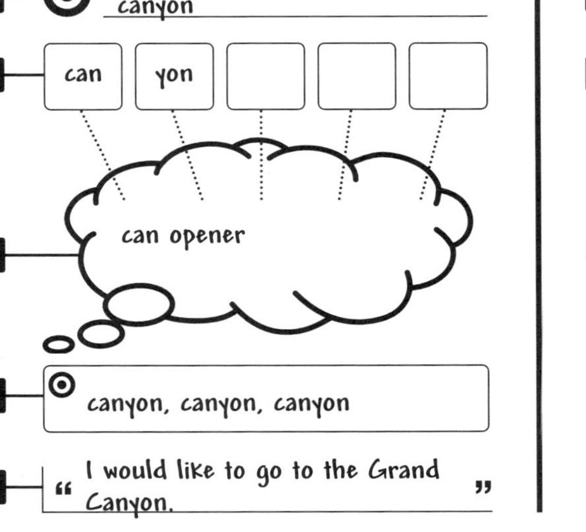
4 channel, channel, channel
5 "We to took a boat down the channel."

1 cliff
2 cliff | | | |
3 Clifford
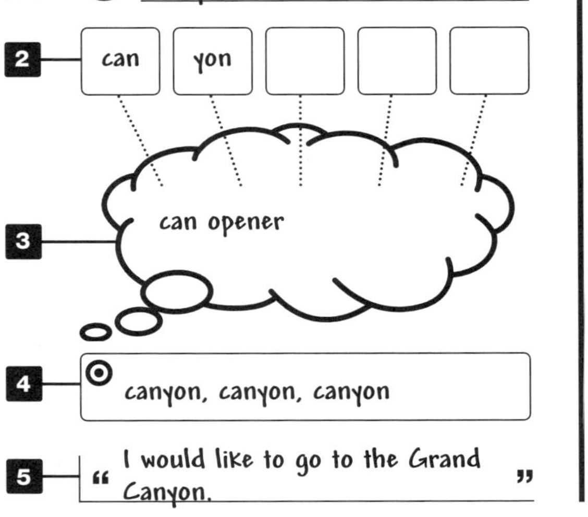
4 cliff, cliff, cliff
5 "I was worried about driving off the cliff."

1 tundra
2 tun | dra | | |
3 tons
4 tundra, tundra, tundra
5 "Tundras are found in Alaska."

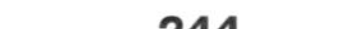

VOCABULARY SUBJECT: COMMUNITY

Objective: To teach learners to apply the syllable-dividing and same-sounds cues to community vocabulary

Instructions: The community vocabulary is presented in the list on this page and embedded in the completed Syllable-Dividing and Same-Sounds Syllable Cue Study Forms that follow. Have the learner practice the selected community vocabulary using the syllable-dividing and same-sounds cue retrieval strategies.

suburb	library	paramedic
neighborhood	city	citizen
mall	stadium	principal
hospital	ball park	librarian

NAME CONTENT AREA Social Studies: Community DATE

1 Target Word
2 Syllable-Dividing
3 Think Same-Sounds Syllable or Familiar-Word Cues
4 Rehearse Target Word as a Unit
5 Rehearse Target Word in a Sentence

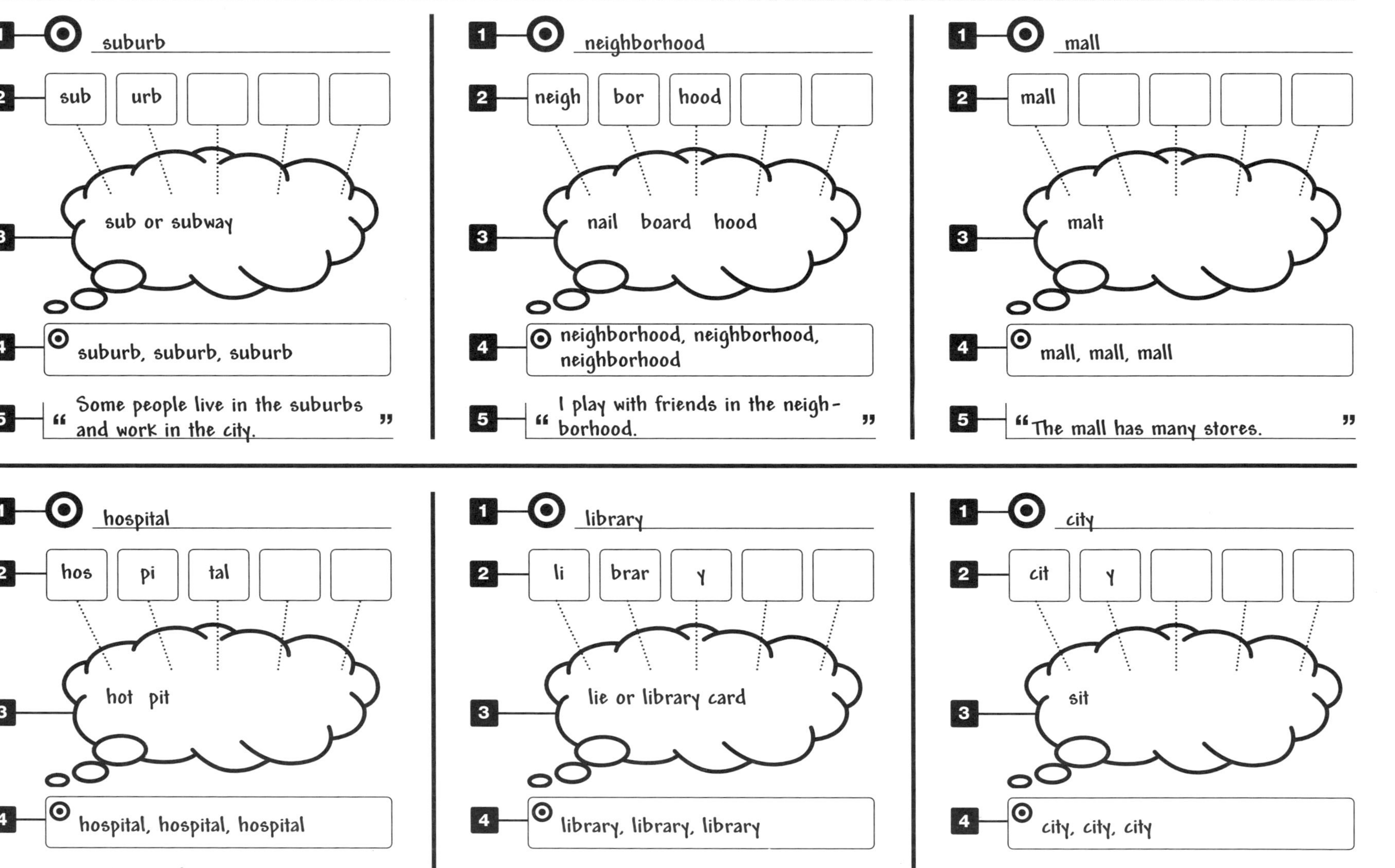

1 suburb
2 sub | urb
3 sub or subway
4 suburb, suburb, suburb
5 "Some people live in the suburbs and work in the city."

1 neighborhood
2 neigh | bor | hood
3 nail board hood
4 neighborhood, neighborhood, neighborhood
5 "I play with friends in the neigh-borhood."

1 mall
2 mall
3 malt
4 mall, mall, mall
5 "The mall has many stores."

1 hospital
2 hos | pi | tal
3 hot pit
4 hospital, hospital, hospital
5 "Doctors and nurses work in a hospital."

1 library
2 li | brar | y
3 lie or library card
4 library, library, library
5 "I get books at the library."

1 city
2 cit | y
3 sit
4 city, city, city
5 "Tall buildings are found in the city."

WFIP–2 SYLLABLE-DIVIDING AND SAME-SOUNDS SYLLABLE CUE STUDY FORM

NAME CONTENT AREA Social Studies: Community DATE

1 Target Word
2 Syllable-Dividing
3 Think Same-Sounds Syllable or Familiar-Word Cues
4 Rehearse Target Word as a Unit
5 Rehearse Target Word in a Sentence

1 stadium
2 sta | di | um | |
3 stay or football stadium
4 stadium, stadium, stadium
5 "I watch sports at the stadium."

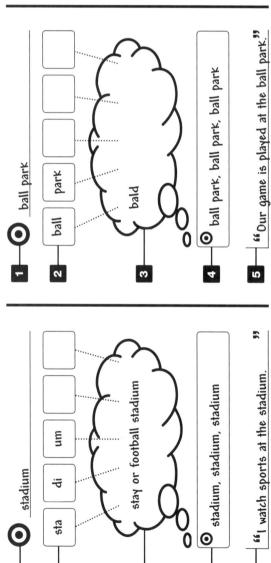

1 ball park
2 ball | park | | |
3 bald
4 ball park, ball park, ball park
5 "Our game is played at the ball park."

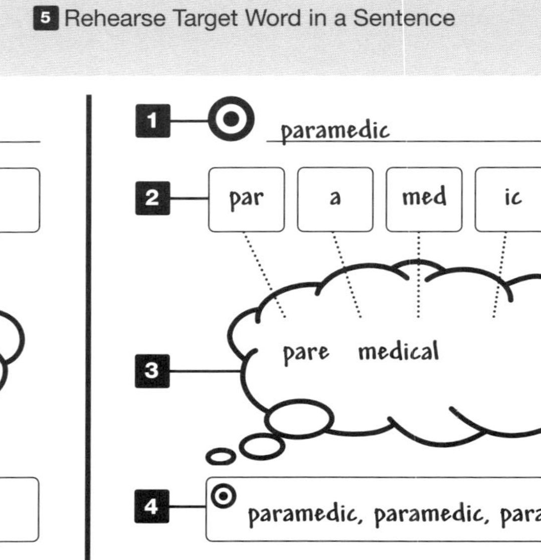

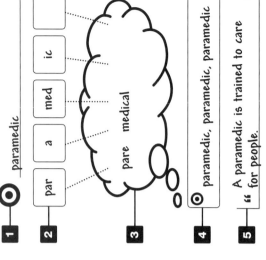

1 paramedic
2 par | a | med | ic |
3 pare medical
4 paramedic, paramedic, paramedic
5 "A paramedic is trained to care for people."

1 citizen
2 cit | i | zen | |
3 sit
4 citizen, citizen, citizen
5 "A citizen can vote in an election."

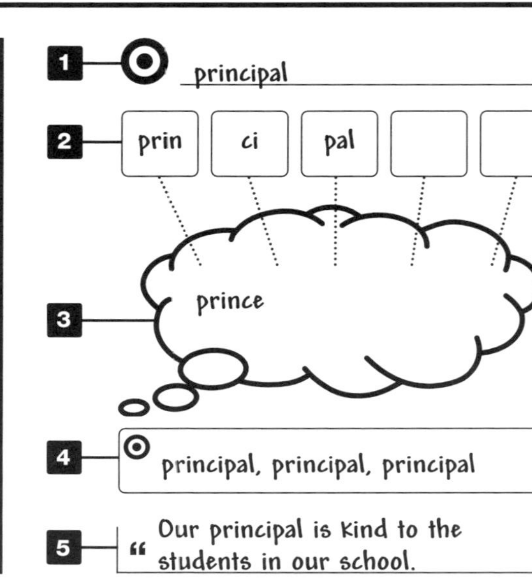

1 principal
2 prin | ci | pal | |
3 prince
4 principal, principal, principal
5 "Our principal is kind to the students in our school."

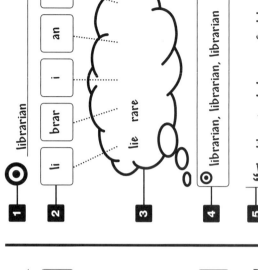

1 librarian
2 li | brar | i | an |
3 lie rare
4 librarian, librarian, librarian
5 "The librarian helps you find books."

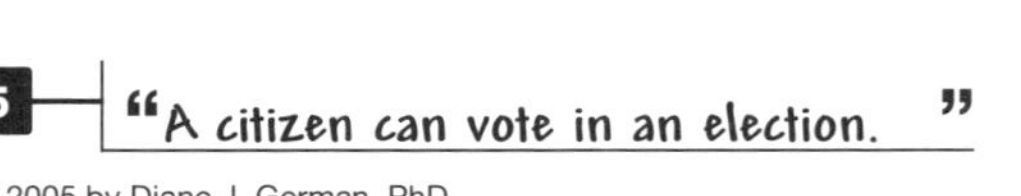

VOCABULARY SUBJECT: GOVERNMENT

Objective: To teach learners to apply the syllable-dividing and same-sounds cues to government vocabulary

Instructions: The government vocabulary is presented in the list on this page and embedded in the completed Syllable-Dividing and Same-Sounds Syllable Cue Study Forms that follow. Have the learner practice the selected government vocabulary using the syllable-dividing and same-sounds cue retrieval strategies.

congress	amendment	governor
executive	constitution	president
judicial	judge	cabinet
legislative	mayor	congressman

WFIP–2 SYLLABLE-DIVIDING AND SAME-SOUNDS SYLLABLE CUE STUDY FORM

NAME ____________ CONTENT AREA *Social Studies: Government* DATE ____________

1 Target Word
2 Syllable-Dividing
3 Think Same-Sounds Syllable or Familiar-Word Cues
4 Rehearse Target Word as a Unit
5 Rehearse Target Word in a Sentence

1 *congress*

2 con | gress | | |

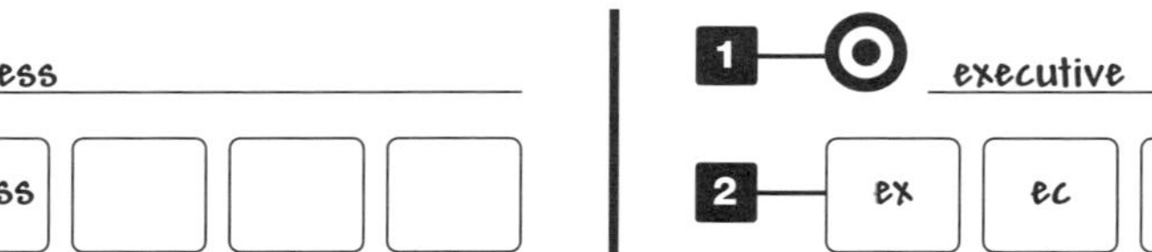

3 *contest*

4 *congress, congress, congress*

5 "*Congress meets in Washington.*"

1 *executive*

2 ex | ec | u | tive |

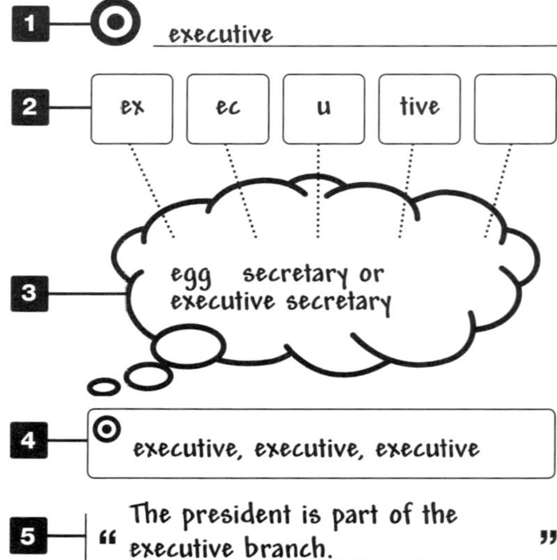

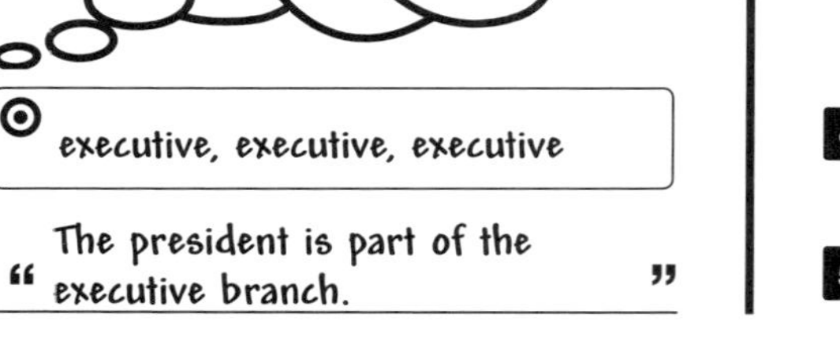

3 *egg secretary or executive secretary*

4 *executive, executive, executive*

5 "*The president is part of the executive branch.*"

1 *judicial*

2 ju | di | cial | |

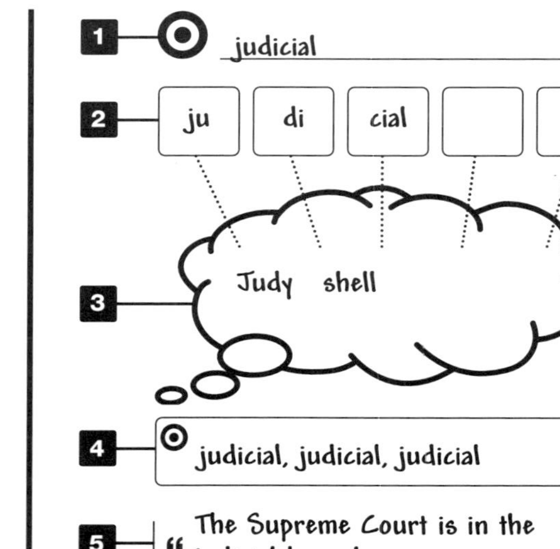

3 *Judy shell*

4 *judicial, judicial, judicial*

5 "*The Supreme Court is in the judicial branch.*"

1 *legislative*

2 leg | is | la | tive |

3 *ledge is late*

4 *legislative, legislative, legislative*

5 "*The legislative branch makes the laws.*"

1 *amendment*

2 a | mend | ment | |

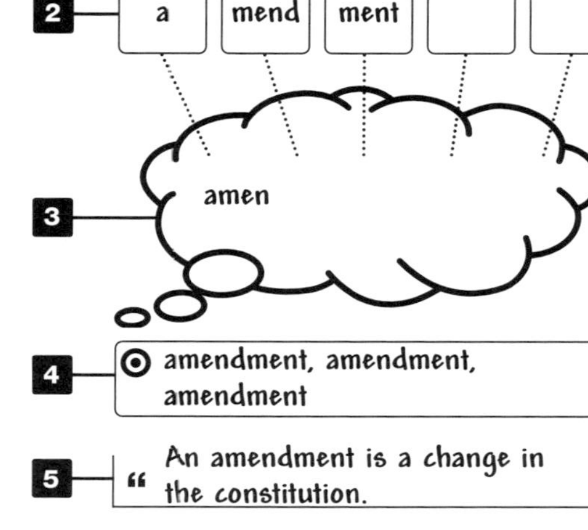

3 *amen*

4 *amendment, amendment, amendment*

5 "*An amendment is a change in the constitution.*"

1 *constitution*

2 con | sti | tu | tion |

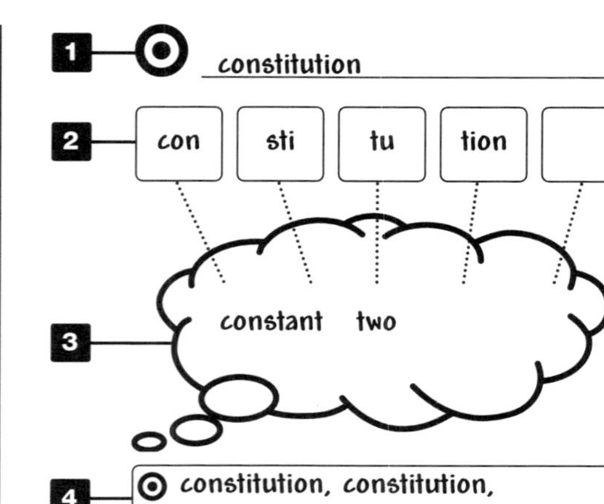

3 *constant two*

4 *constitution, constitution, constitution*

5 "*We study the U.S. Constitution in class.*"

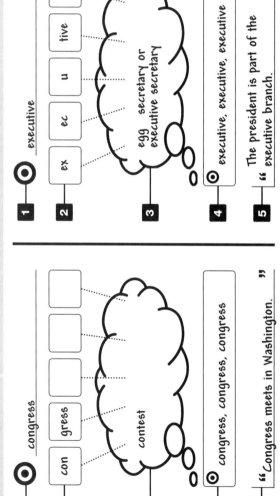

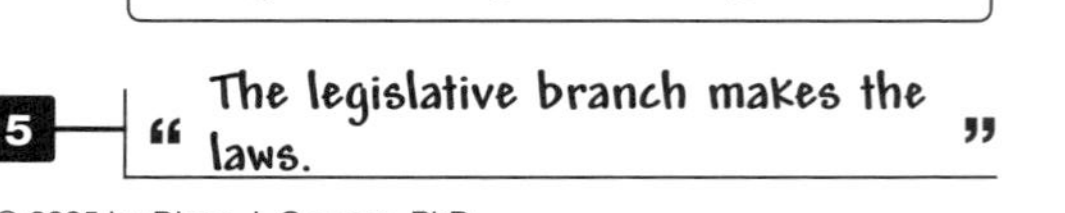

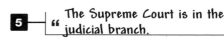

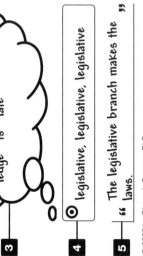

NAME CONTENT AREA *Social Studies: Government* DATE

1 Target Word
2 Syllable-Dividing
3 Think Same-Sounds Syllable or Familiar-Word Cues
4 Rehearse Target Word as a Unit
5 Rehearse Target Word in a Sentence

1 judge

2 judge | | | |

3 Judge Judy or judge the contest

4 judge, judge, judge

5 "The judge presides over the court."

1 mayor

2 may | or | | |

3
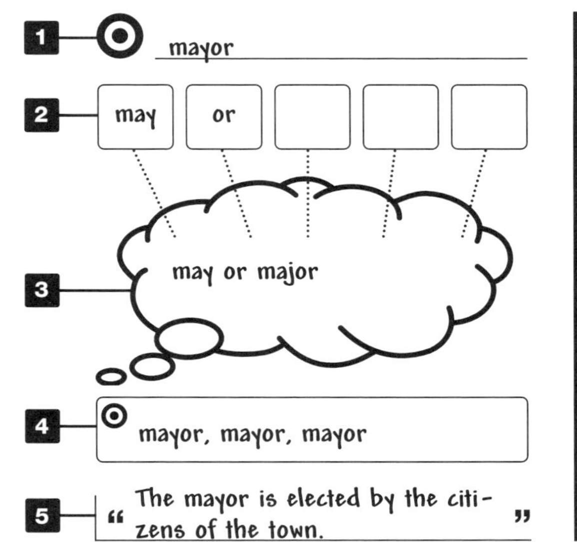

4 mayor, mayor, mayor

5 "The mayor is elected by the citizens of the town."

1 governor

2 gov | er | nor | |

3
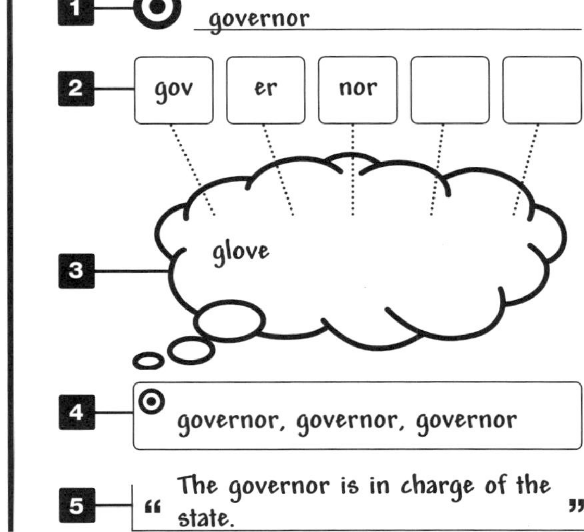

4 governor, governor, governor

5 "The governor is in charge of the state."

1 president

2 pres | i | dent | |

3 press dent

4 president, president, president

5 "The president is elected every four years."

1 cabinet

2 cab | i | net | |

3
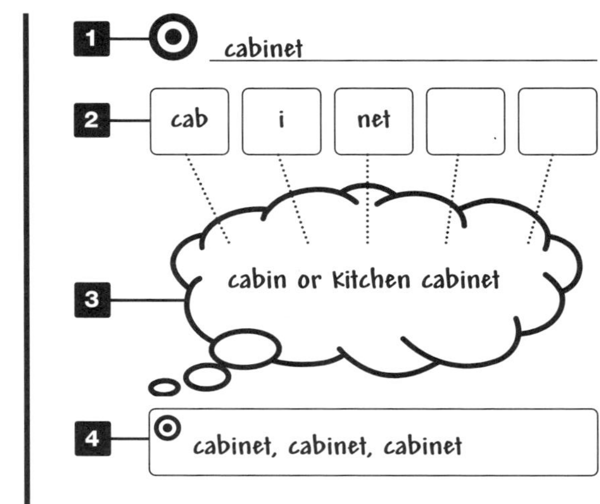

4 cabinet, cabinet, cabinet

5 "He is on the president's cabinet."

1 congressman

2 con | gress | man | |

3
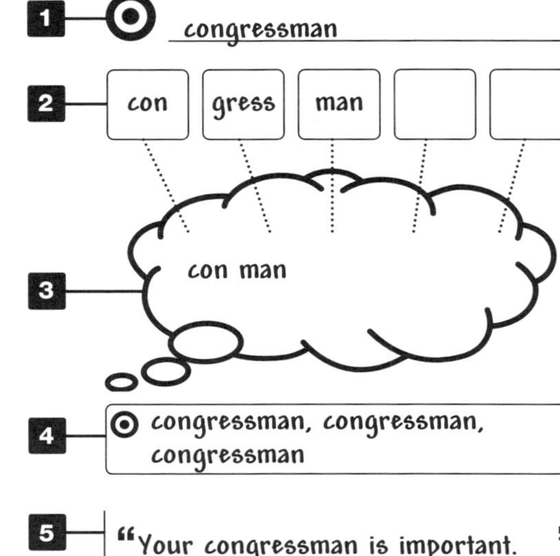

4 congressman, congressman, congressman

5 "Your congressman is important."

VOCABULARY SUBJECT: GLOBAL CONNECTIONS

Objective: To teach learners to apply the syllable-dividing and same-sounds cues to global connections vocabulary

Instructions: The global connections vocabulary is presented in the list on this page and embedded in the completed Syllable-Dividing and Same-Sounds Syllable Cue Study Forms that follow. Have the learner practice the selected global connections vocabulary using the syllable-dividing and same-sounds cue retrieval strategies.

globe	boundary	latitude
atlas	equator	longitude
legend	continent	prime meridian
region	hemisphere	resource

NAME CONTENT AREA *Social Studies: Global Connections* DATE

1 Target Word
2 Syllable-Dividing
3 Think Same-Sounds Syllable or Familiar-Word Cues
4 Rehearse Target Word as a Unit
5 Rehearse Target Word in a Sentence

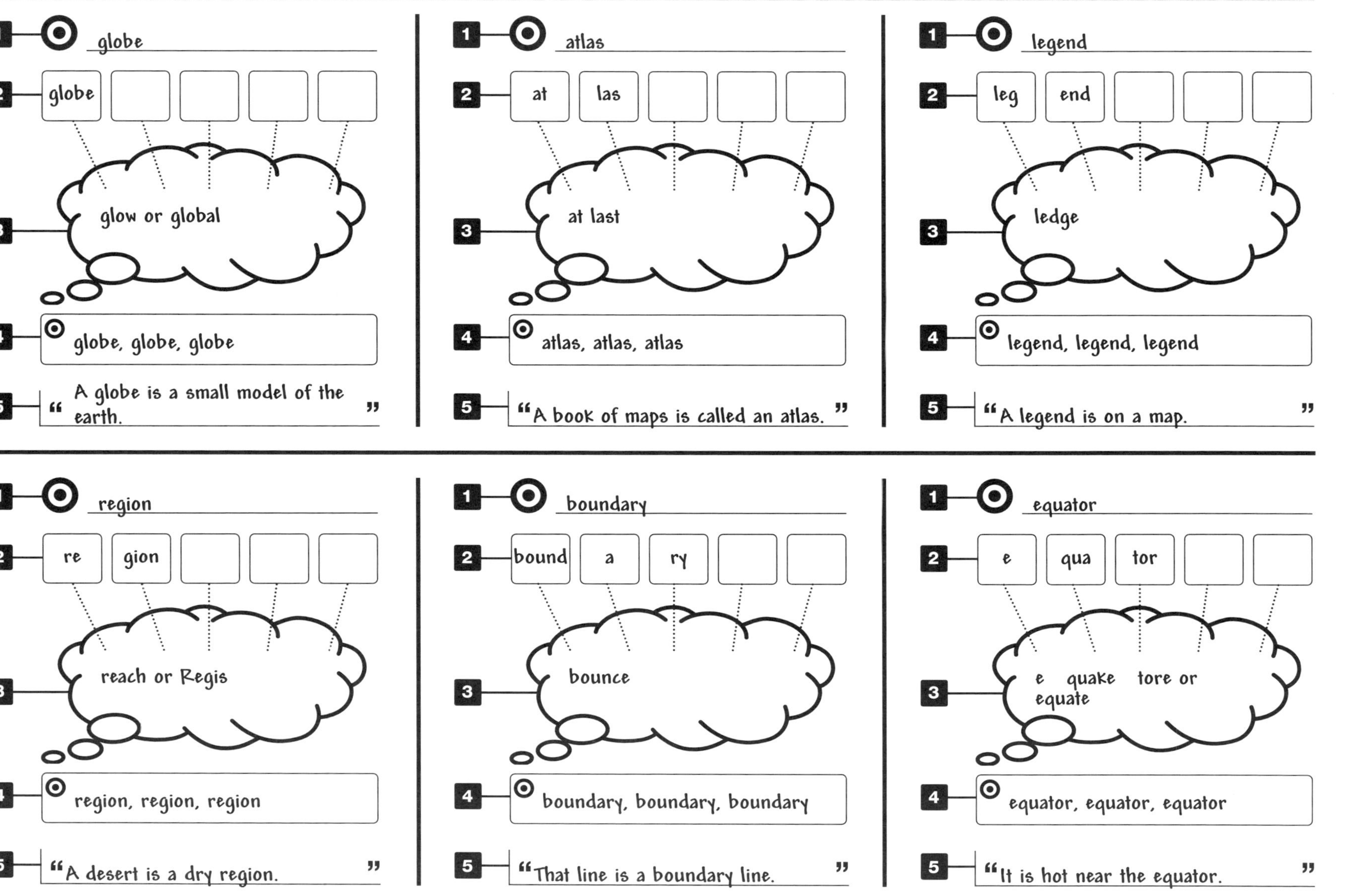
1 globe
2 globe
3 glow or global
4 globe, globe, globe
5 "A globe is a small model of the earth."
1 atlas
2 at | las
3 at last
4 atlas, atlas, atlas
5 "A book of maps is called an atlas."
1 legend
2 leg | end
3 ledge
4 legend, legend, legend
5 "A legend is on a map."
1 region
2 re | gion
3 reach or Regis
4 region, region, region
5 "A desert is a dry region."
1 boundary
2 bound | a | ry
3 bounce
4 boundary, boundary, boundary
5 "That line is a boundary line."
1 equator
2 e | qua | tor
3 e quake tore or equate
4 equator, equator, equator
5 "It is hot near the equator."

WFIP–2 SYLLABLE-DIVIDING AND SAME-SOUNDS SYLLABLE CUE STUDY FORM

NAME   **CONTENT AREA** Social Studies: Global Connections   **DATE**

1 Target Word
2 Syllable-Dividing
3 Think Same-Sounds Syllable or Familiar-Word Cues
4 Rehearse Target Word as a Unit
5 Rehearse Target Word in a Sentence

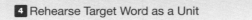

1 continent

2 con | ti | nent | |

3 content or continental di-vide

4 continent, continent, continent

5 “A large area of land is called a continent.”

1 hemisphere

2 hem | i | sphere | |

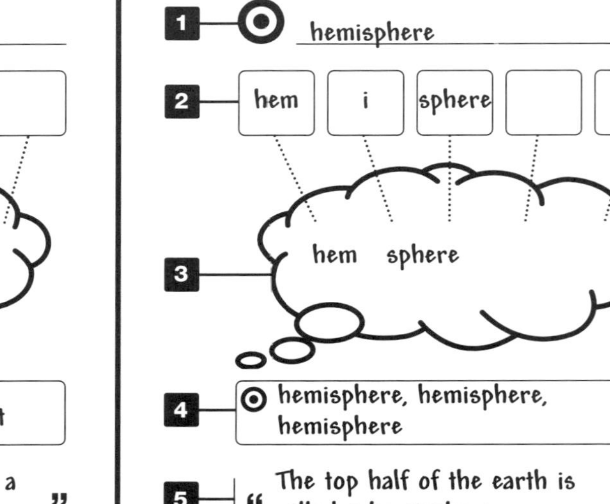

3 hem sphere

4 hemisphere, hemisphere, hemisphere

5 “The top half of the earth is called a hemisphere.”

1 latitude

2 lat | i | tude | |

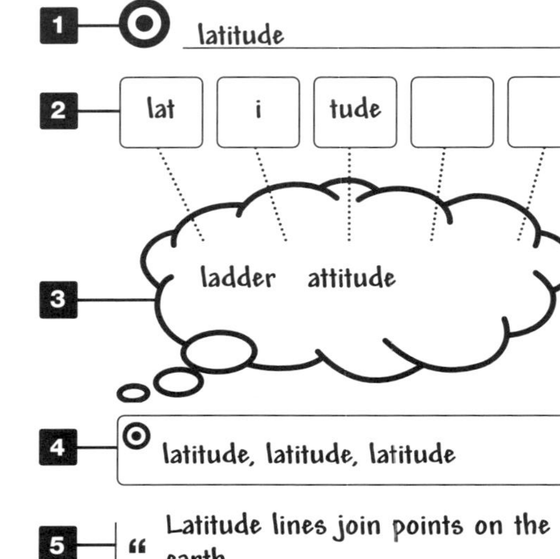

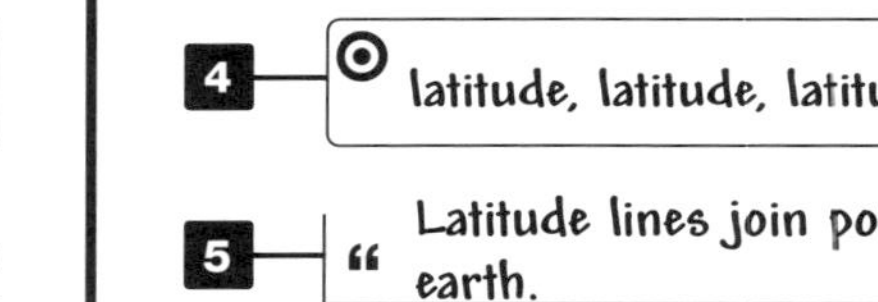

3 ladder attitude

4 latitude, latitude, latitude

5 “Latitude lines join points on the earth.”

1 longitude

2 lon | gi | tude | |

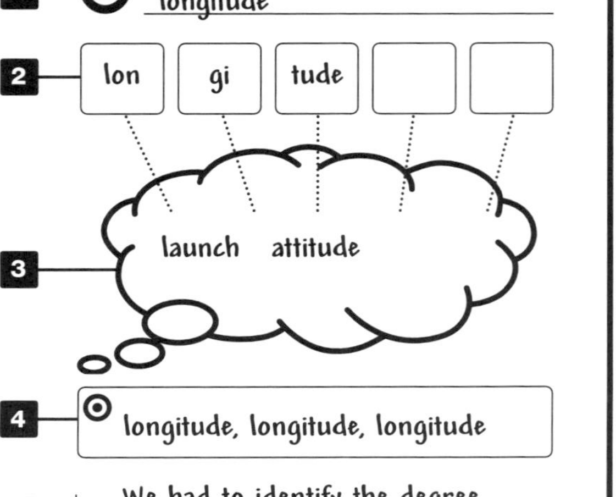

3 launch attitude

4 longitude, longitude, longitude

5 “We had to identify the degree longitude for our city.”

1 prime meridian

2 prime | me | rid | i | an

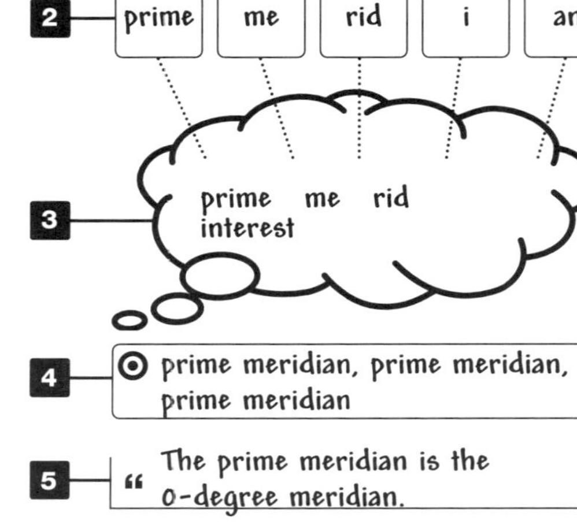

3 prime me rid interest

4 prime meridian, prime meridian, prime meridian

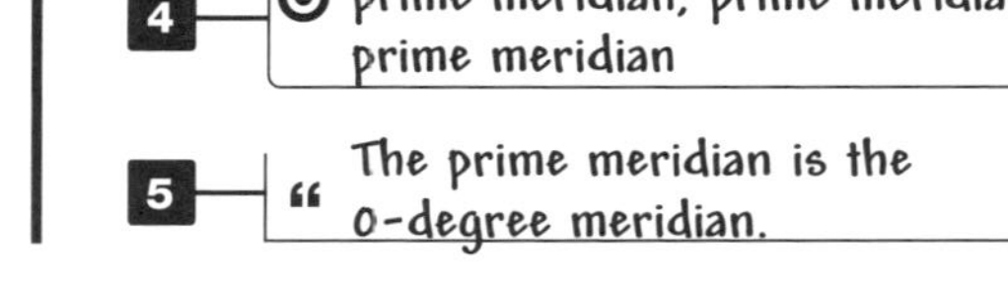

5 “The prime meridian is the 0-degree meridian.”

1 resource

2 re | source | | |

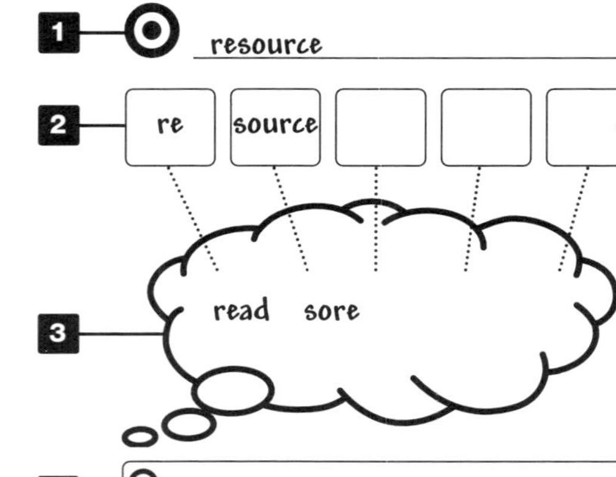

3 read sore

4 resource, resource, resource

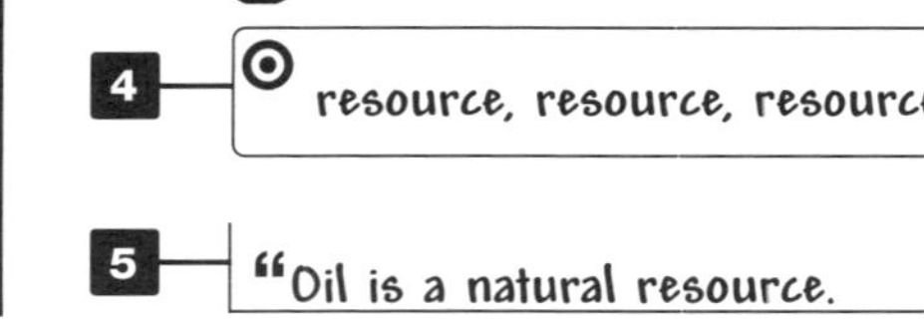

5 “Oil is a natural resource.”

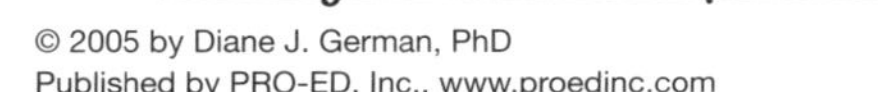

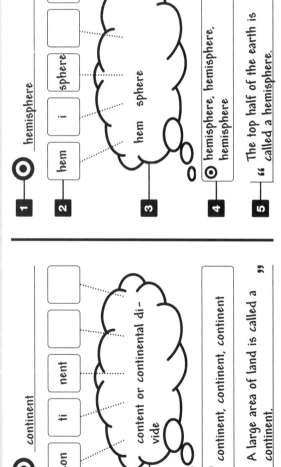

VOCABULARY SUBJECT: MATH

Objective: To teach learners to apply the syllable-dividing and same-sounds cues to math vocabulary

Instructions: The math vocabulary is presented in the list on this page and embedded in the completed Syllable-Dividing and Same-Sounds Syllable Cue Study Forms that follow. Have the learner practice the selected math vocabulary using the syllable-dividing and same-sounds cue retrieval strategies.

calculate	zero	angle
estimate	ones	parallel
formula	hour	degrees
perpendicular	watch	area
even	second	circumference
odd	minute	compass
order	tens	ruler
add	hundreds	metric
subtract	thousand	array
problem	million	congruent
sum	addition	geometry
total	subtraction	polygon
value	multiplication	
place	division	

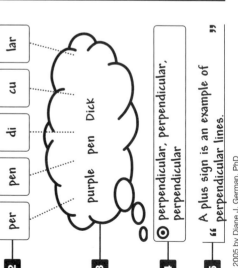

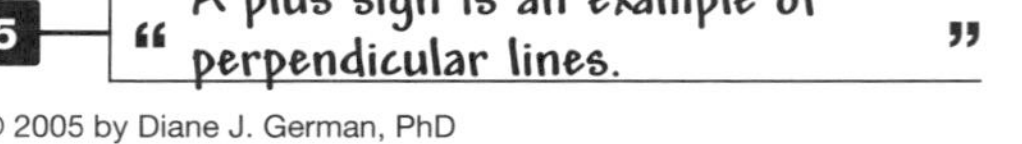

WFIP–2 SYLLABLE-DIVIDING AND SAME-SOUNDS SYLLABLE CUE STUDY FORM

NAME CONTENT AREA Math DATE

1 Target Word
2 Syllable-Dividing
3 Think Same-Sounds Syllable or Familiar-Word Cues
4 Rehearse Target Word as a Unit
5 Rehearse Target Word in a Sentence

1 calculate

2 cal | cu | late | |

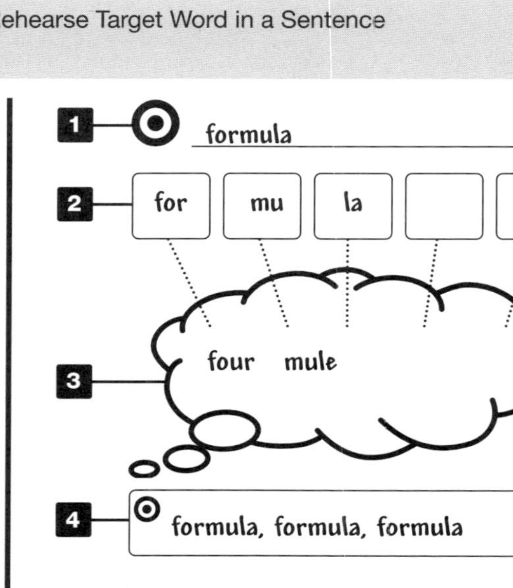

3 calendar cute

4 calculate, calculate, calculate

5 "Calculate the sum for each problem."

1 estimate

2 es | ti | mate | |

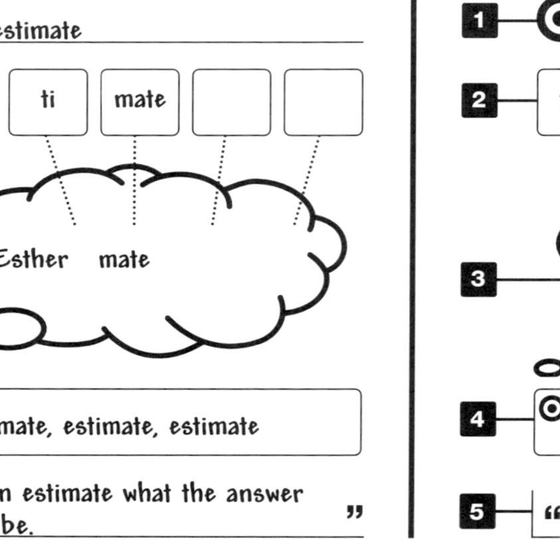

3 Esther mate

4 estimate, estimate, estimate

5 "I can estimate what the answer will be."

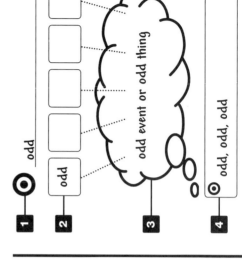

1 formula

2 for | mu | la | |

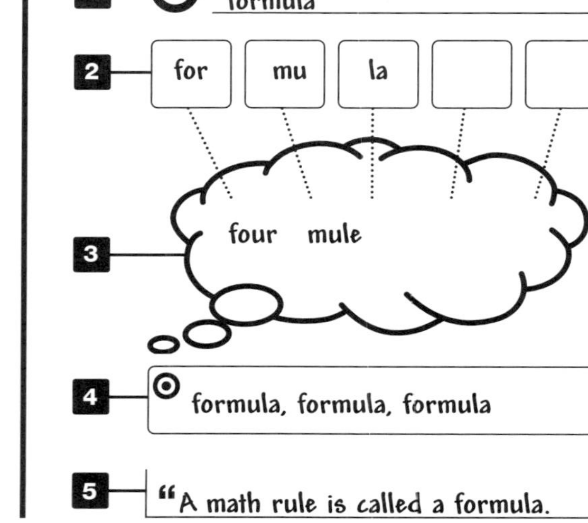

3 four mule

4 formula, formula, formula

5 "A math rule is called a formula."

1 perpendicular

2 per | pen | di | cu | lar

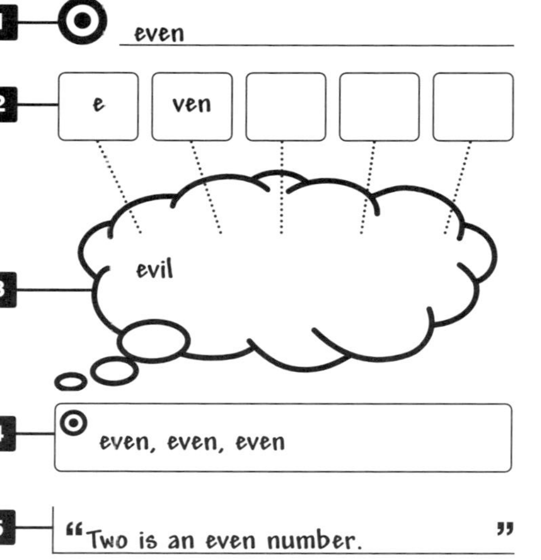

3 purple pen Dick

4 perpendicular, perpendicular, perpendicular

5 "A plus sign is an example of perpendicular lines."

1 even

2 e | ven | | |

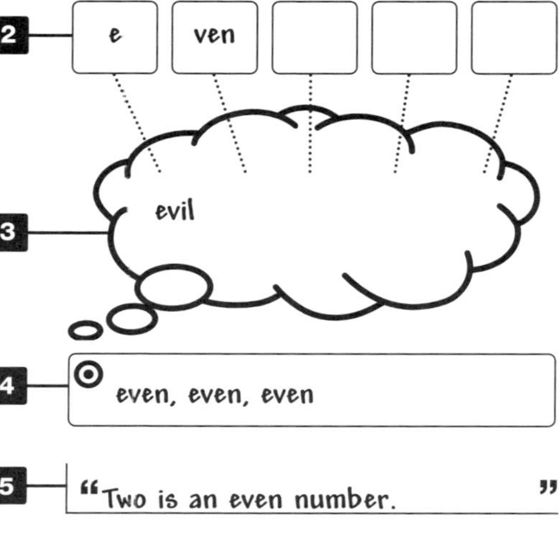

3 evil

4 even, even, even

5 "Two is an even number."

1 odd

2 odd | | | |

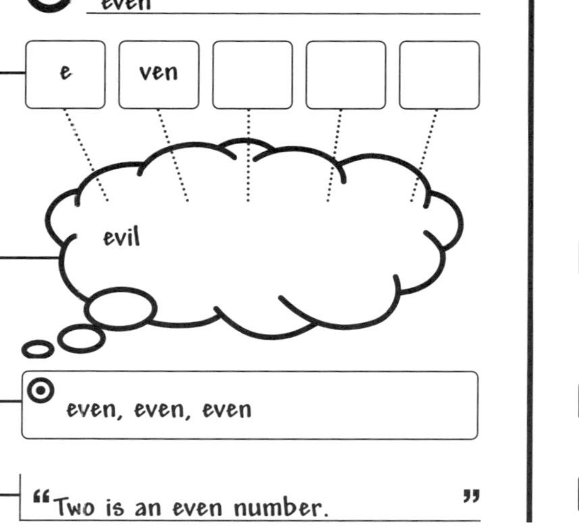

3 odd event or odd thing

4 odd, odd, odd

5 "One is an odd number."

NAME CONTENT AREA Math DATE

1 Target Word
2 Syllable-Dividing
3 Think Same-Sounds Syllable or Familiar-Word Cues
4 Rehearse Target Word as a Unit
5 Rehearse Target Word in a Sentence

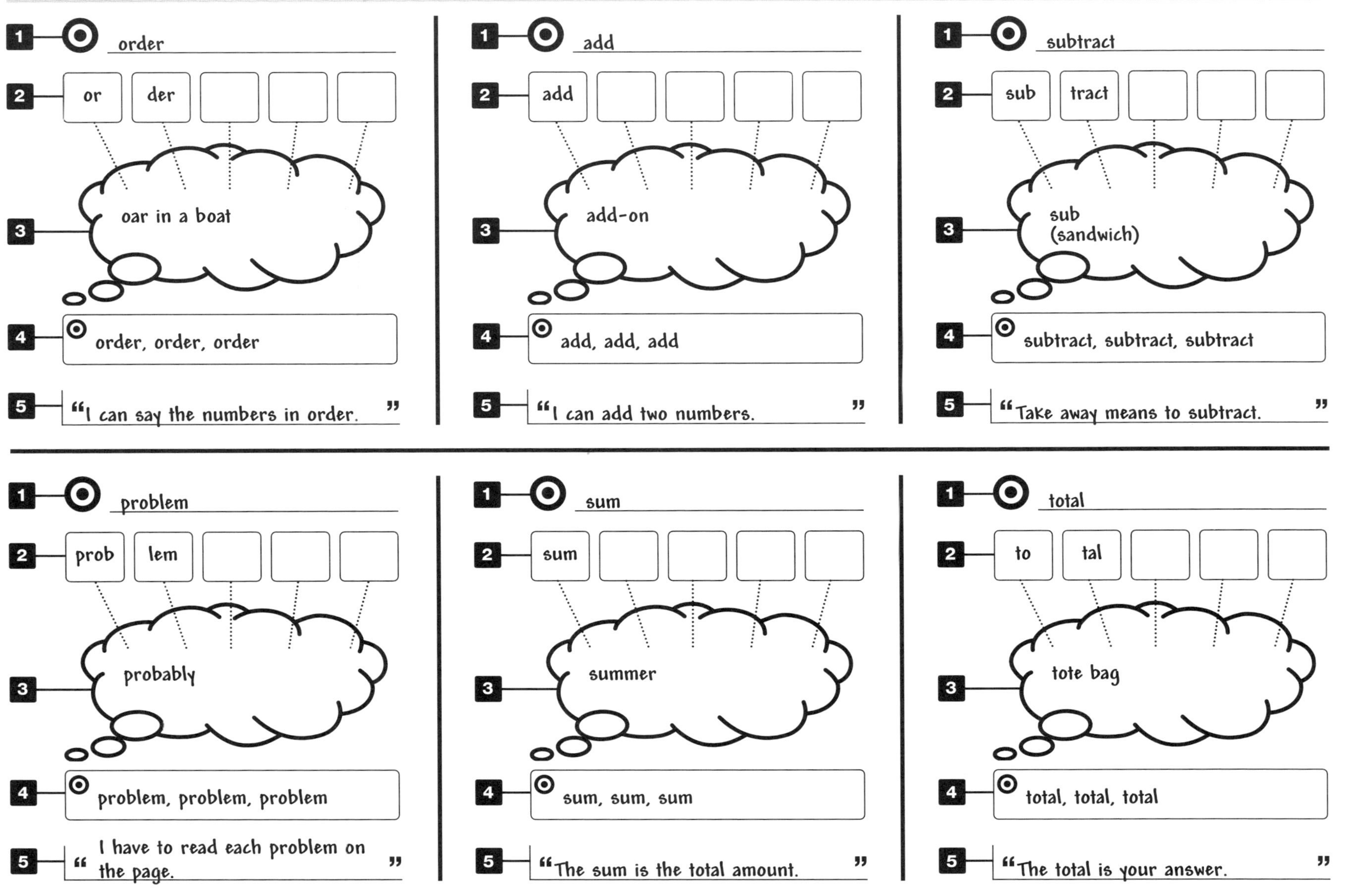
1 order
2 or | der
3 oar in a boat
4 order, order, order
5 "I can say the numbers in order."
1 add
2 add
3 add-on
4 add, add, add
5 "I can add two numbers."
1 subtract
2 sub | tract
3 sub (sandwich)
4 subtract, subtract, subtract
5 "Take away means to subtract."
1 problem
2 prob | lem
3 probably
4 problem, problem, problem
5 "I have to read each problem on the page."
1 sum
2 sum
3 summer
4 sum, sum, sum
5 "The sum is the total amount."
1 total
2 to | tal
3 tote bag
4 total, total, total
5 "The total is your answer."

WFIP–2 SYLLABLE-DIVIDING AND SAME-SOUNDS SYLLABLE CUE STUDY FORM

NAME CONTENT AREA Math DATE

1 Target Word
2 Syllable-Dividing
3 Think Same-Sounds Syllable or Familiar-Word Cues
4 Rehearse Target Word as a Unit
5 Rehearse Target Word in a Sentence

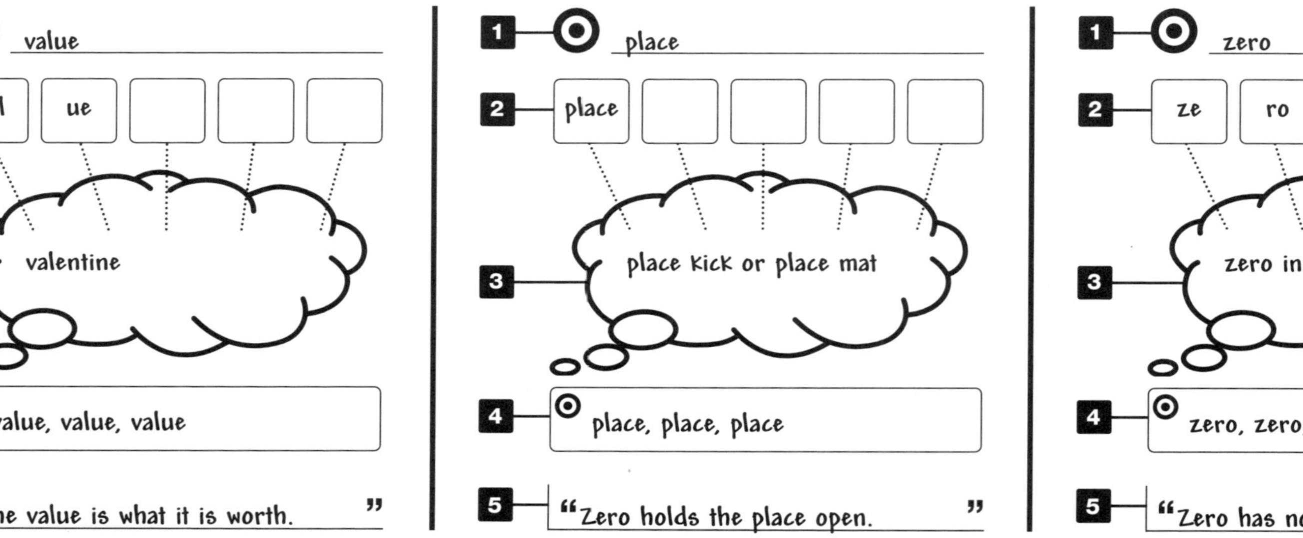
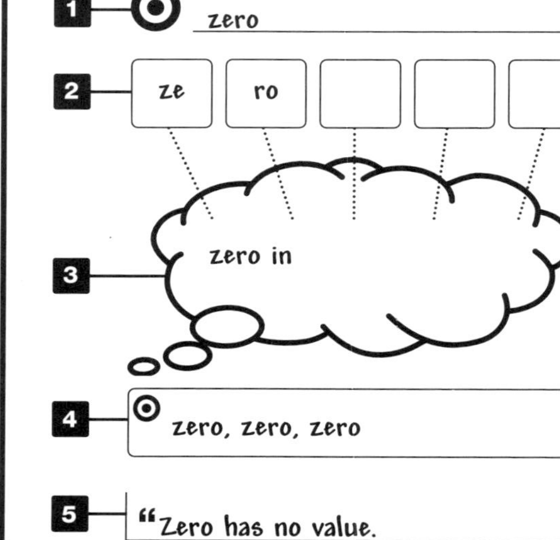
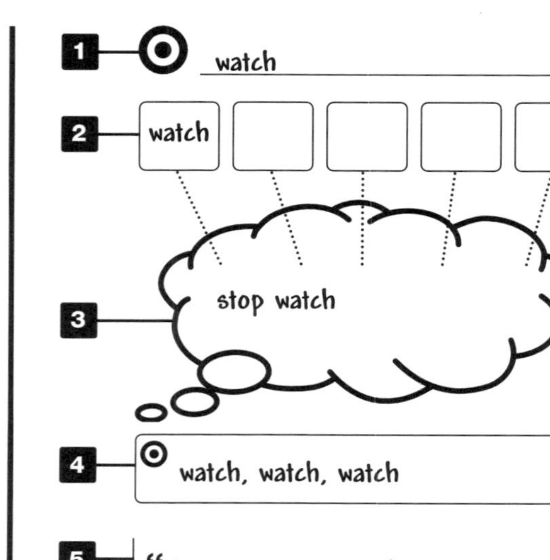

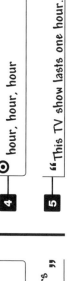

1 value
2 val | ue
3 valentine
4 value, value, value
5 "The value is what it is worth."

1 place
2 place
3 place kick or place mat
4 place, place, place
5 "Zero holds the place open."

1 zero
2 ze | ro
3 zero in
4 zero, zero, zero
5 "Zero has no value."

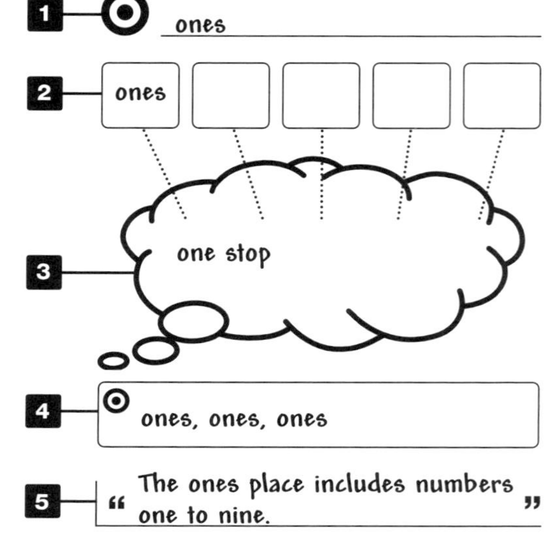
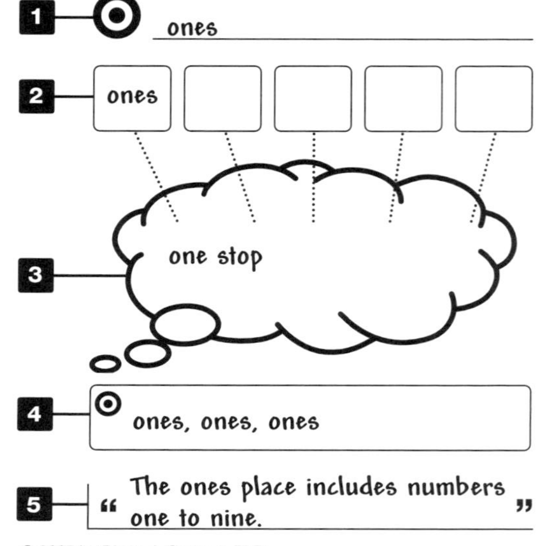
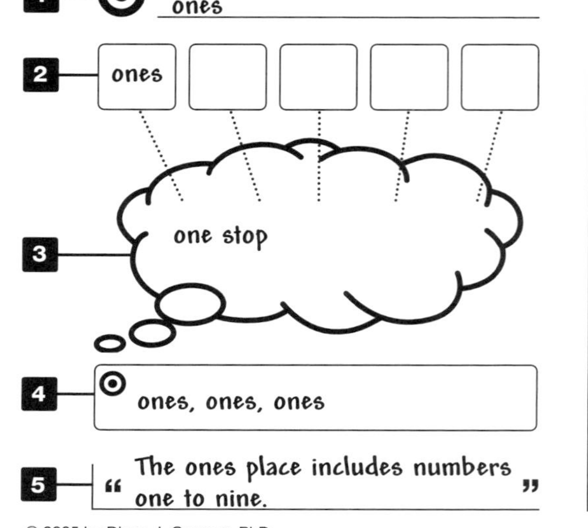
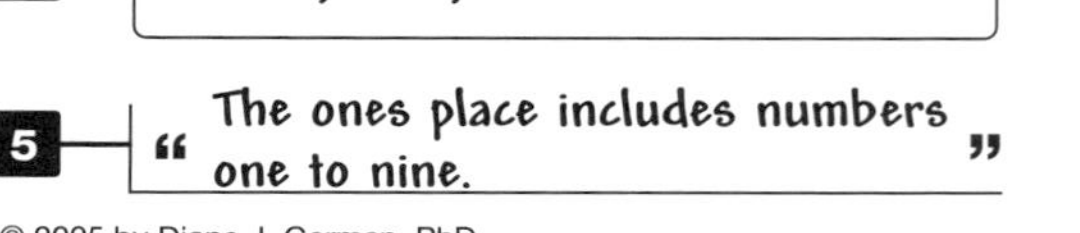

1 ones
2 ones
3 one stop
4 ones, ones, ones
5 "The ones place includes numbers one to nine."

1 hour
2 hour
3 hourglass
4 hour, hour, hour
5 "This TV show lasts one hour."

1 watch
2 watch
3 stop watch
4 watch, watch, watch
5 "You wear your watch on your wrist."

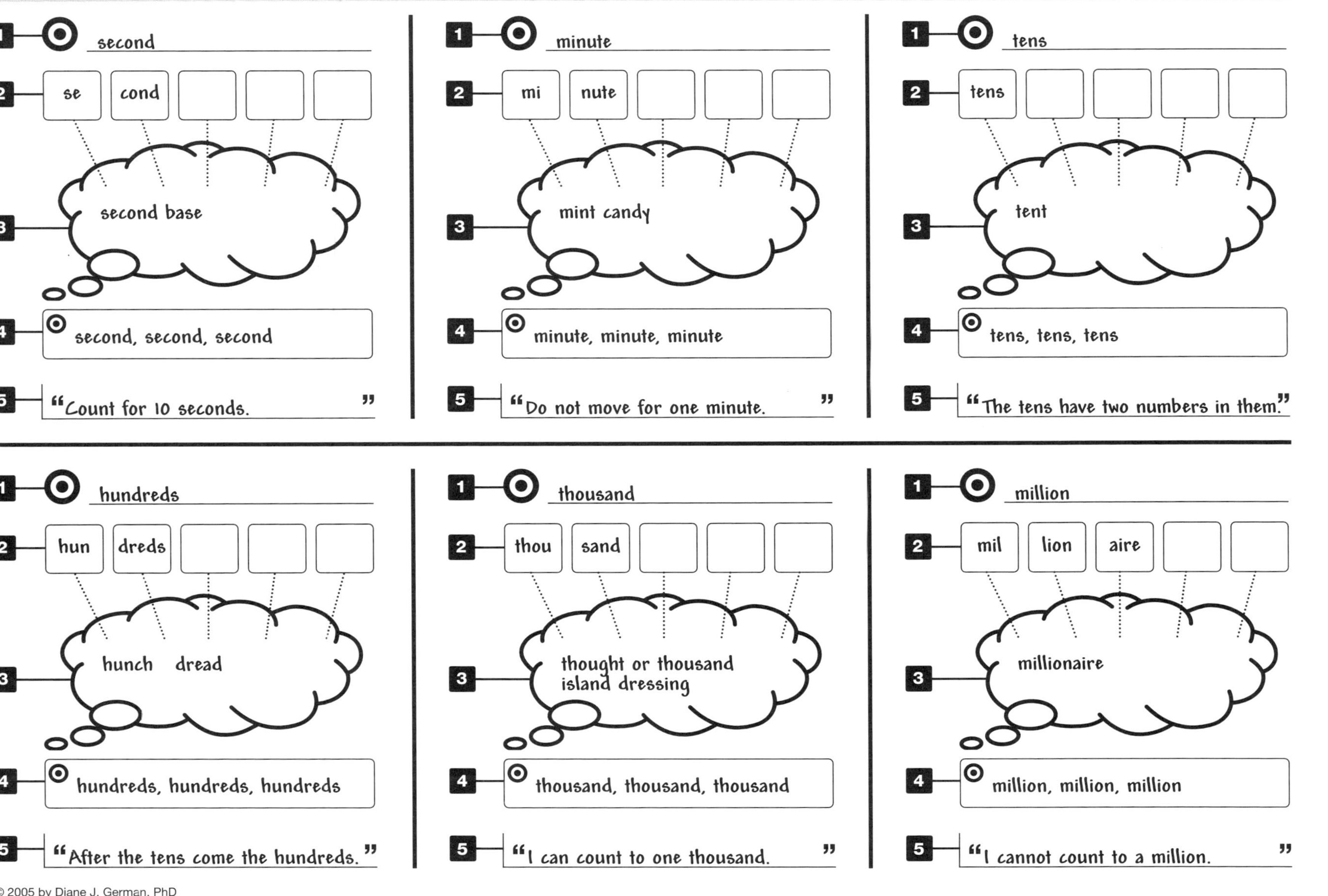

NAME | CONTENT AREA Math | DATE

1 Target Word
2 Syllable-Dividing
3 Think Same-Sounds Syllable or Familiar-Word Cues
4 Rehearse Target Word as a Unit
5 Rehearse Target Word in a Sentence

1 second
2 se | cond
3 second base
4 second, second, second
5 "Count for 10 seconds."

1 minute
2 mi | nute
3 mint candy
4 minute, minute, minute
5 "Do not move for one minute."

1 tens
2 tens
3 tent
4 tens, tens, tens
5 "The tens have two numbers in them."

1 hundreds
2 hun | dreds
3 hunch dread
4 hundreds, hundreds, hundreds
5 "After the tens come the hundreds."

1 thousand
2 thou | sand
3 thought or thousand island dressing
4 thousand, thousand, thousand
5 "I can count to one thousand."

1 million
2 mil | lion | aire
3 millionaire
4 million, million, million
5 "I cannot count to a million."

Published by PRO-ED, Inc., www.proedinc.com

WFIP–2 SYLLABLE-DIVIDING AND SAME-SOUNDS SYLLABLE CUE STUDY FORM

NAME CONTENT AREA Math DATE

1 Target Word
2 Syllable-Dividing
3 Think Same-Sounds Syllable or Familiar-Word Cues
4 Rehearse Target Word as a Unit
5 Rehearse Target Word in a Sentence

1 addition

2 ad | di | tion | |

3 addict

4 addition, addition, addition

5 "Addition is putting things together."

1 subtraction

2 sub | trac | tion | |

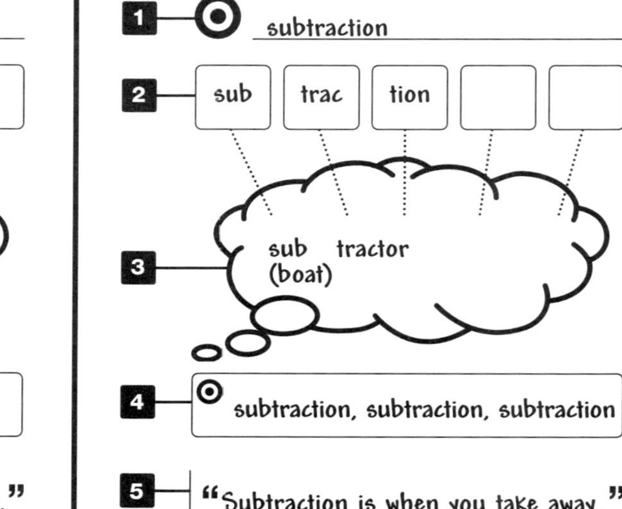

3 sub tractor (boat)

4 subtraction, subtraction, subtraction

5 "Subtraction is when you take away."

1 multiplication

2 mul | ti | pli | ca | tion

3 multiple choice

4 multiplication, multiplication, multiplication

5 "I know my multiplication facts."

1 division

2 di | vi | sion | |

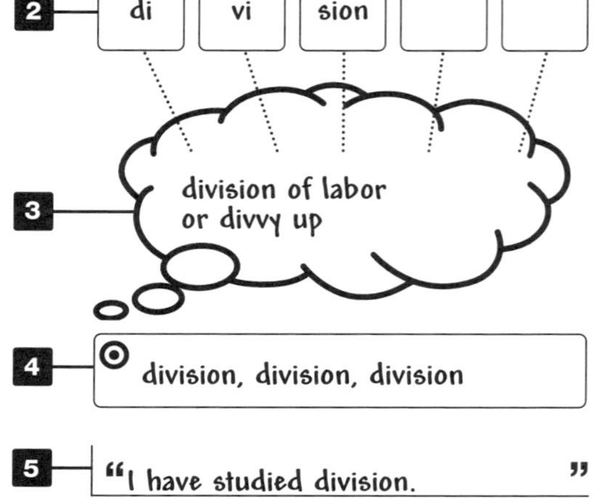

3 division of labor or divvy up

4 division, division, division

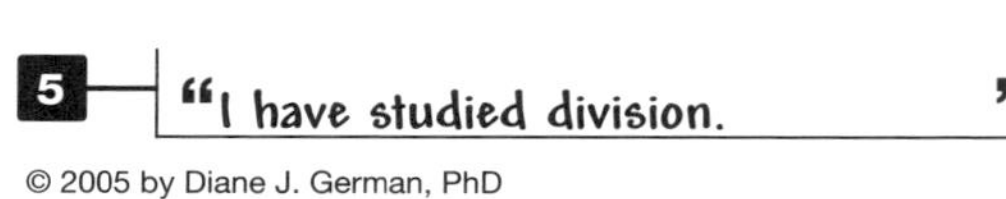

5 "I have studied division."

1 angle

2 an | gle | | |

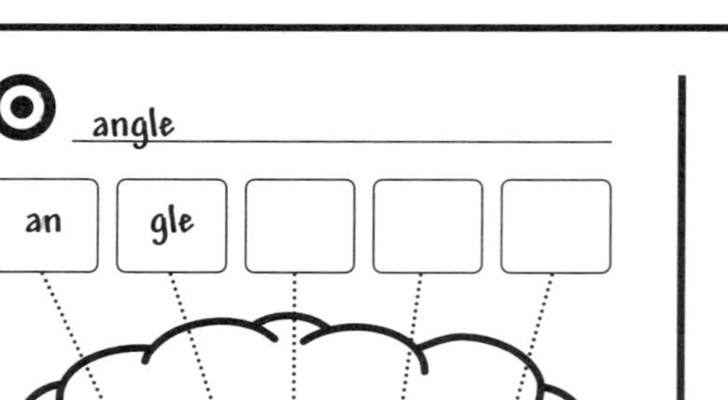

3 angel

4 angle, angle, angle

5 "I need to measure the angle."

1 parallel

2 par | al | lel | |

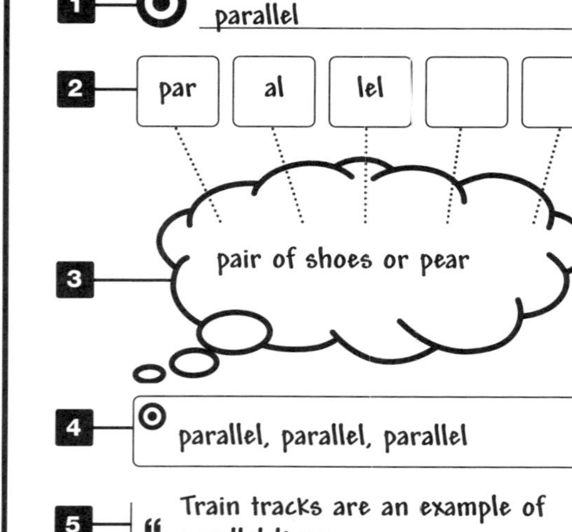

3 pair of shoes or pear

4 parallel, parallel, parallel

5 "Train tracks are an example of parallel lines."

NAME CONTENT AREA Math DATE

1 Target Word
2 Syllable-Dividing
3 Think Same-Sounds Syllable or Familiar-Word Cues
4 Rehearse Target Word as a Unit
5 Rehearse Target Word in a Sentence

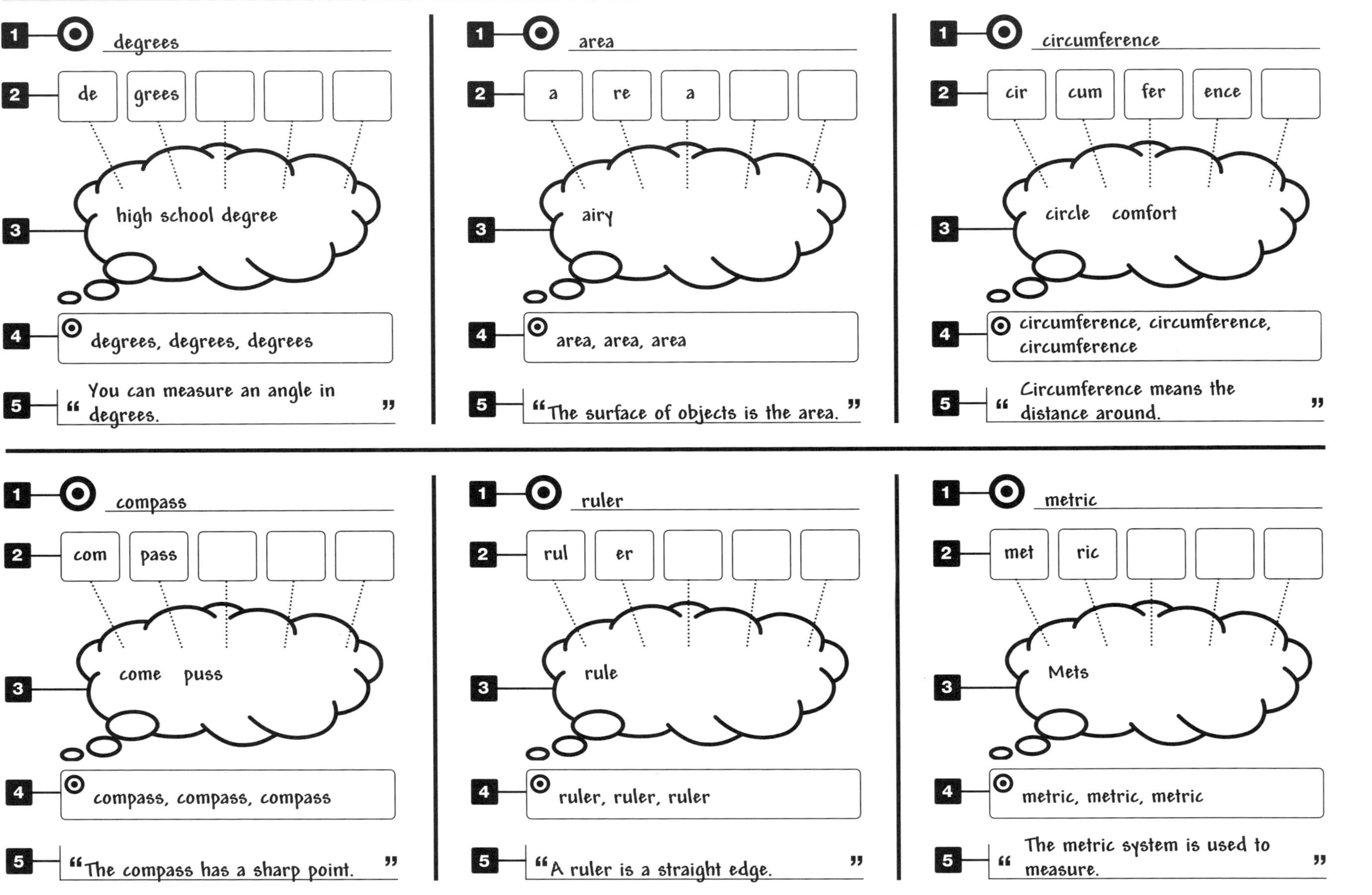

1 degrees
2 de | grees
3 high school degree
4 degrees, degrees, degrees
5 "You can measure an angle in degrees."

1 area
2 a | re | a
3 airy
4 area, area, area
5 "The surface of objects is the area."

1 circumference
2 cir | cum | fer | ence
3 circle comfort
4 circumference, circumference, circumference
5 "Circumference means the distance around."

1 compass
2 com | pass
3 come puss
4 compass, compass, compass
5 "The compass has a sharp point."

1 ruler
2 rul | er
3 rule
4 ruler, ruler, ruler
5 "A ruler is a straight edge."

1 metric
2 met | ric
3 Mets
4 metric, metric, metric
5 "The metric system is used to measure."

Published by PRO-ED, Inc., www.proedinc.com

WFIP–2 SYLLABLE-DIVIDING AND SAME-SOUNDS SYLLABLE CUE STUDY FORM

NAME CONTENT AREA Math DATE

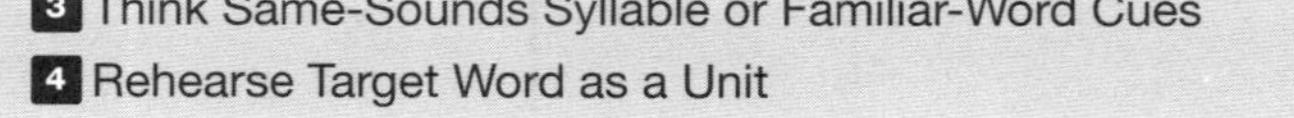

1 Target Word
2 Syllable-Dividing
3 Think Same-Sounds Syllable or Familiar-Word Cues
4 Rehearse Target Word as a Unit
5 Rehearse Target Word in a Sentence

1. array
2. ar | ray | | |
3. arrest
4. array, array, array
5. "An array is an arrangement of objects in rows."

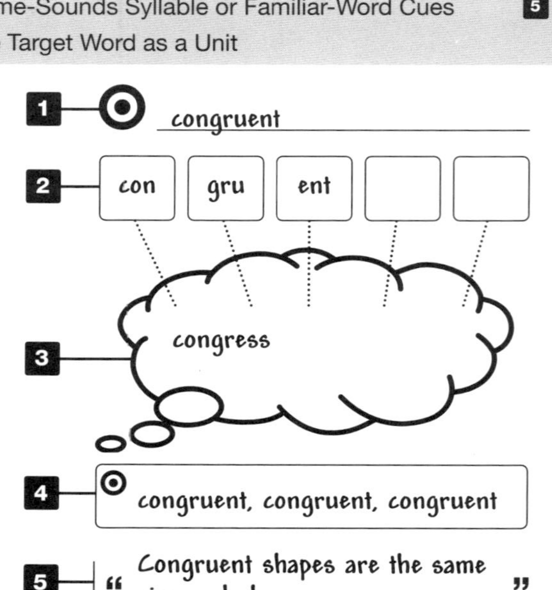

1. congruent
2. con | gru | ent | |
3. congress
4. congruent, congruent, congruent
5. "Congruent shapes are the same size and shape."

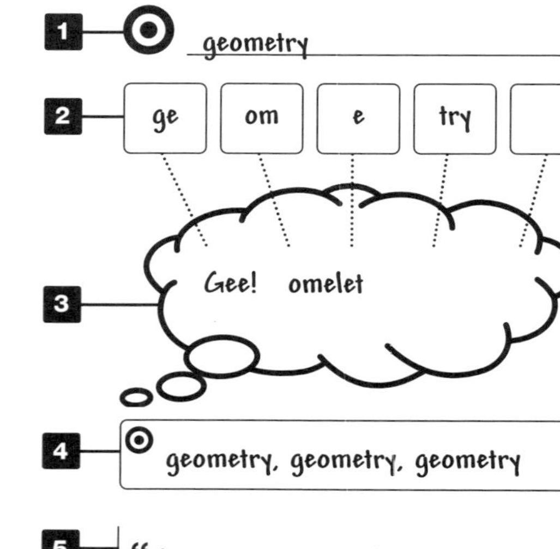

1. geometry
2. ge | om | e | try |
3. Gee! omelet
4. geometry, geometry, geometry
5. "Geometry is a study of shapes."

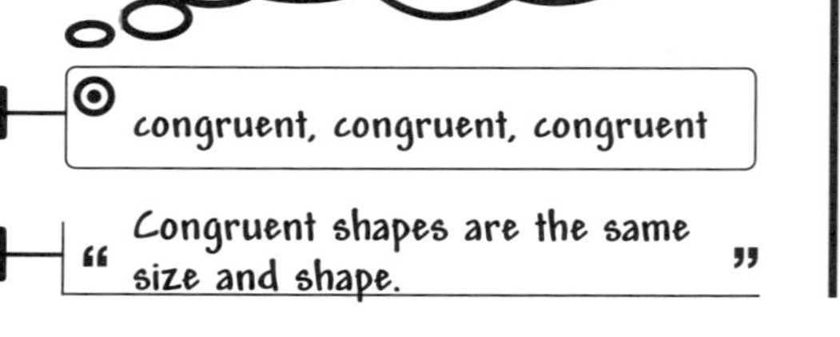

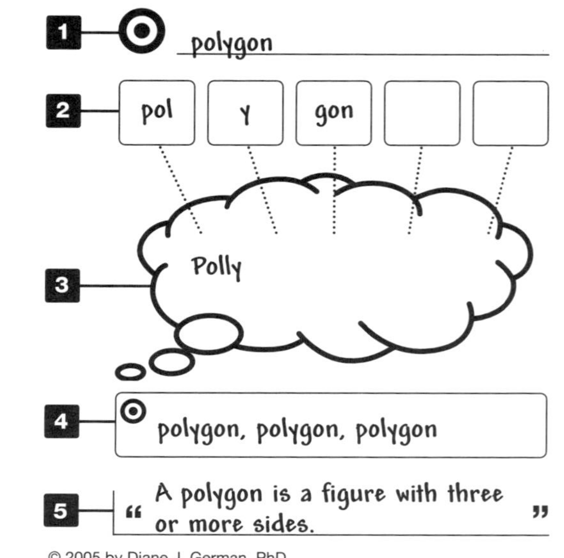

1. polygon
2. pol | y | gon | |
3. Polly
4. polygon, polygon, polygon
5. "A polygon is a figure with three or more sides."

Additional Words

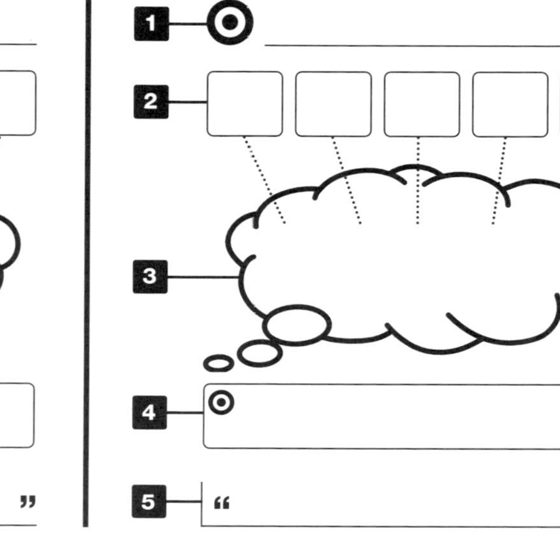

1.
2.
3.
4.
5. " "

Additional Words

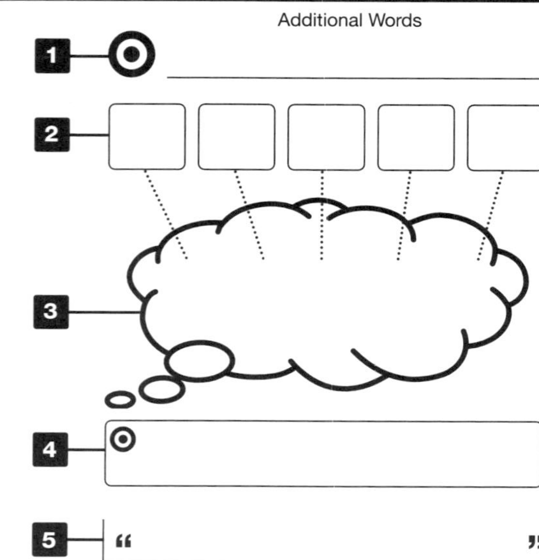

1.
2.
3.
4.
5. " "

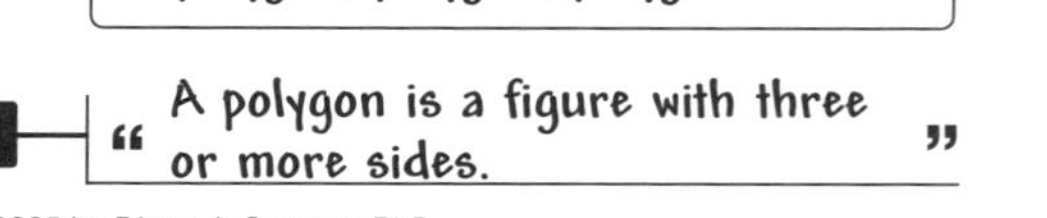

MODEL SENTENCES FOR SELECTED WFIP–2 VOCABULARY

Instructions: Following are selected vocabulary lists embedded in sentences and grouped by subject. Review these lists with the learner, following three basic steps for each vocabulary subject:

1. From the sentences given, select sentences for each of five target words. Read those sentences to the learner.

2. Ask the learner to develop three sentences of his or her own for each target word using the sentence that you read as a model, or after you have read the sentences aloud, have the learner repeat each sentence three times.

3. Select sentences for five additional target words and repeat Steps 1 and 2.

Vocabulary Subject: Social Studies

1. Delegates to *Congress* debate important issues.
   Congress is made up of delegates from every state in the union.
   It was the 23rd session of *Congress*.

2. The president is part of the *executive* branch.
   The president is the head of the *executive* department.
   The *executive* branch of the government enforces the law.

3. The *judicial* branch of the government explains the law.
   The Supreme Court is in the *judicial* branch.
   Judges have *judicial* power.

4. The *legislative* branch of the government makes the laws.
   Writing proposed laws is a *legislative* position.
   A delegate is elected to a *legislative* position.

5. An *amendment* is a change to the constitution.
   Laws can be improved by passing a new *amendment.*
   The 26th *amendment* improves democracy.

6. The *constitution* tells the laws of a nation or state.
   The preamble is an introduction to the *constitution.*
   The *Constitution* of the United States was written in Philadelphia.

7. The *judge* presides over the court.
   Decisions of the court are made by the *judge.*
   The bench is a special name for the seat of a *judge.*

8. The office of *mayor* is the highest city office.
   The *mayor* is elected by the citizens of the town.
   City council meetings are presided over by the *mayor.*

9. The *governor* is in charge of the affairs of the state.
   The chief executive of a state is the *governor.*
   The *governor* is elected by the citizens who live in the state.

10. The *president* governs the affairs of the country.
    The chief executive officer of the United States is the *president.*
    The *president* is elected every four years.

11. The president's *cabinet* is made up of people he has chosen.
    It is the job of a *cabinet* member to advise the president.
    A *cabinet* member is the head of an executive department.

12. A *congressman* works in Congress and may be a congresswoman.
    A *congressman* will be a member of the house of representatives or the senate.
    It is necessary to be elected to the position of *congressman.*

13. A small model of the earth is called a *globe.*
    A *globe* is usually the size of a basketball.
    The earth rotates, so a *globe* should turn.

14. A book of maps is called an *atlas.*
    An *atlas* can be a very large book of maps.
    Every library should have a world *atlas.*

15. A list of symbols on a map is called a *legend.*
    A *legend* on a map may also be called a key.
    Symbols in the *legend* explain the map.

16. An area having a common feature is called a *region.*
    A desert is an example of a dry *region.*
    We have to find the *region* on the map.

17. The line that shows the border of a region is called a *boundary* line.
    A *boundary* is also called a border line.
    The eastern *boundary* of that state is the Muddy River.

18. An imaginary line running east and west is called the *equator.*
    The *equator* divides the earth into the northern half and the southern half.
    The climate near the *equator* is usually hot.

19. A large land area is called a *continent.*
    A *continent* may be one of seven land areas on earth.
    Several different landforms may be found on one *continent.*

20. The top or bottom half of the earth is called a *hemisphere.*
    The equator divides the southern *hemisphere* from the north.
    The North Pole is in the northern *hemisphere.*

21. I want to climb to the top of that *mountain.*
    The *mountain* has snow at the top.
    A *mountain* is taller than a hill.

22. The low land between mountains is called a *valley.*
    We will follow the trail to the *valley* below.
    The stream runs down to the grassy *valley.*

23. The *desert* is hot and dry.
    There is very little rainfall in the *desert.*
    In a *desert* the ground is sand, not soil.

24. An *island* is land that is surrounded by water.
    The sailor saw a small *island* in the distance.
    They found no one living on the deserted *island.*

25. A *river* is moving water that is larger than a stream.
    The steamboat chugged up the *river.*
    The water in a *river* is muddy and dark.

26. The water in a *lake* is usually clear.
    A *lake* is water that is surrounded by land.
    A *lake* is not as large as a sea or ocean.

27. A *suburb* is a smaller town outside of the city.
    Some people work in the city and live in a *suburb.*
    Workers commute from the *suburb* to the city.

28. An *ocean* is a larger body of salty water.
    Ocean liners are built to carry things across the *ocean.*
    The *ocean* has a tide coming in and going out.

29. The *mall* has many stores under one roof.
    I shop with my parents in the *mall.*
    The *mall* has places to eat and rest.

30. A *hospital* is a place where sick and injured people go for care.
    Doctors and nurses work at a *hospital.*
    An ambulance can take you to the *hospital* quickly.

31. A *library* is a place with shelves where books are kept.
    I like to check out interesting books at the *library.*
    I use my *library* card to check out books.

32. A *paramedic* is trained to care for people in an emergency.
    A fireman is often taught to be a *paramedic.*
    The *paramedic* helps to save lives before going to the hospital.

33. A *citizen* is a person who lives in a town or a city or a country.
    A *citizen* can vote in an election.
    Some people from other lands want to become American *citizens.*

34. The *principal* of a school is the head person.
    The secretary said, "The *principal* is in his office."
    Our *principal* is kind to all of the children in the school.

35. A *librarian* checks your books out.
    The manager of a library is called a *librarian.*
    The *librarian* asks to see your library card.

Vocabulary Subject: Baseball

1. A *bat* is made out of wood.
   The ball is hit with a *bat.*
   The *bat* is heavy.

2. The catcher wears a *glove.*
   The *glove* protects his hand.
   The *glove* is made from leather.

3. The fans sit in the *stands.*
   The *stands* are seats at the baseball game.
   People watch the game from the *stands.*

4. The players are sitting in the *dugout.*
   A *dugout* is where players rest.
   The players wait for their turn in the *dugout.*

5. The *catcher* plays behind the batter.
   The pitcher works with the *catcher.*
   The *catcher* tries to tag you out.

6. The *pitcher* throws the ball to the batter.
   The *pitcher* stands in the middle.
   The *pitcher* tries to strike you out.

7. If you miss the ball it is called a *strike.*
   After the third *strike,* you're out.
   It is not good to get a *strike.*

8. It's a *home run* when a player runs around all of the bases.
   A point is scored with a *home run.*
   If you hit the ball out of the park, you'll get a *home run.*

9. A ball that goes outside the line is a *foul ball.*
   Sometimes a *foul ball* goes over your head.
   A *foul ball* counts as a strike.

10. A *runner* races around the bases.
    The players try to get the *runner* out.
    A *runner* may slide into a base.

11. The player in the field is called a *fielder.*
    The *fielder* throws the ball back to the base man.
    A *fielder* must go after the ball.

12. The *umpire* called it a foul ball.
    The players argue with the *umpire.*
    An *umpire* is like a judge.

13. The sun made it hard to catch the high *fly ball.*
    A *fly ball* is hit high.
    The fielder caught the high *fly ball.*

14. The best fielder on a team is usually the *shortstop.*
    The *shortstop* stands between second and third base.
    A *shortstop* can help win the game.

15. The *batboy* helps the players.
    The *batboy* returns the bats to a special place.
    The *batboy* is usually a teenager.

Vocabulary Subject: Football

1. The building where the game is played is called a *stadium.*
   A *stadium* has hundreds of seats for fans.
   You can buy your tickets at the *stadium.*

2. The *goalpost* is at the end of the field.
   The upright bars are called a *goalpost.*
   He kicks the ball through the *goalpost.*

3. The *scoreboard* says "Home" and "Visitors."
   To see who's winning, look at the *scoreboard.*
   The *scoreboard* shows the score.

4. Pulling a player to the ground is called a *tackle.*
   Everyone tries to *tackle* the player with the football.
   A *tackle* may cause players to get hurt.

5. The players *huddle* to make their plans.
   The players talk secretly when they are in a *huddle.*
   They make a circle and listen in the *huddle.*

6. One period of play is called a *quarter.*
   It is very exciting during the last *quarter.*
   Halftime comes between the second *quarter* and third quarter.

7. A football game begins with a *kickoff.*
   A *kickoff* is made at the beginning of the game and after halftime.
   A good *kickoff* makes the ball go high and far.

8. The game will go into *overtime* if the score is tied.
   More time to play at the end of the fourth quarter is called *overtime.*
   The team won in *overtime.*

9. The boundary marked at the side of the field is the *sideline.*
   A player must stay inside the *sideline.*
   Fans cannot go on the *sideline.*

10. The scoring area of the field is called the *end zone.*
    Touchdowns are scored in the *end zone.*
    The playing field has an *end zone* at each end of the field.

11. If the ball is dropped by a player, it is called a *fumble.*

    A player is angry with himself if he loses the ball because of a *fumble.*

    If you *fumble* the ball, the other team may get it.

12. If a player can catch a pass that was intended for another player, it is called an *interception.*

    The other team takes possession of the ball after an *interception.*

    The pass was not completed because of the *interception.*

13. A player who often receives and runs the ball is called a *halfback.*

    A *halfback* stands behind the quarterback.

    A *halfback* can run quickly around the side.

Vocabulary Subject: Math

1. Write the numbers in consecutive *order.*

   Division has several steps that are done in *order.*

   The *order* of the numbers shows their value.

2. I can *estimate* what the answer will be.

   An approximate answer is an *estimate.*

   We *estimate* the answer before working the problem out.

3. A math rule is called a *formula.*

   Use a *formula* to find the distance around a circle.

   A *formula* to find area is $A = L \times W$.

4. A plus sign is an example of *perpendicular* lines.

   A street intersection is an example of *perpendicular* lines.

   Perpendicular lines make four 90° angles.

5. The distance around a circle is its *circumference.*

   Circumference means the distance around.

   Measure the *circumference* of the circle.

6. A *compass* draws intersections of a line.

   I need a pencil for this *compass.*

   This *compass* has a sharp point.

7. A *ruler* is a straight edge.
   One tool for measuring is called a *ruler.*
   Most students use a 12-inch *ruler.*

8. The *metric* system is used to measure.
   Ten is the base in the metric system.
   Metric is a good system of measurement.

9. An *angle* is measured in degrees.
   The corner of a book is a right *angle.*
   Two lines that cross form an *angle.*

10. In *division,* you are dividing things.
    You need a divisor and a dividend for a *division* problem.
    In math class, we studied *division.*

11. *Subtraction* is taking things away.
    We use *subtraction* to find the remainder.
    A minus sign means the operation is *subtraction.*

12. I know all of the *multiplication* tables.
    Division is the opposite of *multiplication.*
    The times sign means to use *multiplication.*

13. *Addition* is putting things together.
    My favorite operation in math is *addition.*
    Addition is the opposite of subtraction.

14. Two is an *even* number.
    I can divide a number that is *even.*
    Numbers can be odd or *even.*

15. Numbers can be even or *odd.*
    One, three, and five are *odd* numbers.
    Seven, nine, and eleven are also *odd* numbers.

16. I can *add* two numbers together.
    Two and three *add* up to five.
    A plus sign means to *add* the numbers.

17. I can *subtract* a smaller number from a larger number.
    Take away means to *subtract* the numbers.
    I *subtract* to get the remainder.

18. $3 + 3 = 6$ is an addition *problem.*
    $6 - 3 = 3$ is a subtraction *problem.*
    Read each *problem* on the page.

19. The *sum* of four plus four is eight.
    I add numbers to find their *sum.*
    The *sum* is the total amount.

20. The sum is the *total* amount.
    Write the *total* below the line.
    The *total* is your answer.

21. Ten has more *value* than six.
    Hundreds shows a place *value.*
    The *value* shows what it is worth.

22. The position of a number is its *place* value.
    Zero holds the *place* open.
    We call zero a *place* holder.

23. *Zero* has no value.
    Capital *O* looks like the number *zero.*
    The word *zero* starts with a *z.*

24. The first place value is the *ones* place.
    The *ones* are from one to nine.
    Tens come right after the *ones.*

25. When I count, one *second* is the time between numbers.
    It happened in a split *second.*
    My watch has a *second* hand.

26. Sixty seconds make a *minute.*
    It is one *minute* before 3 o'clock.
    I'll be with you in just a *minute.*

DUAL-FOCUS VOCABULARY INSTRUCTION FORM

Vocabulary	Comprehension Strategies (Vocabulary Meaning)	Metalinguistic and Mnemonic Retrieval Strategies				
		Syllable Dividing	Same-Sounds Cues	Familiar-Word Cue	Synonym or Category Alternate	Rehearsal

Note. Adapted from *Best Practice for Students with Word Finding Difficulties: Handbook for Classroom Teachers,* by D. German, 1996.

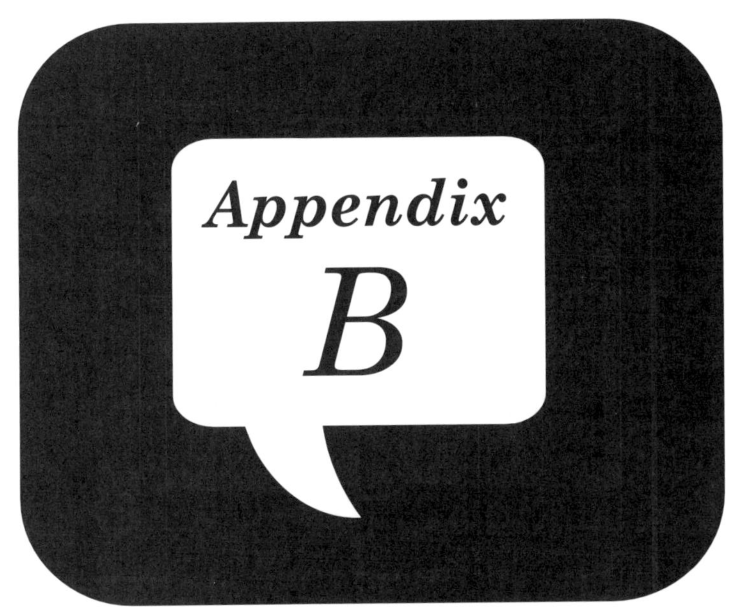

Word-Finding Self-Advocacy Instruction Form

*S*pecialists and teachers may copy this form for use with the WFIP–2.

WORD-FINDING SELF-ASSESSMENT SURVEY

Purpose: The purpose of the Word Finding Self-Assessment Survey is to help learners identify those influences that impact both positively and negatively on their word-finding skills (such as the language setting, language circumstances, retrieval context, the academic subject, and the nature of the target word syntax, frequency of occurrence, length, and phonological complexity.) *The self-reflection required in this analysis may be difficult for some younger learners. Therefore, specialists and teachers should feel free to use only those portions of the survey they feel their learners will be able to complete.*

Instructions: Follow the instructions in the self-advocacy lesson plans, and in Chapter 4, that focus on the self-assessment of the learner's word-finding skills. Review the portions of the survey under consideration and help the learner rate his or her word-finding skills on a scale from 1 to 3 with 1 representing little difficulty, 2 representing moderate difficulty, and 3 representing significant difficulty.

Learner's Name ______________________ Specialist: ______________________

Date ____________ Grade ____________ Teacher(s) ______________________

Part 1: Language Settings

Language Setting	Difficulty Rating			Comments
	1	2	3	
School				
Science				
Reading				
Social studies				
Math				
Languages				
Computers				
Writing				
Home and Community				
Dinner table conversation				
Telephone				
Sports-related activities				
Clubs or organizations				
Religious school				
E-mail				
Electronic chat				

Part 2: Language Circumstances

Language Setting	Individual (One-to-One) Difficulty Rating			Small or Large Group Difficulty Rating			Comments
	1	2	3	1	2	3	
School Conversations							
Teachers							
Principals/administrators							
Peers							
Home Conversations							
Parents							
Siblings							
Relatives							
Friends							
School Assignments							
Giving an oral report							
Answering questions							
Oral reading							
School projects							

Part 3: Retrieval Contexts

Language Setting	Retrieving Specific Words or Names Difficulty Rating			Relating an Experience (Narrative or Discourse) Difficulty Rating			Comments
	1	2	3	1	2	3	
School							
Teachers							
Principals/administrators							
Peers							
Cooperative groups							
Home							
Parents							
Siblings							
Relatives							
Friends							
School Assignments							
Answering questions							
Examinations (writing)							
Homework							
Computer assignments							

Part 4: Subject of the Vocabulary

Vocabulary Subject	Difficulty Rating			Comments
	1	2	3	
People (Names or Titles)				
Friends				
Teachers				
Family members				
TV personalities and characters				
Sports figures				
Literary characters				
Government figures				
Social Studies (Names)				
Government offices				
Cities, states, and countries				
Geography (rivers, lakes)				
Science and Math (Terms and Concepts)				
Vocabulary				
Symbols				
Equipment				
Formulas				
Processes or operations				

Part 5: Nature of the Target Word (Lexical Factors)

Nature of the Target Word (Lexical Factors)	Difficulty Rating			Comments
	1	2	3	
Syntax				
Nouns and proper nouns				
Action words (verbs)				
Adjectives				
Prepositions				
Frequency of Occurrence				
Rare words				
Common words				
Length				
Short words				
Long words				
Phonological Complexity				
One-syllable words				
Multisyllabic words				
Polysyllabic words				
Compound words				

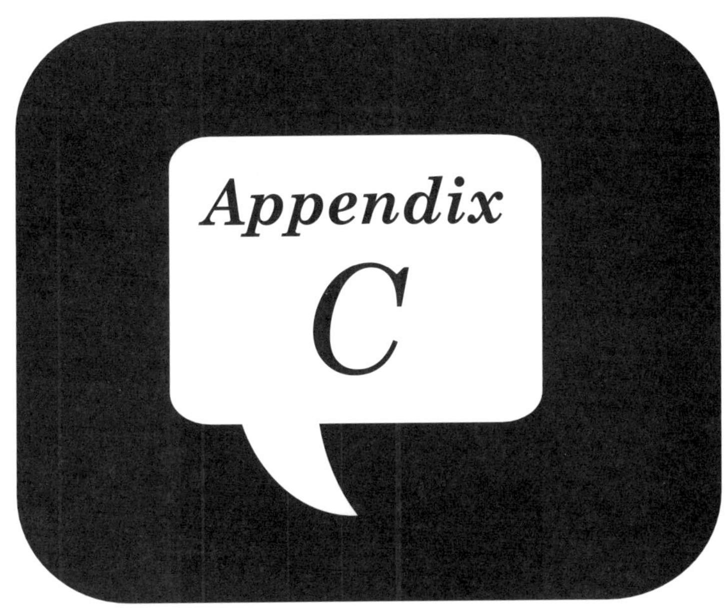

Word-Finding Accommodations Forms

Specialists and teachers may copy this form for use with the WFIP–2.

CLASSROOM OBSERVATION FORM

Learner's Name ______________________ Grade ____________ Date ______________

Observer's Name ______________________ Teacher's Name ______________________

Instructions: Using the boxes, indicate the methods presently used in the classroom. Mark an ✗ in the box to the left of each high-retrieval-load instructional practice being used. Mark a ✓ in the box to the left of each low-retrieval-load instructional practice being used. Mark a + in the box to the left of each supportive technology used in the classroom.

Activity	✗ High Retrieval Load	✓ Low Retrieval Load	✓ Supportive Technology
Classroom discussion or other oral classroom work	☐ Oral questioning ☐ Group work ☐ Math / spelling drills ☐ Oral reports		☐ Presentation software
Written classroom work	☐ Short answer ☐ Fill in the blank ☐ Note taking ☐ Essay	☐ Circle or select the answer	☐ Word-processing software ☐ Word-prediction software ☐ Electronic spell check ☐ Electronic dictionary
Homework assignments	☐ Note taking ☐ Short answer ☐ Essay ☐ Fill in the blank	☐ Circle or select the answer	☐ Internet sites
Evaluations	☐ Recall of facts ☐ Essay ☐ Fill in the blank	☐ True–false ☐ Multiple-choice ☐ Open book	☐ Portfolio assessment ☐ Digital video projects ☐ Electronic resource files

RECOMMENDED WORD-FINDING ACCOMMODATIONS FORM

Learner'sName ______________________ Specialist ______________________

Date ____________ Grade ____________ Teacher ______________________

Instructions: Use this form to indicate word-finding accommodations recommended for the learner's classroom. Check (✓) the recommended accommodation for each content area selected.

		Content Area							
			Reading						
Activity	**Recommended Accommodations or Support Materials**	**Math**	**Oral**	**Silent Comp.**	**Social Studies**	**English**	**Science**	**Computers**	**Other**
Classroom Discussion									
Oral questions	Cue with initial consonant and vowel or syllable of the target word								
	Multiple-choice frames								
	Volunteer participation								
	Yes–no or true–false response								
	Prime the learner with a question								
	Give additional time								
Open-ended sentence frames	Multiple-choice frames								
Group work	Co-presentations with peers								

Activity	Recommended Accommodations or Support Materials	Content Area							
			Reading						
		Math	Oral	Silent Comp.	Social Studies	English	Science	Computers	Other
Oral classroom work									
Oral reading	Silent reading Choral reading								
Oral math drills	Multiple-choice frames								
Computation	Calculator								
	Software with multiple choice								
	Yes–no or true–false response								
Oral reports	Presentation software								
	Transparencies or other visual aids								
	Substitute or augment with prerecorded audio or video tapes								
	Note cards								
Other									
Written Classroom Work									
Worksheets requiring short answers	Multiple-choice frames								
Reading comprehension questions	Multiple-choice frames								

Activity	Recommended Accommodations or Support Materials	Content Area							
			Reading						
		Math	Oral	Silent Comp.	Social Studies	English	Science	Computers	Other
	Find and underline answer in text								
	Yes–no or true–false								
	Circle or mark answer								
Note taking	Teacher-provided outline and/or lecture notes.								
	Electronic note sharing between students								
Essay	Word processor								
	Develop outline using book								
	Answer multiple-choice questions								
Other									
Homework									
Note taking	Word processing								
	Develop resource notebook								
Answering questions	Indicate page number of questions								
	Underline answer in copy of text								
	Match answers to questions								

Activity	Recommended Accommodations or Support Materials	Content Area							
			Reading						
		Math	Oral	Silent Comp.	Social Studies	English	Science	Computers	Other
Essay	Develop resource outline using book								
Evaluation									
Recall of facts	Resource notebook (electronic or hardcopy)								
	Open-book exam								
	Take-home exam								
	Multiple-choice								
	Yes–no or true–false response								
	Matching								
	Identification of topic-related Internet sites								
Essay	Open-book exam								
	Take-home exam								
	Use word processor								
	Inspiration software								
	Objective format (multiple-choice, matching, true–false)								
	Digital videos								

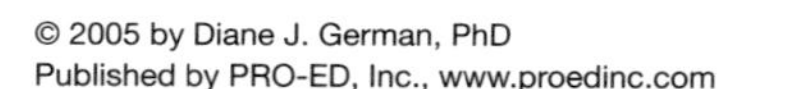

Activity	Recommended Accommodations or Support Materials	Content Area							
			Reading						
		Math	Oral	Silent Comp.	Social Studies	English	Science	Computers	Other
Short answer	Multiple-choice; underline answer								
	Extended time								
	Identify Internet sites								

REFERENCES

Bellingrath, E., & Lisicia, R. (1992). *Cognitive rehabilitation of memory: A practical guide.* Gaithersburg, MD: Aspen.

Bierwisch, M., & Schreuder, R. (1991). From concepts to lexical items. In W. J. M. Levelt (Ed.), *Lexical access in speech production* (pp. 23–60). Cambridge, MA: Blackwell.

Bjork, R., & Bjork, L. (1992). A new theory of disuse and an old theory of stimulus fluctuation. In A. F. Healy, S. M. Kosslyn, & R. M. Shiffrin (Eds.), *From learning processes to cognitive processes: Essays in honor of William K. Estes* (Vol. 2, pp. 35–67). Hillsdale, NJ: Erlbaum.

Blachman, B. A. (1994). What we have learned from longitudinal studies of phonological processing and reading, and some answered questions: A response to Torgesen, Wagner, and Rashotte. *Journal of Learning Disabilities, 27,* 287–291.

Bowers, P. G, & Swanson, L. B. (1991). Naming speed deficits in reading disability: Multiple measures of a singular process. *Journal of Experimental Child Psychology , 51,* 195–219.

Brown, A. S. (1991). A review of the "tip of the tongue" phenomenon. *Journal of Verbal Learning and Verbal Behavior, 5,* 325–337.

Burke, D. M., MacKay, D. G., Worthley, J. S., & Wade, E. (1991). On the tip of the tongue: What causes word-finding failures in young and older adults? *Journal of Memory and Language, 30,* 542–579.

Caramazza, A., & Hillis, A. E. (1990). Where do semantic errors come from? *Cortex, 26,* 95–122.

Catts, H. (1999). Phonological awareness: Putting research into practice. *Language Learning and Education Newsletter, 6*(1), 26–29.

Catts, H., & Kamhi, A. (1999). Causes of reading difficulties. In H. W. Catts & A. G. Kamhi (Eds.), *Language and reading disabilities* (pp. 95–127). Boston: Allyn & Bacon.

Cazden, C. (1988). *Classroom discourse: The language of teaching and learning.* Portsmouth, NH: Heinemann.

Cermak, L. S. (1975). Imagery as an aid to retrieval for Korsakoff patients. *Cortex, 11,* 160–169.

Conca, L. (1989). Strategy choice by LD children with good and poor naming ability in a naturalistic memory situation. *Learning Disabilities Quarterly, 12,* 92–106.

Dapretto, M., & Bjork, E. L. (2000). The development of word retrieval abilities in the second year and its relation to early vocabulary growth. *Child Development, 71,* 635–648.

Denckla, M. B., & Rudel, R. G. (1976). Naming of object drawing by dyslexic and other learning disabled children. *Brain and Language, 3,* 1–15.

Drummond, S., & Rentschler, G. (1981). The efficacy of gestural cueing in dysphasic word-retrieval responses. *Journal of Communication Disorders, 14,* 287–298.

Elbers, L., (1985). A tip-of-the tongue experience at age two? *Journal of Child Language, 12,* 353–365.

Garrett, M. (1991). Disorders of lexical selection. In W. J. M. Levelt (Ed.), *Lexical access in speech production* (pp. 143–180). Cambridge, MA: Blackwell.

German, D. J. (1989). *Test of Word Finding.* Austin, TX: PRO-ED.

German, D. J. (1990). *Test of Adolescent/Adult Word Finding.* Austin, TX: PRO-ED.

German, D. J. (1991). *Test of Word Finding in Discourse.* Austin, TX: PRO-ED.

German, D. J. (1993). *Word finding intervention program: Remediation, compensatory modification, and self-advocacy.* Austin, TX: PRO-ED.

German, D. J. (1996). *Best practice for students with word finding difficulties: Handbook for classroom teachers.* Unpublished manuscript.

German, D. J. (2000a). *Test of Word Finding* (2nd ed.). Austin, TX: PRO-ED.

German, D. J. (2000b, October). *Formulate a second hypothesis: Word finding (WF) based oral reading (OR) errors.* Presentation at the Illinois Dyslexia Association (IIDA), Oak Park, IL.

German, D. J. (2000c, November). *Word finding (WF) sensitive oral reading (OR) analysis.* Poster session presented at the American Speech-Language-Hearing Association (ASHA), Washington, DC.

German, D. J. (2001). *It's on the tip of my tongue: Word-finding strategies to remember names and words you often forget.* Chicago: Word Finding Materials.

German, D. J. (2002). A phonologically based strategy to improve word-finding abilities in children. *Communication Disorders Quarterly, 23,* 179–192.

German, D. J., & Gellar, M. (2002, November). *What you should know about word finding and reading.* Presentation at the International Dyslexia Association (IDA), Atlanta, GA.

German, D. J., & Gellar, M. (2003, February). *The impact of word-finding difficulties on oral reading assessment.* Presentation at the Learning Disabilities Association (LDA), Chicago, IL.

German, D. J., & German, A. E. (1992). *Word finding referral checklist.* Chicago: Word Finding Materials.

German, D. J., & Newman, R. S. (2004). The impact of lexical factors on children's word finding errors. *Journal of Speech, Language, and Hearing Research, 47*(3) 624–636.

German, D. J., & Schwanke, J. (November, 2003). *Tele-health: Word-finding intervention using video conferencing technologies.* Presentation at the American Speech-Language-Hearing Association (ASHA), Chicago, IL.

Gordon, B. (1997). Models of naming. In H. Goodglass & A. Wingfield, (Eds.), *Anomia neuroanatomical and cognitive correlates* (pp. 31–64). San Diego, CA: Academic Press.

Graham, S., & Harris, K. (2002). The road less traveled: Prevention and intervention in written language. In K. Butler & E. Silliman (Eds.), *Speaking, reading, and writing in children with language learning disabilities* (pp.199–218). Mahwah, NJ: Erlbaum.

Hallahan, D. P., & Kauffman, J. M. (2000). *Exceptional learners: Introduction to special education* (8th ed.). Boston: Allyn & Bacon.

Hanson, M. (1996). Self-management through self-monitoring. In K. Jones & T. Charlton (Eds.), *Overcoming learning and behaviour difficulties: Partnership with pupils* (pp.173–191). London: Routledge.

Harrell, M., Parenté, F., Bellingrath, E., & Lisicia, R. (1992). *Cognitive rehabilitation of memory: A practical guide.* Gaithersburg, MD: Aspen.

Higbee, K. L. (1993). *Your memory: How it works and how you improve it.* New York: Paragon House.

Hillis, A. E., & Caramazza, A. (1995). Converging evidence for the interaction of semantic and sublexical phonological information in accessing lexical representation for spoken output. *Cognitive Neuropsychology, 12,* 187–227.

Hudson, J., & Fivush, R. (1991). As time goes by: Sixth graders remember a kindergarten experience. *Applied Cognitive Psychology, 5,* 347–360.

James, L. E., & Burke, D. M. (2000). Phonological priming effects on word retrieval and tip-of-the-tongue experiences in young and older adults. *Journal of Experimental Psychology: Learning, Memory & Cognition, 26,* 1378–1392.

Johnson, D., & Myklebust, H. (1967). *Learning disabilities: Educational principles and practices.* San Diego, CA: Grune & Stratton.

Katz, R. B. (1986). Phonological deficiencies in children with reading disabilities: Evidence from an object-naming task. *Cognition, 22,* 225–257.

Lahey, M., & Edwards, J. (1999). Naming errors of children with specific language impairment. *Journal of Speech and Hearing Research, 42*(1), 195–205.

Lesser, R. (1989). Some issues in the neuropsychological rehabilitation of anomia. In X. Seron & G. Deloche (Eds.), *Cognitive approaches in neuropsychological rehabilitation.* Hillsdale, NJ: Erlbaum.

Levelt, W. J. M. (1989). *Speaking, from intention to articulation.* Cambridge, MA: MIT Press.

Levelt, W. M. J. (1991). *Lexical access in speech production.* Cambridge, MA: Blackwell.

Levelt, W. J. M., Roelofs, A., & Meyer, A. S. (1999). A theory of lexical access in speech production. *Behavioral and Brain Sciences, 22,* 1–75.

MacArthur, C. A. (2000). New tools for writing: Assistive technology for students with writing difficulties. *Topics in Language Disorders, 20*(4), 85–100.

Masterson, J. J., Apel, K., & Wood, L. A. (2002). Technology and literacy: Decisions for the new millennium. In K. Butler & E. Silliman (Eds.), *Speaking, reading, and writing in children with language learning disabilities* (pp.199–218). Mahwah, NJ: Erlbaum.

Mastropieri, M. A., Sweda, J., & Scruggs, T. E. (2000). Teacher use of mnemonic strategy instruction. *Learning Disabilities Research and Practice, 15,* 69–74.

McBride-Chang, C., & Franklin, R. (1996). Structural invariance in the associations of naming speed, phonological awareness, and verbal reasoning in good and poor readers: A test of the double deficit hypothesis. *Reading and Writing: An Interdisciplinary Journal, 88*(4), 323–339.

McGregor, K. K. (1994). Use of phonological information in word-finding treatment for children. *Journal of Speech and Hearing Research, 37,* 1381–1393.

McGregor, K. K., & Appel, A. (2002). On the relation between mental representation and naming in a child with specific language impairment. *Clinical Linguistics & Phonetics, 16*(1), 1–20.

McGregor, K. K., & Windsor, J. (1996). Effects of priming on the naming accuracy of preschoolers with word-finding deficits. *Journal of Speech and Hearing Research, 39,* 1048–1058.

McNamara, J. K., & Wong, B. (2003). Memory for everyday information in students with learning disabilities. *Journal of Learning Disabilities, 36*(5), 394–406.

McNamara, T. P., & Healy, A. F. (1988). Semantic, phonological, and mediated priming in reading and lexical decisions. *Journal of Experimental Psychology: Learning Memory and Cognition, 14,* 398–409.

Meyer, A. S., & Bock, J. K. (1992). The tip of the tongue phenomenon: Blocking or partial activation? *Memory and Cognition, 20,* 715–726.

Murphy, L. A., Pollatsek, A., & Well, A. D. (1988). Developmental dyslexia and word retrieval deficits. *Brain and Language, 35,* 1–23.

Nelson, N. (1998). *Childhood language disorders in context: Infancy through adolescence* (2nd ed.). Columbus, OH: Merrill.

Nichols, L. M. (1996). Pencil and paper versus word processing: A comparative study of creative writing in the elementary school. *Journal of Research on Computing in Education, 29*(2), 159–166.

Ornstein, P. A., Naus, M. J., & Liberty, C. (1975). Rehearsal and organizational processes in children's memory. *Child Development, 76,* 818–830.

Owston, R. D., & Wideman, H. H. (1997). Word processors and children's writing in a high-computer-access setting. *Journal of Research on Computing in Education, 30*(2), 202–220.

Paul, R. (2001). *Language disorders from infancy through adolescence* (2nd ed.). Philadelphia: Mosby.

Pease, D., & Goodglass, H. (1978). The effects of cueing on picture naming in aphasia. *Cortex, 14,* 178–189.

Rubin, H., Berstein, S., & Katz, R. G. (1989). Effects of cues on object naming in first grade good and poor readers. *Annals of Dyslexia, 33,* 111–120.

Rubin, H., & Liberman, I. (1983). Exploring the oral and written language errors made by language disabled children. *Annals of Dyslexia, 33,* 110–120.

Scott, C. M. (2002). A fork in the road less traveled: Writing intervention based on language profile. In K. Butler & E. Silliman (Eds.), *Speaking, reading, and writing in children with language learning disabilities* (pp.219–237). Mahwah, NJ: Erlbaum.

Scott, C., & Windsor, J. (2000). Central language performance measures in spoken and written narrative and expository discourse of school-age children with language learning disabilities. *Journal of Speech Language and Hearing Research, 43,* 324–339.

Smith, C. R. (1991). *Learning disabilities: The interaction of learner, task, and setting.* Boston: Allyn & Bacon.

Smith, C. R. (2004). Learning disabilities: The interaction of students and their environments (5th ed.). Boston: Allyn & Bacon.

Snowling, M., & Stackhouse, J. 1(996). *Dyslexia speech and language: A practitioner's handbook*. London: Whurr.

Snowling, M., Wagtendonk, B., & Stafford, C. (1988). Object-naming deficits in developmental dyslexia. *Journal of Research in Reading, 11,* 67–85.

Snyder, I. (1993). The impact of computers on students' writing: A comparative study of the effects of pens and word processors on writing context, process and product. *Australian Journal of Education, 37*(1), 5–25.

Thompson, C. K., Hall, H., & Sison, C. (1986). Effects of hypnosis and imagery training on naming behavior in aphasia. *Brain and Language, 28,* 141–153.

Toglia, P., Shlechter, M., & Chevalier, S. (1992). Memory for directly and indirectly experienced events. *Applied Cognitive Psychology, 6,* 293–306.

Torgesen, J. K., Wagner, R. K., & Rashotte, C. A. (1994). Longitudinal studies of phonological processing and reading. *Journal of Learning Disabilities, 27,* 276–286.

Uberti, H. Z., Scruggs, T. E., & Mastropieri, M. A. (2003). Keywords make the difference! Mnemonic instruction in inclusive classrooms. *Teaching Exceptional Children, 10*(3), 56–61.

VanKleeck, A. (1990). Emergent literacy: Learning about print before learning to read. *Topics in Language Disorders, 10,* 25–45.

VanKleeck, A., Gillam, R., & McFadden, T. (1998). A study of classroom-based phonological awareness training for preschoolers with speech and/or language disorders. *American Journal of Speech–Language Pathology, 7,* 65–76.

Vitevitch, M. S. (2002). The influence of phonological similarity neighborhoods on speech production. *Journal of Experimental Psychology: Learning, Memory & Cognition, 28,* 735–747.

Wagner, R., Torgesen, J., & Rashotte, C. (1994). Development of reading-related phonological processing abilities: New evidence of bidirectional causality from a latent variable longitudinal study. *Developmental Psychology, 30,* 73–87.

Wiig, E. H., & Becker-Caplan, L. (1984). Linguistic retrieval strategies and word-finding difficulties among children with language disabilities. *Topics in Language Disorders, 4,* 1–18.

Wiig, E. H., & Semel, E. M. (1984). *Language assessment and intervention for the learning disabled* (2nd ed.). Columbus, OH: Merrill.

Wimmer, H., (1993). Characteristics of developmental dyslexia in a regular writing system. *Applied Psycholinguistics, 14*(1), 1–33.

Wing, C. S. (1990). A preliminary investigation of generalization to untrained words following two treatments of children's word-finding problems. *Language, Speech, and Hearing Services in Schools, 21,* 151–156.

Wolf, M. (1980). The word-retrieval process and reading in children and aphasics. *Children's Language, 3,* 437–490.

Wolf, M. (1986). Rapid alternating stimulus naming in the developmental dyslexias. *Brain and Language, 27,* 360–379.

Wolf, M., & Bowers, P. (2000). Naming-speed deficits in developmental reading disabilities: An introduction to the special series on the double-deficit hypothesis. *Journal of Learning Disabilities, 33*(4), 322–324.

Wolf, M., & Goodglass, H. (1986). Dyslexia, dysnomia, and lexical retrieval: A longitudinal investigation. *Brain and Language, 28,* 154–168.

Wolf, M., & Segal, D. (1992). Word finding and reading in the developmental dyslexias. *Topics in Language Disorders, 13*(1), 51–65.

Wood, L., & Masterson, J. (1999). Use of technology to facilitate language skills in school-age children. *Seminars in Speech and Language, 2*(3), 219–232.

Woolard, G. (2004). *Keywords for fluency—Intermediate.* Hove, East Sussex, England: Language Teaching Publications.

ABOUT THE AUTHOR

Diane J. German is a professor in the National College of Education at National-Louis University, Chicago, Illinois. She is holder of the Ryan Endowed Chair in Special Education, which is funded to support her research in word finding. She has also been selected as a fellow of the International Academy for Research in Learning Disabilities. She has conducted research in word finding; published articles, presented technical papers; and conducted numerous state, national, and international seminars in the area of word finding. She is the author of the standard assessments in word-finding: the *Test of Word Finding–Second Edition* (TWF–2), the *Test of Adolescent/Adult Word Finding* (TAWF), and the *Test of Word Finding in Discourse* (TWFD). Further, she has authored *It's on the Tip of My Tongue: Word Finding Strategies to Remember Names and Words You Often Forget,* a user-friendly self-help book about word finding. Dr. German invites you to contact her at www.wordfinding.com or www.word-finding.com with questions about word-finding assessment or intervention.